DATE DUE

S

Xenobiotics and Inflammation

Xenobiotics and Inflammation

Edited by

Lawrence B. Schook
Department of Veterinary PathoBiology
University of Minnesota
St. Paul, Minnesota

Debra L. Laskin
Program in Toxicology
Rutgers University
Piscataway, New Jersey

Academic Press
San Diego   New York   Boston   London   Sydney   Tokyo   Toronto

Academic Press, Inc.
A Division of Harcourt Brace & Company
525 B Street, Suite 1900, San Diego, California 92101-4495

United Kingdom Edition published by
Academic Press Limited
24-28 Oval Road, London NW1 7DX

Library of Congress Cataloging-in-Publication Data

Xenobiotics and inflammation / edited by Lawrence B. Schook, Debra L.
   Laskin.
         p.   cm.
      Includes bibliographical references and index.
      ISBN 0-12-628930-1
      1. Immunotoxicology.   2. Xenobiotics--Immunology.
   3. Inflammation--Mediators.   4. Cytokines--Pathophysiology.
   5. Growth factors--Pathophysiology.   I. Schook, Lawrence B.
   II. Laskin, Debra L.
   RC582.17.X46   1994
   616.07'9--dc20   93-48067
                                                          CIP

PRINTED IN THE UNITED STATES OF AMERICA
94   95   96   97   98   99   BC   9   8   7   6   5   4   3   2   1

Contents

1

Immunotoxicity and Inflammation: An Overview
Gary J. Rosenthal and Michael I. Luster

2

The Inflammatory Process
Elizabeth J. Kovacs and Michelle R. Frazier-Jessen

3

Inflammatory Cytokines: An Overview

Mary E. Brandes and Sharon M. Wahl

4

Induction of Inflammation: Cytokines and Acute-Phase Proteins

C. D. Richards and J. Gauldie

5

Role of Tumor Necrosis Factor α in Acute and Chronic Inflammatory Responses: Novel Therapeutic Approaches

Carl K. Edwards, III, Shawn M. Borcherding, Jun Zhang, and David R. Borcherding

6

Bone Marrow Phagocytes, Inflammatory Mediators, and Benzene Toxicity
Laureen MacEachern and Debra L. Laskin

7

Dimethylnitrosamine-Associated Inflammation: Induction of Cytokines Affecting Macrophage Differentiation and Functions
Lawrence B. Schook, Alice L. Witsell, John F. Lockwood, and Michael J. Myers

8

Effects of Metals on Lymphocyte Development and Function

Michael J. McCabe, Jr., and David A. Lawrence

9

Xenobiotic-Induced Skin Toxicity

Jeffrey D. Laskin and Diane E. Heck

10

Pathogenesis of Atherosclerosis: A Cytokine Hypothesis

George Ku and Richard L. Jackson

11

Ozone-Induced Inflammatory Response in Pulmonary Cells

Hillel S. Koren, Robert B. Devlin, and Susanne Becker

12

Pulmonary Fibrosis Induced by Silica, Asbestos, and Bleomycin
Pierre F. Piguet

13

Nonparenchymal Cells, Inflammatory Mediators, and Hepatotoxicity
Debra L. Laskin

14

Central Nervous System: Viral Infection and Immune-Mediated Inflammation

Georgia Schuller-Levis, Piotr B. Kozlowski, and Richard J. Kascsak

Contributors

Numbers in parentheses indicate the pages on which the authors' contributions begin.

Susanne Becker (249), Alliance Technologies, Inc., Chapel Hill, North Carolina 27514

David R. Borcherding (97), Department of Chemistry, Marion Merrell Dow Research Institute, Marion Merrell Dow, Inc., Kansas City, Missouri 64134

Shawn M. Borcherding (97), Worldwide Medical Affairs, Procter and Gamble, Cincinnati, Ohio 45241

Mary E. Brandes (33), Laboratory of Immunology, National Institute of Dental Research, National Institutes of Health, Bethesda, Maryland 20892

Robert B. Devlin (249), Human Studies Division, Health Effects Research Laboratory, United States Environmental Protection Agency, Research Triangle Park, North Carolina 27711

Carl K. Edwards, III (97), Department of Immunology, Marion Merrell Dow Research Institute, Marion Merrell Dow, Inc., Kansas City, Missouri 64134

Michelle R. Frazier-Jessen (17), Department of Cell Biology, Neurobiology, and Anatomy, Loyola University, Maywood, Illinois 60153

J. Gauldie (71), Molecular Virology and Immunology Programme, Department of Pathology, McMaster University, Hamilton, Ontario, Canada L8N 3Z5

Diane E. Heck (217), Department of Environmental and Community Medicine, University of Medicine and Dentistry of New Jersey, Robert Wood Johnson Medical School, Piscataway, New Jersey 08854

Richard L. Jackson (233), Marion Merrell Dow Research Institute, Cincinnati, Ohio 45215

Richard J. Kascsak (321), New York State Institute for Basic Research in Developmental Disabilities, Staten Island, New York 10314

Hillel S. Koren (249), Human Studies Division, Health Effects Research Laboratory, United States Environmental Protection Agency, Research Triangle Park, North Carolina 27711

Elizabeth J. Kovacs (17), Department of Cell Biology, Neurobiology, and Anatomy, Loyola University, Maywood, Illinois 60153

Piotr B. Kozlowski (321), New York State Institute for Basic Research in Developmental Disabilities, Staten Island, New York 10314

George Ku (233), Marion Merrell Dow Research Institute, Cincinnati, Ohio 45215

Debra L. Laskin (149, 301), Department of Pharmacology and Toxicology, Rutgers University, Piscataway, New Jersey 08854

Jeffrey D. Laskin (217), Department of Environmental and Community Medicine, University of Medicine and Dentistry of New Jersey, Robert Wood Johnson Medical School, Piscataway, New Jersey 08854

David A. Lawrence (193), Department of Pharmacology and Toxicology, Albany Medical College, Albany, New York 12208

John F. Lockwood (173), Laboratory of Molecular Immunology, Department of PathoBiology, University of Minnesota, St. Paul, Minnesota 55108

Michael I. Luster (1), National Institute of Environmental Health Sciences, National Institutes of Health, Research Triangle Park, North Carolina 27709

Laureen MacEachern (149), Department of Pharmacology and Toxicology, Rutgers University, Piscataway, New Jersey 08854

Michael J. McCabe, Jr. (193), Department of Toxicology, Karolinska Institutet, Stockholm 104 01, Sweden

Michael J. Myers (173), United States Food and Drug Administration, Division of Veterinary Medical Research, Beltsville, Maryland 20705

Pierre F. Piguet (283), Département de Pathologie, Université de Genève, CH 1211 Genève 4, Switzerland

C. D. Richards (71), Molecular Virology and Immunology Programme, Department of Pathology, McMaster University, Hamilton, Ontario, Canada L8N 3Z5

Gary J. Rosenthal (1), National Institute of Environmental Health Sciences, National Institutes of Health, Research Triangle Park, North Carolina 27709

Lawrence B. Schook (173), Laboratory of Molecular Immunology, Department of PathoBiology, University of Minnesota, St. Paul, Minnesota 55108

Georgia Schuller-Levis (321), New York State Institute for Basic Research, Staten Island, New York 10314

Sharon M. Wahl (33), Laboratory of Immunology, National Institute of Dental Research, National Institutes of Health, Bethesda, Maryland 20892

Alice L. Witsell (173), Laboratory of Molecular Immunology, Department of Animal Sciences, University of Illinois, Urbana, Illinois 61801

Jun Zhang (97), Department of Immunology, Marion Merrell Dow Research Institute, Marion Merrell Dow, Inc., Kansas City, Missouri 64134

Foreword

There has been an explosion of interest in inflammation in the past 10 years. The likely causes of this excitement are developments in molecular biology that have enabled structural identification of cytokines, their functions, and the genes that regulate their expression and activities. Concurrently, there has also been a heightened awareness of xenobiotics and their ubiquitous presence in the environment, as well as their toxic potential. This book is particularly timely because it relates developments in both areas and presents an informative and enlightening discussion of recent developments.

Inflammation has been defined as a localized protective reaction of tissue to irritation, injury, or infection that is characterized by pain, redness, swelling, and sometimes loss of function (*American Heritage Dictionary*, 3rd Ed., Houghton Mifflin, 1992). This condition also has been defined as a pathological process consisting of a dynamic complex of cytological and histological reactions that occur in blood vessels and tissue in response to an abnormal stimulation caused by a chemical, biological, or physical agent (modified from *Stedman's Medical Dictionary*, 12th Ed., William & Wilkins, 1961). Thus, inflammation has an inherent duality of function: protection and injury.

The cells that constitute the inflammatory response, and the factors they secrete, are responsible not only for the injury suffered by various organs but also for the host protection associated with inflammation.

This book is organized into overviews of the basic elements of inflammation (i.e., cytokine structure and function) and of xenobiotic bioactivity, particularly in relation to the immune system. Inflammation can occur in any tissue. Chapters in this book deal with accumulation and activity of inflammatory cells in various organs, including the lung, liver, and skin. However, the text clearly indicates that inflammatory cell production and interaction do not necessarily lead to injury.

The feature common to all inflammatory responses is the elaboration of cytokines. Local and systemic responses are independent of the type of inflammatory stimulus. Chapter 3 presents an overview of inflammatory cytokines; other chapters discuss particular cytokines, as well as their induction and regulation by xenobiotics, in greater detail. The selection of xenobiotic agents for discussion includes, among others, metals, oxidative air toxicants, organics, and pesticides.

Inflammation functions to restrict damage to tissue and to neutralize the toxic agent. The questions of primary interest are: How does inflammation differ with various irritating xenobiotics? Do cytokine profiles in inflammation differ depending on the xenobiotic? A provocative answer to this question is provided in Chapter 1. Xenobiotics may inhibit transcription of cytokines in macrophages (corticosteroids) or inhibit early activating events. It is apparent that the nature of the xenobiotic affects the type of cytokine produced as well as its regulation. Metals, drugs, organometallics, and ultraviolet radiation influence the patterns of cytokine production. The immunosuppressant FK 506 influences early activating events and suppresses growth-promoting cytokines.

Do tissues differ in their responses to a particular xenobiotic? If so, what is the molecular basis for the difference in response? What is the role of local tissue components in the inflammatory response? Are local components independent of the type of inflammation stimulus? These questions and many more are addressed in this excellent volume.

Inflammation is a highly regulated process. Several chapters are concerned with the regulation of the injurious potential of inflammatory cells while others deal with the accumulation of inflammatory cells in the various organs. Injury results from a collection of events that appear to be highly regulated and that include the nature of the substrate with which the cells interact, the combination and temporal sequence of stimuli, and the rates of accumulation and removal of cells. Under the appropriate conditions, the cells mediate damage largely by liberation of oxygen metabolites, cations, and proteases. Inhibitors and inactivators of each class of compounds are present in tissues. The net result is a balance of factors.

Occasionally, the xenobiotic is antigenic, resulting in the recruitment of lymphocytes. Leukocytes produce protein, lipid, and peptide mediators, including cytokines. Cytokines can modulate every stage of the inflammatory response, from initial recruitment to resolution of injury. Cytokines that have been recognized and are discussed include the interleukins, tumor necrosis factor, interferon, macrophage inflammatory protein, transforming growth factor, and colony stimulating factor. The cells that produce the cytokines include the inflammatory infiltrate as well as resident cells. Cytokines may be preexisting or newly synthesized. The biochemistry and biology of cytokines are reviewed in Chapter 3, in conjunction with discussion of regulatory elements controlling cytokines and transcription factors.

The overlapping and synergistic roles of cytokines are addressed in Chapter 3 as well. Regulation occurs among the complexity of mediators. Cells control the order in which cytokines are produced. Their production is transient even in the presence of a continual stimulus. Regulation may occur at one or more stages of cytokine production or activity: at transcription, translation, or release. Cytokine function may require accompanying cell surface activation or activation of the cytokine following its release from the cells. Other modes of regulation are possible. Regulation may be by extracellular proteins that limit the activity of secreted cytokines or by structures such as cell junctions and matrices.

The chapters on xenobiotic-induced inflammatory responses (Chapters 7–14) appropriately build on the information and knowledge presented in the first half of the book. Comparisons of pulmonary inflammation and cytokine induction by ozone, for example, with that induced in the same organ by bleomycin are particularly enlightening.

With the explosion within the past several years of information related to cytokines and their production, activity, and regulation, this book is unique in its focus on xenobiotic-induced inflammation and should be found in personal libraries of all those interested in xenobiotic toxicity.

Meryl Karol
University of Pittsburgh

Preface

In recent years, it has become evident that inflammatory cytokines not only are involved in the response of the host to xenobiotics, but also are associated with xenobiotic-induced changes in immune responsiveness (immunotoxicity). This newfound knowledge clearly indicates a need for a book that addresses not only the role of cytokines in inflammation but also the way in which chemicals that affect different organs activate specific cytokine cascades. Moreover, the use of this information could lead to novel strategies for designing drugs to control cytokine induction or biological activity.

This book is organized to provide the reader with an introduction to cytokines, xenobiotics, and the inflammatory process, including the induction of acute-phase proteins. Examples of specific xenobiotics and their effects on different organ systems, which clearly demonstrate the need to improve our understanding of the unique nature of organ-specific inflammatory responses, are included.

The first chapter, by Rosenthal and Luster, provides an excellent overview of chemically induced changes in the inflammatory process. The authors provide examples of chemicals that affect the lung and skin and the specific cytokines involved in the response of these tissues. Chapter 2, by Kovacs and Frazier-Jessen, provides the reader with a general overview of the cells and mediators involved in both acute and chronic inflammation. The third chapter is an excellent review of the biochemical and biological features of inflammatory cytokines. In this chapter, Brandes and Wahl also provide the reader with an important perspective on the interplay between cytokine cascades. In the fourth chapter, Richards and Gauldie focus on the induction of acute-phase proteins and their regulation by the inflammatory cytokines, interleukin 1 and interleukin 6. This chapter also provides a discussion of how exposure to xenobiotics such as bleomycin, chloride, and metals can lead to altered levels of cytokines in various disease states. The first portion of the book ends with a comprehensive review of a specific cytokine, tumor necrosis factor, and its role in various pathophysiological processes. This contribution, by Edwards, Borcherding, Zhang, and Borcherding, provides the reader with a clear understanding of how elevated levels of tumor necrosis factor, which occur in various disease states, can contribute to the sequelae associated with sepsis and inflammatory diseases such as arthritis.

The second portion of the book begins with a review by MacEachern and Laskin on the potential role of mature bone marrow macrophages and neutrophils in benzene-induced hematotoxicity. This chapter provides an in-depth description of how *in vivo* exposure to benzene modifies bone marrow phagocyte oxidative metabolism, cytokine production, and the regulation of bone marrow cell proliferation. Chapter 7, by Schook, Witsell, Lockwood, and Myers, follows with a review of how the hepatotoxic chemical dimethylnitrosamine can induce alterations in macrophage functioning. According to these authors, elevated production of inflammatory cytokines in the liver can affect macrophage differentiation from bone marrow stem cells and subsequent functional responsiveness, including cytokine production. McCabe and Lawrence contribute a chapter in which the effects of metals on B and T cell development are discussed. Thus, exposure to heavy metals can lead to changes in regulatory circuits controlling host responses. The chapter by Laskin and Heck addresses the role of keratinocytes and inflammatory cells that migrate into the skin in tissue injury induced by dermal irritants. These authors describe studies that clearly demonstrate that keratinocytes can acquire macrophage-like activity following exposure to inflammatory mediators. In the next chapter, Ku and Jackson speculate on the role cytokines play in the pathogenesis of atherosclerosis. The following chapter by Koren, Devlin, and Becker, is an excellent in-depth review that addresses the role that cytokines and inflammatory mediators play in ozone-induced lung injury. This chapter is followed by one by Piguet on pulmonary fibrosis induced by bleomycin, silica, and asbestos. This presentation, which contains many examples of how chronic exposure to these agents leads to elevated cytokine production associated with fibrosis, is a much needed discussion of the effects of long-term elevated cytokine activity. The chapter by Laskin focuses on the potential role of nonparenchymal cells in liver injury induced by hepatotoxicants. Data presented document how the inhibition of macrophage functioning and mediator production abrogates liver injury. The last chapter (Schuller-Levis, Kozlowski, and Kascsak) provides the reader with an interesting hypothesis on the role of various inflammatory cells and mediators in the pathogenesis and progression of central nervous system injury induced by viral pathogens.

We hope that the introductory chapters, followed by numerous examples of specific target organ responses, will give the reader a full appreciation for the many roles that cytokines play in xenobiotic-induced inflammation. The editors greatly appreciate the opportunity to work with all the authors on this project. Our excitement about the significance of their contributions is highlighted in the Foreword by Meryl Karol. To each of the contributors, we extend our gratitude, and to the readers, our hope that they will learn as much as we have about cytokines and the plethora of roles they play in xenobiotic-induced tissue injury.

Debra L. Laskin
Lawrence B. Schook

1

Immunotoxicity and Inflammation: An Overview

Gary J. Rosenthal and Michael I. Luster

I. Introduction

When broken down to its component Greek roots, the term "xenobiotic" defines a foreign entity relative to a particular form of life. If the organism is a human, the term xenobiotic refers to any substance, whether man-made or natural, that by nature is foreign to the human. Considering the increasing number of xenobiotics introduced to the human environment, and the elaborate systems devised by the body to deal with these foreign invaders, the growth in visibility within the past decade of the discipline of toxicology in general, and of immunotoxicology in particular, is understandable. Often defined as the reaction of tissues to injury, inflammation is a common manifestation of xenobiotic toxicity. Any organ, including lymphoid organs, is capable of responding to xenobiotic insult via inflammation. However, an underlying common feature of organ inflammation, whether the kidney, liver, or lung, is the initiation of nonspecific or specific immune responses. These immune responses may be directed at the xenobiotic itself (e.g., viruses, lipopolysaccharide), at the tissue damage caused by the xenobiotic (e.g., irradiation or ozone damage), or at a combination of both chemical and tissue factors (e.g., asbestos and metal effects). Although the overall immune response can be quite complex, involving soluble proteins and cellular and chemical components, a primary immunological response shared by xenobiotics inducing inflammation is the elaboration of various cytokines.

Although xenobiotics represent all foreign substances, immunotoxicology is defined as the study of adverse effects on the immune system resulting from occupational, inadvertent, or therapeutic exposure to chemical or certain biological materials. These materials include products or by-products used in the pharmaceutical, farming, chemical, and consumer product industries, food additives, and natural products such as mycotoxins. The types of effects shown to occur are often chemical specific as well as species specific, and include immunosuppression targeting systemic or local immunity (e.g., lung or skin), hypersensitivity disease manifested as respiratory tract allergies or contact dermatitis, and, in certain instances, autoimmunity. An increasing emphasis has been placed on assessing xenobiotics common to the indoor environment. Among the so-called "bioacrosols" are viruses, bacteria, fungi, algae, and protozoa and their products. Most bioaerosols have the potential to act as sensitizing agents in susceptible hosts, whereas some cause infectious disease. In contrast, multiple chemical sensitivity (MCS, chemical hypersensitivity, etc.), although of considerable concern, has no consensus definition; insufficient evidence exists to classify this as an immune-mediated condition. Instead, MCS refers to a syndrome reflecting a constellation of adverse symptoms alleged to result from exposure to molecular organic chemicals at levels below those normally considered safe in the population, and will not be discussed further in this chapter.

II. General Mechanisms of Xenobiotic Immunotoxicity Relating to Inflammation

A. Systemic Immunosuppression

Suppression of the immune response, as evidenced by studies in experimental animals, is characteristic of a number of xenobiotics (Table I) although the precise mechanism(s) of immunosuppression for most chemicals remains largely unknown. From an experimental standpoint, the most extensively studied class of environmental pollutants is that of the halogenated aromatic hydrocarbons, including chlorinated dibenzo-p-dioxins, dibenzofurans, napthalenes, benzenes, and biphenyls as well as polybrominated biphenyls (PBB; reviewed by Vos and Luster, 1989). Chronic low-level human exposure to polychlorinated biphenyls (PCBs) has occurred on a large scale because of the wide use and long half-life of this chemical, but whether PCB is associated with adverse health effects is unclear. A study in rhesus monkeys demonstrating that chronic low-level PCB exposure induced slight alterations in certain immune parameters, most notably decreasing antibody response and CD4:CD8 ratios (Tryphonas et al., 1989), is of particular significance since the studies were designed to simulate likely human exposures. Accidental exposures in China and Japan to relatively high concentrations of PCB and furan mixtures have resulted from consumption of contaminated rice oil. In certain exposed Japanese individuals, a toxic syndrome referred to as "Yusho" disease was reported that included chloracne and greater susceptibility to respiratory infections (Shigematsu et al., 1978).

2,3,7,8-Tetra chlorodibenzo-p-dioxin (TCDD) is an extremely immunotoxic chemical in mice, with an acute ED_{50} of 1–2 μg/kg body weight for

Table I Xenobiotics Reported to Inhibit Immune Function and Decrease Host Resistance[a]

Class	Examples[b]
Polyhalogenated aromatic hydrocarbons	TCDD, PCB, PBB
Metals	Lead, cadmium, arsenic
Aromatic hydrocarbons	Benzene, toluene
Polycyclic aromatic hydrocarbons	DMBA, B(a)P, MCA
Pesticides	Trimethyl phosphorothioate, carbofuran, chlordane
Organotins	Dibutyltin chloride
Aromatic amines	Benzidine, acetylaminofluorene
Oxidant gases	NO_2, O_3, SO_2
Particulates	Asbestos, silica, beryllium
Drugs	Cyclosporin, methotrexate, azothioprine, dexamethosone

[a] Adapted from Luster et al. (1990), with permission.
[b] Abbreviations: TCDD, tetrachlorodibenzo-p-dioxin; PCB, polychlorinated biphenyls; PBB, polybrominated biphenyls; DMBA, dimethylbenzanthracene; B(a)p, benz(a) pyrene; MCA, methylcholanthrene.

some effects. Many of the immunological effects associated with this class of compounds are mediated through the intracellular Ah receptor, a steroidlike receptor that can be found in numerous tissues including macrophages and lymphocytes, although reports have suggested that non-Ah receptor-mediated events also may be involved. One of the most potent immunological effects associated with TCDD exposure in animals is suppression of the antibody response. Snyder et al. (1991) demonstrated that this suppression was reversible by treating animals with interferon γ (IFNγ). Although no explanation for this phenomenon is available, note that IFNγ also acts as an antagonist of TCDD-induced cytochrome P-450 mixed function oxidase (MFO) activity, a measure of cellular enzyme induction. Cytokine modulation, specifically tumor necrosis factor (TNF) and interleukin 1 (IL-1) induction, has been shown to occur in macrophages after TCDD exposure (Steppan and Kerkvliet, 1991). The marked pathological changes in liver by TCDD (Jones and Grieg, 1975), in addition to the ability of this compound to induce endotoxin hypersensitivity (Vos et al., 1978; Rosenthal, 1989), have implicated that TCDD-induced cytokine production, particularly production of tumor necrosis factor, may be a primary mechanism for some of the toxicities associated with TCDD (Taylor, 1992). In addition, TCDD can alter either the release of or the response to a variety of soluble mediators in nonimmune cells, including epidermal growth factor (EGF) and transforming growth factor α (TGFα) in keratinocytes, an effect that has been postulated to be involved in TCDD toxicity and carcinogenicity (Choi et al., 1991). Evidence also suggests that a common mechanism responsible for many of the effects on soluble mediators is the ability of TCDD to alter tyrosine kinase activity (Clark *et al.*, 1991), which is known to help regulate the response to many cytokines.

Polycyclic aromatic hydrocarbons (PAHs), another extensively studied class of compounds, are formed as products of incomplete combustion of fossil fuels and subsequently are found as environmental contaminants in tobacco smoke, coke, and automobile exhausts. Several PAHs that produce immunosuppression are also carcinogenic, including benzo(a)pyrene, 7,12-dimethylbenzathracene (DMBA), and 3-methylcholanthrene (MCA), although the causative nature of this correlation remains to be determined. Work by House *et al.* (1987,1989) has documented the selective effects of DMBA on T cell functions, specifically on IL-2 release. These studies suggest that DMBA targets T-helper cell functions, which can be reversed by addition of exogenous IL-2 or of untreated T-helper cells (House *et al.*, 1987). Additional studies have implicated defective T-cell antigen recognition as another mechanism of action for this compound (House *et al.*, 1989). Ladics *et al.* (1991) have shown that DMBA metabolites generated from splenic tissue can account for DMBA immunotoxicity; the 3,4-diol metabolite is 65 times more potent than the parent compound in suppressing antibody responses. In studies with benzo(*a*)pyrene, IL-1 production has been reported to be inhibited after *in vivo* exposure in mice (Lyte and Bick, 1988), although this observation has not been confirmed and, alternatively, has been linked to impaired antigen presentation (Myers *et al.*, 1987).

Inorganic heavy metals such as lead, cadmium, mercury, and nickel have been studied both *in vitro* and *in vivo* using experimental animals. These studies have uncovered fairly divergent effects, ranging from suppression or enhancement of the immune response to no effect, and, for some metals such as mercury chloride, induction of autoimmune disease (reviewed by Luster *et al.*, 1990). Studies show that lead exposure in animals appears to mimic clinical observations in humans, because a reduction in nucleated bone marrow cells, including stem cells and lymphoid cells, occurs (Shlick *et al.*, 1982). This and other experiments with cadmium (Hays and Margaretten, 1985) and mercury (Strom *et al.*, 1979) suggest that the bone marrow may be a sensitive indicator of metal toxicity and may be integral to the immunosuppressive effects observed for some of these compounds. The influence of metals on cytokine production has been evaluated only recently and will be examined comprehensively in Chapter 7.

B. Hypersensitivity

Numerous environmental chemicals have the ability to produce a hypersensitivity response after inadvertent and, more commonly, occupational exposure. A partial list of compounds known or presumed to produce an allergic response is given in Table II. Although hypersensitivity diseases are common, affecting millions of Americans, the incidence associated with

Table II   Industrial Materials Known or Presumed to Cause Allergic Problems

Material	Industry
Platinum salts	Metal refining
Cotton dust	Textile manufacturing
Formaldehyde	Garment, laboratory
Grain, flour	Farming, baking, milling
Ethylenediamine, phthalic and trimellitic anhydride, toluene diisocyanate (TDI, HDI)	Chemical, plastic, rubber manufacturing
Phenylglycine acid chloride, sulfone chloramides, amprolium hydrochloride, antibiotic dust	Pharmaceutical
Wood dust	Wood milling, carpentry
Vegetable gums	Printing
Organophosphate insecticides	Farming
Pyrrolysis products of polyvinyl chlorides	Meat wrapping

environmental or occupational exposure is unknown, but has been estimated to be 5–10% of all cases. The characteristic that distinguishes allergic responses from immune mechanisms involved in host defense is the excessive nature of the reaction, which often leads to tissue damage. Chemically induced hypersensitivities usually fall into two responses distinguished not only mechanistically but temporally: (1) delayed-type hypersensitivity (DTH), a cell-mediated response that occurs within 24–48 hr, and (2) immediate hypersensitivity, which is mediated by immunoglobulin, most commonly IgE, and is manifested within minutes of exposure to an allergen. The type of immediate hypersensitivity response elicited (anaphylactic, cytotoxic, Arthus, or immune complex) depends on the interaction of a sensitizing antigen or structurally related compound with antibody. DTH responses are characterized by T lymphocytes bearing antigen-specific receptors which, on contact with macrophage-associated antigen, respond by secreting cytokines that mediate the DTH response. Almost any organ can be targeted by hypersensitivity reactions, including the gastrointestinal tract, blood elements and vessels, joints, kidneys, central nervous system, and thyroid, although the skin and lung, which demonstrate urticaria and asthma, respectively, are the most common targets.

Chemically induced hypersensitivity is a widely recognized problem, both environmentally and occupationally, and is the subject of many reviews (e.g., Chan-Yeung and Lam, 1986; Menne et al., 1987). As a chemical class, metals stand out in their capacity to elicit both contact hypersensitivity and immunological lung disease. Beryllium, mercury, cobalt, nickel, platinum, chromium, and gold are representative of metals that can induce the spectrum of hypersensitivity responses, from delayed-onset to immediate. Nickel is considered a medium-to-strong contact sensitizer in humans based on studies by Vanderberg and Epstein (1963) and Kligman (1966), who sensitized 9 and 48% of subjects, respectively, using different experimental designs. Chronic pulmonary exposure to nickel has been associated with respiratory cancer (Nieboer and Sanford, 1985), although this phenomenon does not appear to be linked to hypersensitivity. Beryllium is associated with both skin and lung hypersensitivity (berylliosis). The pulmonary inflammation induced by beryllium is a frequently fatal granulomatous hypersensitivity response to a beryllium oxide–protein conjugate. The intensity of the granulomatous response is partly regulated by interactive circuitries of T lymphocytes and by cytokines produced from these cells. Although beryllium-induced neoplastic development in humans is disputable, development of osteocarcinoma and adenocarcinoma has been substantiated in experimental animal studies after administration of beryllium oxide and beryllium sulfate, respectively (Gardner and Heslington, 1946; Vorwald *et al.*, 1955). Clinically, beryllium exposure is associated with T lymphocyte blast transformation from cells obtained in either bronchoalveolar lavage fluid or peripheral blood. Cutaneous hypersensitivity induced by beryllium can be diagnosed by a positive patch test. Reeves and Pruess (1985) have suggested that beryllium hypersensitivity is mediated through the production of chemotactic factors that hinder the mobility of granuloma-forming cells, presumably macrophages and lymphocytes, in the presence of antigen. Although a molecular understanding of metal immunotoxicity is just beginning, the ability of metals to serve as cofactors in adenylate cyclase-mediated phosphorylation of proteins (Engalbert, 1988) suggests an underlying mechanism for cellular activation.

Toluene diisocyanate (TDI), a widely used member of the group of commercial isocyanates used in production of plastics and resins, causes both immediate and DTH responses. Occupational exposure to this low molecular weight hapten has been associated with asthma and contact dermatitis. Studies by Karol *et al.* (1980) have demonstrated that a threshold concentration is required for TDI vapor to produce lung sensitization in guinea pigs. Trimellitic anhydride (TMA) is another xenobiotic of occupational origin capable of inducing both DTH and immediate hypersensitivity responses. Widely used as intermediates in the paint and plastic industry, TMA induces TMA-specific antibodies and elicits at least three distinct syndromes in exposed individuals, including IgE-mediated asthmarhinitis, late-respiratory systemic syndrome, and pulmonary disease anemia (Zeiss *et al.*, 1983).

C. Immune and Inflammatory Responses in the Lung

Occupational and environmental exposure to inflammatory xenobiotics has achieved considerable attention, since such exposure can be controlled and consequently lessened, thereby avoiding adverse biological responses. For instance, occupational exposure to the inflammatory effects of beryllium, carbon tetrachloride, silica, benzene, and heavy metals has prompted much scientific and regulatory activity. The adverse responses or toxicities associated with these and other occupational compounds are most often associated with inflammatory responses in the lung or skin.

Considering the relevance of the respiratory route of exposure, considerable attention has been directed to the immunological effects associated with inhaled pollutants. Examples of such xenobiotics studied include, but are not limited to, gases such as ozone, nitrogen dioxide, and sulfur dioxide and particulates such as asbestos and silica (Table III). These compounds have been examined for their effects on both systemic and local (i.e., lung) immunity.

The term "pneumoconioses," originally applied to lung diseases caused by dust inhalation, is now more widely used to include all disorders caused by the inhalation of any aerosol. Although many individuals consider pneumoconioses to be occupational disorders, direct occupational exposure is not always necessary, particularly for individuals living near an industrial source. Occupationally, pneumoconioses are most often associated with coal dust (i.e., coal worker's pneumoconiosis). However, less common pneumoconioses exist, including berylliosis, those produced by less irritating dusts [e.g., iron dust (siderosis), tin dust (stannosis)], and those pro-

Table III Toxicants Thought to Have an Immunological or Inflammatory Component in Their Associated Diseases

Chemical	Disease
Asbestos, silica	Fibrosis, mesothelioma
Coal	Coal worker's pneumoconiosis
Cotton dust	Byssinosis
Beryllium	Berylliosis
Mercury	Hypersensitivity pneumonitis
Formaldehyde	Pulmonary hypersensitivity, asthma
Platinum salts	Hypersensitivity pneumonitis, asthma
Trimellitic anhydride	Pulmonary disease–anemia syndrome
Iron dust	Siderosis
Tin dust	Stannosis
Cedar dust	Asthma
Toluene diisocyanate	Hypersensitivity pneumonitis, asthma
Gallium arsenide	Fibrosis
Bleomycin	Fibrosis
Methotrexate	Fibrosis
Paraquat	Fibrosis
Ozone	Pulmonary edema, increased infections
NO_2	Pulmonary edema, increased infections
Heavy metals	Hypersensitivity, cancer
Cigarette smoke	Cancer, emphysema

duced by the inhalation of organic dusts [e.g., cotton (byssinosis), red cedar (asthma)]. Immune mechanisms appear to play a major role in the pathogenesis of these inflammatory disorders. For example, alveolar macrophages obtained from individuals with silicosis, asbestosis, or coal worker's pneumoconiosis spontaneously release increased amounts of fibronectin and other mediators that act synergistically to signal fibroblast proliferation (Rom et al., 1987). Occupationally, cotton workers have experienced pulmonary hypersensitivity (byssinosis) and other symptoms common to organic dusts such as grain or vegetable dust (Pernis et al., 1961; Rylanden, 1990). Studies by Ryan and Karol (1991) have shown that cotton dust inhalation in guinea pigs induces a prodigious quantity of tumor necrosis factor measurable in both lavage fluid and alveolar macrophage cultures.

Although occupational diseases associated with inhalation of cotton and other grain dusts may be associated with endotoxin from gram-negative bacteria, apparently the form of endotoxin [bacteria-associated versus purified lipopolysaccharide (LPS)] is an important parameter in the activation of macrophages. In this respect, cells of the mononuclear phagocyte lineage (e.g., macrophages, Langerhans cells, Kupffer cells) play a major role in the local response via the postactivational release of numerous cytokines including, among others, IL-1 and platelet derived growth factor (PDGF). Evidence for this role is provided by studies demonstrating not only the increased release of cytokines following inhalation of particulates (Driscoll et al., 1990) but also the presence of high affinity cytokine receptors in lung fibroblasts (Chin et al., 1987). Pulmonary inflammation associated with idiopathic pulmonary fibrosis (Khalil et al., 1991) or bleomycin-induced fibrosis (Khalil et al., 1989) has correlated with expression of transforming growth factor β (TGFβ) mRNA in alveolar macrophages and type II cells.

D. Immune and Inflammatory Responses in the Skin

In addition to contact hypersensitivity reactions, some xenobiotics can modulate immune responses and inflammatory processes in the skin. Immune cells and active components (e.g., antibody–antigen complexes) are readily recruited to the skin from the circulatory system in response to stimuli initiated by xenobiotic–epidermal cell interactions. Additionally, certain immune cells permanently reside in the skin, including Langerhans cells, bone marrow-derived monocytes that are responsible for antigen processing, and dendritic T lymphocytes. The disappearance of Langerhans cells from the skin or loss of their function occurs in response to exogenous factors such as ultraviolet (UV) light (Fan et al., 1959; Applegate et al., 1989) and certain toxic chemicals including DMBA (Halliday et al., 1988). Subsequently, the ability to induce contact hypersensitivity responses at the site of exposure is lost. At considerably higher exposures to these exogenous factors, systemic immunosuppression may occur by mechanisms that are unclear, but may be associated with the induction of antigen-specific suppressor T cells (Kripke, 1990). Growing evidence suggests that exogenous interference with skin immunity (e.g., UV radiation) is associated with the development of skin cancers and possibly with other clinical effects (Table IV).

The keratinocyte, which represents the vast majority of cells that compose the epidermis (>95%), is the source of immunologically active cytokines. Researchers have postulated that the release of these cytokines in response to various stimuli orchestrates many of the immunological and inflammatory responses observed to occur in the skin after exposure to dermatotoxins (Stenn, 1989; Barker *et al.*, 1991). In this respect, the pathogenesis of psoriasis, a chronic skin disease characterized by excessive keratinocyte proliferation and inflammatory cell infiltrates, is closely associated with altered regulation of keratinocyte-produced cytokines (Nickoloff *et al.*, 1991) and may serve as a model for chemical-induced dermatotoxicity. The mechanisms and events by which these processes occur are currently major areas of research. Some of the cytokines known or presumed to be products of keratinocytes include, among others, IL-1α and β, granulocyte–macrophage colony stimulating factor (GM-CSF), IL-6, IL-8, TGFα and β, TNFα, and IL-3. Based on several lines of *in vitro* and *in vivo* evidence, a cytokine network theory has been proposed that, at present, has not been definitively proven (Barker *et al.*, 1991). In this model, environmental stimuli, which include contact allergens, UV light, and certain dermatotoxic chemicals, can act directly on epidermal keratinocytes, resulting in the release of IL-1 and TNFα as well as the expression of ICAM-1, an adhesion ligand for lymphocytes. The secretion of IL-1 and TNFα leads to the expression of surface leukocyte adhesion molecules on dermal endothelial cells (e.g., VCAM-1). TNFα and/or IL-1 may also serve in an autocrine fashion and eventually can result in the release of keratinocyte-derived IL-8, a potent attractant for T lymphocytes and polymorphonuclear leukocytes (PMNs). When the initial environmental stimulant is antigenic, as in the case of NiSO$_4$, the response involves increased apposition of mononuclear cells with subsequent involvement of sensitized T cells. Such interactions lead to IFNα and TNFα release and an increase in intensity and prolongation of the response.

Table IV   Possible Clinical Effects of
Ultraviolet Radiation and Other Skin Toxicants

Development of nonmelanoma skin cancer
Development of infectious disease
Potential role in autoimmune disease
Inhibition of contact hypersensitivity

E. Autoimmunity

Several environmental chemicals, particularly drugs, produce autoimmune responses that in some cases lead to autoimmune diseases in experimental animal models and humans (reviewed by Bigazzi, 1988; Kammuller et al., 1989). Development of autoimmunity is a complex process involving multiple factors. Whether environmental chemicals actually play a cofactor role in autoimmunity is unknown; however, several mechanisms for such a role have been proposed (Table V). Evidence for drug-induced autoimmunity is more compelling, or at least more complete, than that for those that are environmentally related, as exemplified by numerous reports on penicillamine-, procainamide-, and hydrazine-induced lupus erythematosus. Hydrazine-induced lupus is of particular interest since it occurs in a fairly restricted population (i.e., slow acetylators) and the compound is found in various natural products including tobacco, mushrooms, and alfalfa seeds. Other drugs have been reported to produce autoimmune hemolytic anemia or thrombocytopenia, the most notable being methyldopa (Gordon-Smith, 1983). Similar responses have also been reported in patients receiving chlorpropamide, procainamide, carbamazepine, and interferon therapy (reviewed by Bigazzi, 1988). Other work has focused on lymphoproliferative reactions induced by diphenylhydantoin (Krueger, 1989), the development of thyroid antibodies in patients receiving lithium, and drug-induced hepatitis in association with halothane, nitrofurantoin, or isoniazid treatment.

In contrast to drug-induced autoimmune phenomena, evidence of autoimmunity induced by environmental chemicals, particularly in humans, is limited. Occupational or inadvertent exposure to vinyl chloride, quartz, or trichloroethylene has been linked to a disorder resembling scleroderma which, in the case of vinyl chloride, like idiopathic scleroderma, shows a prevalence for individuals with HLA-DR5. Certain metals such as mercury cause immune-complex glomerulonephritis in humans (Tubbs et al., 1982). Low levels of mercury administered to susceptible strains of mice and rats result in immune-complex glomerulonephritis and nuclear autoantibodies (Druet et al., 1978). An "autoimmune-like" disorder has also been reported

Table V Proposed Mechanisms by Which Chemicals Can Influence Autoimmune Disease

Mechanism	Chemical
Estrogenic activity	Kepone, mirex, diethylstilbestrol
Chemical thymectomy	Cyclosporin A
Immune regulation	Mercury
Tissue damage	CCL_4, asbestos

in a large population of Spanish residents who inadvertently digested aniline-adulterated rapeseed oil; this condition was referred to as toxic oil syndrome (TOS; Kammuller *et al.*, 1988). The immunological symptoms associated with TOS are similar to those observed in some humans receiving hydantoin-related compounds. Definitive studies with TOS would be difficult since the exact chemical composition of the adulterated oil is unknown.

III. Immunotoxicity of Drugs

Although the primary focus of this book involves xenobiotic-induced inflammation, several compounds, particularly pharmaceuticals, have the capacity to inhibit the inflammatory process. Indeed, the pharmacological inhibition of cytokines has numerous therapeutic applications in inflammatory diseases including arthritis, granulomas, and fibrosis. Subsequently, considerable efforts are being devoted to studying highly specific inhibitors of cytokine release or cytokine action. Corticosteroids such as dexamethasone are well known for their immunosuppressive activities (Cupps and Fauci, 1982), one of which inhibits the transcription and consequently the production of inflammatory cytokines from macrophages (Knudsen *et al.*, 1987). Cytokine inhibition need not be limited to macrophages, as exemplified by the cyclosporins, which have been used successfully to treat the host-mediated immune response to transplanted tissues or organs. The effectiveness of cyclosporin A (CsA) is mediated at least partly through the inhibition of lymphokines required for the generation of target-specific cytotoxic T lymphocytes, which are integral to the development of a host-mediated attack on the implanted tissue. Evidence indicates that new candidates for immunosuppressive therapy, such as the macrolide antibiotic FK-506 (isolated from cultures of *Streptomyces tsukubanensis*) or rapamycin (isolated from *Streptomyces hygroscopicus*), may be 10- to 100-fold more potent than CsA (Morris and Shorthouse, 1990). Studies by Dumont *et al.* (1990) have shown that FK-506, like CsA, affects T cells through inhibition of early activating events and suppression of growth-promoting cytokines (e.g., IL-2 and IL-4) whereas rapamycin inhibits T cell proliferation by impeding the response of T cells to growth-promoting cytokines.

Although these therapeutics have as their mechanism of action the capacity to inhibit inflammation, certain drugs have adverse consequences that result in the induction of inflammation. Acetaminophen and bleomycin, which induce liver and lung inflammation, respectively, provide classical examples of drug toxicity that is not simply a manifestation of exaggerated pharmacological action but an inflammatory response.

The immunotoxicity of abused drugs also has been explored, although such studies have generally been at the level of cellular effects. The natural cannabinoids, unique to the *Cannabis sativa* plant, have been shown to be immunosuppressive (for review, see Holsapple and Munson, 1985); both the psychoactive and the nonpsychoactive components possess immuno-modulatory properties. *In vitro* exposure of murine or human lymphocytes to the major psychoactive component of marijuana, delta-9-tetrahydrocan-nabinol (THC), can result in decreased lymphocyte blast transformation (Klein *et al.*, 1985; Spector *et al.*, 1990) whereas *in vivo* exposure increases the mortality rate of mice in response to a dual challenge of Friend leukemia virus and herpes simplex virus (Spector *et al.*, 1991). Another abused drug, with an estimated 10 million chronic users in the United States alone (Isaacs *et al.*, 1987), is cocaine, a member of the tropane family of alkaloids. Immu-notoxicological assessment following *in vivo* cocaine exposure has generally been equivocal, showing suppression, stimulation, and no effect (reviewed by Watzl and Watson, 1990). However, studies by Di Francesco *et al.* (1990) have shown that cocaine administration results in marked suppression of cell-mediated immunity in mice. Animals treated for 1 or 7 days with as little as 1 mg/kg had deficient cytotoxic T lymphocyte responsiveness that correlated with increased susceptibility to influenza virus infections. Al-though the mechanism(s) responsible for immune defects following cocaine exposure is unknown, evidence would support a critical neuroendocrine influence (Watzl and Watson, 1990).

IV. Summary

Within the area of immunotoxicology, examination of the ability of xeno-biotics to modulate cytokines and, consequently, specific and nonspecific inflammatory processes is becoming an integral component of routine test-ing and regulatory assessment. Already many compounds that modulate cell-specific cytokine production have been tentatively identified (Table VI). Without question, an understanding of the mechanisms by which xenobiotics modulate cytokine responses will increasingly be included by regulatory agencies for risk determination. Future work in immunotoxicol-ogy will see a number of descriptive studies with previously unexamined or newly developed compounds. As the actions of chemicals on immune function become apparent, researchers will need to assess the combined effects of chemicals, particularly the "recreational" or "life-style" toxicants such as alcohol and cigarettes, and occupational and environmental pollut-ants. Similarly, although difficult to study mechanistically, complex mix-tures such as drinking water and air pollutants will have to be evaluated to provide adequate immunotoxicology risk assessment. As methods of bioassays and chemical determinations evolve, a better understanding of complex cytokine patterns will make determination of disease or mecha-nism of toxic action more quantitative. Emphasis will shift from examination of individual cytokines to studies of entire batteries of relevant cytokines

Table VI Selected Examples of Xenobiotics Demonstrated to Modulate Cytokine Production

Xenobiotic	Cytokine-producing target
Environmental/occupational	
Ozone	Macrophages
Asbestos	Macrophages, fibroblasts
Benz(a)pyrene	Macrophages
Dimethylbenzanthracene	Macrophages, T cell
Benzene	Bone marrow stromal cells
Coal	Macrophages
Carbon tetrachloride	Kupffer's cells
Nitrosamines	Macrophages
Drugs	
Cyclosporin A	T cells
Corticosteroids	Macrophages, T cells, B cells
Platinum salts	T cells, B cells
FK-506	T cells
Bleomycin	Macrophages, T cells
Acetaminophen	Kupffer's cells
Pentamidine	Macrophages
Naturally occurring	
Ultraviolet light	Langerhans cells
Viruses, bacteria, fungi	Infected target cells
Wood dust	Macrophages
Ozone	Macrophages
Nitrogen dioxide	Macrophages

and their interaction messengers. Such determinations will aid in the mechanistic understanding of toxicities and should enable development of more rational therapeutic intervention.

References

Applegate, L. A., Ley, R. D., Alcalay, J., and Kripke, M. L. (1989). Identification of the molecular target for the suppression of contact hypersensitivity by ultraviolet radiation. *J. Exp. Med.* **170**, 1117–1131.

Barker, J. N. W. N., Mitra, R. S., Griffiths, C. E. M., Dixit, V. M., and Nickoloff, B. J. (1991). Keratinocytes as initiators of inflammation. *Lancet* **337**, 211–214.

Bekesi, J. G., Holland, J. F., Anderson, H. A., Fischbein, A. S., Rom, W., Wolff, M. S., and Selikoff, I. J. (1978). Lymphocyte function of Michigan dairy farmers exposed to polybrominated biphenyls. *Science* **199**, 1207–1209.

Bigazzi, P. E. (1988). Autoimmunity induced by chemicals. *Clin. Toxicol.* **26**, 125–156.

Chan-Yeund, M. I., and Lam, S. (1986). Occupational asthma. *Am. Rev. Resp. Dis.* **133**, 686–703.

Chin, J., Camron, P., Rupp, E., and Schmidt, J. (1987). Identification of a high affinity receptor for native IL-1β and IL-1α on normal human lung fibroblasts. *J. Exp. Med.* **165**, 70–86.

Choi, E. J., Toscano, D. G., Ryan, J. A., Riedel, N., and Toscano, W. A., Jr. (1991). Dioxin induces transforming growth factor-α in human keratinocytes. *J. Biol. Chem.* **266(15)**, 9591–9597.

Clark, G. C., Blank, J. A., Germolec, D. R., and Luster, M. I. (1991). 2,3,7,8-Tetrachlorodibenzo-*p*-dioxin (TCDD) stimulates protein phosphorylation and tyrosine kinase activity in B-lymphocytes. *Mol. Pharmacol.* **39**, 495–501.

Cupps, T. R., and Fauci, A. S. (1982). Corticosteroid-mediated immunoregulation in man. *Immunol. Rev.* **65**, 156–159.

Di Francesco, P., Pica, F., Crocey, C., Favalli, C., Tubano, E., and Garaci, E. (1990). Effect of acute or daily cocaine administration of cellular immune responses and virus infection in mice. *Nat. Immun. Cell Growth Regul.* **9**, 397–405.

Driscoll, K., Linderschmidt, R., Maurer, J., Higgens, J., and Ridder, G. (1990). Pulmonary response to silica or titanium dioxide: Inflammatory cells, alveolar macrophage derived cytokines and histopathology. *Am. J. Resp. Cell Mol. Biol.* **2**, 381–390.

Druet, P., Druet, E., Potdevin, F., and Sapin, C. (1978). Immune type glomerulonephritis induced by $HgCl_2$ in the Brown–Norway rat. *Ann. Immunol. (Paris)* **129C**, 777–792.

Dumont, F., Melino, M., Staruch, M., Koprak, S., Fisher, P., and Sigal, N. (1990). The immunosuppressive macrolides FK506 and rapamycin act as reciprocal antagonists in murine cells. *J. Immunol.* **41**, 4812–4820.

Engalbert, A. (1988). Membrane receptors and mechanisms of transduction. *Med. Sci.* Special No. 1, 40–48.

Fan, J., Schoenfeld, R. J., and Hunter, R. (1959). A study of the epidermal clear cells with special reference to their relationship to the cells of Langerhans. *J. Invest. Dermatol.* **32**, 445.

Gardner, L., and Heslington, H. F. (1946). Osteo-sarcomata from intravenous beryllium compounds in rabbits. *Fed. Proc.* **5**, 221.

Gordon-Smith, E. S. (1983). Immune drug-induced blood dyscrasias. *In* "Immunotoxicology" (G. G. Gibson, H. Hubbard, and D. V. Parke, eds.), pp. 161–184. Academic Press, New York.

Halliday, G. M., Cavanagh, L. L., and Muller, H. K. (1988). Antigen presented in the local lymph node by cells from dimethylbenzanthracene-treated murine epidermis activates suppressor cells. *Cell. Immunol.* **117**, 289–302.

Hays, E. F., and Margaretten, N. (1985). Long-term oral cadmium produces bone marrow hypoplasia in mice. *Exp. Hematol.* **13**, 229–236.

Holsapple, M., and Munson, A. (1985). Immunotoxicity of abused drugs. *In* "Immunotoxicology and Immunopharmacology" (J. Dean, M. Luster, A. Munson, and H. Amos, ed.), pp. 381–392. Raven Press, New York.

House, R. V., Laver, L. D., Murray, M. J., and Dean, J. H. (1987). Suppression of T-helper cell function in mice following exposure to the carcinogen 7,12-dimethylbenzanthracene and its restoration by interleukin 2. *Int. J. Immunopharmacol.* **9**, 89–97.

House, R. V., Pallardy, M. J., and Dean, J. H. (1989). Suppression of immune cytotoxic T-lymphocyte induction following exposure to 7,12-dimethylbenzanthracene: Dysfunction of antigen recognition. *Int. J. Immunopharmacol.* **11**, 207–215.

Isaacs, S. O., Martin, P., and Willoughby, J. (1987). "Crack" abuse: A problem of the eighties. *Oral Surg. Oral Med. Oral Pathol.* **63**, 12–37.

Jones, G., and Grieg, J. (1975). Pathological changes in the liver of mice given 2,3,7,8-tetrachlorodibenzo(*p*)dioxin. *Experientia* **31**, 1315.

Kammuller, M. E., Bloksma, N., and Seinen, W., eds. (1989). "Autoimmunity and Toxicology." Elsevier, Amsterdam.

Kammuller, M. E., Bloksma, N., and Seinen, W. (1988). Chemical-induced autoimmune reactions and Spanish Toxic Oil Syndrome. Focus on hydantoins and related compounds. *Clin. Toxicol.* **26**, 157–174.

Karol, M. H., Dixon, C., Brody, M., and Alarie, Y. (1980). Immunologic sensitization and pulmonary hypersensitivity by repeated inhalation of aromatic isocyanates. *Toxicol. Appl. Pharmacol.* **53**, 260–269.

Khalil, N., Bereznay, O., Sporn, M., and Greenberg, A. (1989). Macrophage production of TGF-β and fibroblast collagen synthesis in chronic pulmonary inflammation. *J. Exp. Med.* **170**, 727–737.

Khalil, N., O'Conner, R., Unruh, H., Warren, P., Flanders, K., Kemp, A., Berznay, O., and Greenberg, A. (1991). Increased production and immunohistochemical localization of transforming growth factor-β in idiopathic pulmonary fibrosis. *Am. J. Resp. Cell. Mol. Biol.* **5**, 155–162.

Klein, T. W., Newton, C., Widen, R., and Friedman, H. (1985). The effect of delta-9-tetrahydrocannabinol and 11-hydroxy-delta-9-tetrahydrocannabinol on T-lymphocyte and B-lymphocyte mitogen responses. *J. Immunopharmacol.* **7**, 451–466.

Kligman, A. M. (1966). Identification of contact allergies by human assay. III. Maximization test. A procedure for screening and rating contact sensitizers. *J. Invest. Dermatol.* **47**, 393–409.

Knudsen, P. J., Dinarello, C. A., and Strom, T. B. (1987). Glucocorticoids inhibit transcriptional and post-transcriptional expression of IL-1 in U937 cells. *J. Immunol.* **139**, 4129–4133.

Kripke, M. L. (1990). Effects of UV radiation on tumor immunity. *J. Natl. Cancer Inst.* **82**, 1392–1396.

Krueger, G. R. F. (1989). The pathology of diphenylhydantoin-induced lymphoproliferative reactions in animals. *In* "Autoimmunity and Toxicology" (M. E. Kammuller, N. Bloksma, and W. Seinen, eds.), p. 391. Elsevier, Amsterdam.

Ladics, G., Kawabata, T., and White, K. L. (1991). Suppression of the *in vitro* numosal immune response of mouse splenocytes by 7,12-dimethylbenz(a)anthracene metabolites and inhibition of immunosuppression by α-napthoflavon. *Toxicol. Appl. Pharmacol.* **110**, 31–44.

Luster, M. I., Weirda, D., and Rosenthal, G. J. (1990). Environmentally related disorders of the hematologic and immune systems. *Med. Clin. North Am.* **74**, 425–439.

Lyte, M., and Bick, P. H. (1988). Modulation of interleukin-1 production by macrophages following benzo(a)pyrene exposure. *Int. J. Immunopharmacol.* **8**, 377–381.

Menne, T., Christopherson, J., and Maibach, H. I. (1987). Epidemiology of contact sensitization. *In* "Epidemiology of Major Diseases" (H. D. Schlomberger, ed.), pp. 131–161. Karger, Basel.

Morris, R., and Shorthouse, R. (1990). A study of the contrasting effects of cyclosporin A, FK506 and rapamycin on the suppression of allograft rejection. *Transplant. Proc.* **24**, 13–61.

Myers, M., Schook, L. B., and Bick, P. H. (1987). Mechanisms of benzo(a)pyrene-induced modulation of antigen presentation. *J. Pharmacol. Exp. Therapeut.* **242(2)**, 399–404.

Nickoloff, B. J., Karabin, G. D., Barker, J. N. W. N., Griffiths, C. E. M., Sarma, V., Mitra, R. S., Elder, J. T., Kunkel, S. L., and Dixit, V. M. (1991). Cellular localization of interleukin-8 and its inducer, tumor necrosis factor-alpha in psoriasis. *Am. J. Pathol.* **138**, 129–140.

Nieboer, E., and Sanford, W. (1985). Essential toxic and therapeutic functions of metals. *Rev. Biochem. Toxicol.* **7**, 205–245.

Pernis, B., Vigiani, C., Cavagna, C., and Finolli, M. (1961). The role of bacterial endotoxins in occupational diseases caused by inhaling vegetable dusts. *Br. J. Ind. Med.* **18**, 120–129.

Reeves, A. L., and Pruess, O. P. (1985). The immunotoxicity of beryllium. *In* "Immunotoxicology and Immunopharmacology" (J. Dean, M. Luster, A. Munson, and H. Amos, eds.), p. 441. Raven, New York.

Reuter, R., Tessars, G., Vohr, H. W., Gleichmann, E., and Luhrmann, R. (1989). Mercuric chloride induces autoantibodies against U3 small nuclear ribonucleoprotein in susceptible mice. *Proc. Natl. Acad. Sci. USA* **86**, 237–241.

Rom, W. N., Bittaman, P. B., Rennard, S. I., Cantin, A., and Crystal, R. G. (1987). Characterization of the lower respiratory tract inflammation of non-smoking individuals with interstitial lung disease associated with the chronic inhalation of organic dusts. *Am. Rev. Resp. Dis.* **136**, 1229–1243.

Rosenthal, G. J., Lebetkin, E., Thigpen, J. E., Wilson, R., Tucker, A., and Luster, M. I. (1989). Characteristics of 2,3,7,8-tetrachlorodibenzo(*p*)dioxin induced endotoxin hypersensitivity: Association with hepatotoxicity. *Toxicology* **56**, 239–251.

Ryan, L., and Karol, M. (1991). Release of TNF in guinea pigs upon acute inhalation of cotton dusts. *Am. J. Resp. Cell. Mol. Biol.* **5**, 93–98.

Rylanden, R. (1990). Health effects of cotton dust exposure. *Am. J. Ind. Med.* **26**, 314–321.

Schlick, E., and Freidberg, K. D. (1982). Bone marrow cells in mice under the influence of low lead doses. *Arch. Toxicol.* **49**, 227–232.

Shigematsu, N., Ishmaru, S., Saito, R., Ikeda, T., Matsuba, F., Sigiyams, K., and Masuda, Y. (1978). Respiratory involvement in PCB poisoning. *Environ. Res.* **16**, 92–100.

Snyder, N. K., Kramer, C. M., and Holsapple, M. P. (1991). Characterization of murine interferon-gamma antagonism of 2,3,7,8-TCDD-induced humoral immune suppression. *Immunopharmacol.* (*in press*).

Spector, S., Lancz, G., and Hazelden, J. (1990). Marijuana and immunity—Tetrahydrocannabinol-mediated inhibition of lymphocyte blastogenesis. *Int. J. Immunopharmacol.* **12**, 261–267.

Spector, S., Lancz, G., Wistrich, G., and Freidman, H. (1991). Delta-9-tetrahydrocannabinol augments murine retroviral induced immunosuppression and infection. *Int. J. Immunopharmacol.* **13**, 411–417.

Stenn, K. (1989). Production of cytokines by epithelial tissues. *Am. J. Dermatopathol.* **11**, 69–73.

Steppan, L. B., and Kerkvliet, N. I. (1991). Influence of 2,3,7,8-tetrachlorodibenzo(*p*)dioxin on the production of inflammatory cytokine mRNA by C57Bl/6 macrophages. *Toxicologist* **11**, 35.

Strom, S., Johnson, R. L., and Uyeki, E. M. (1979). Mercury toxicity to hematopoietic and tumor colony forming cells and its reversal by selenium *in vitro*. *Toxicol. Appl. Pharmacol.* **49**, 431.

Taylor, M. J., Lucier, G. W., Mahler, J. F., Thompson, M., Lockhart, A. C., and Clark, G. C. (1992). Inhibition of acute TCDD toxicity by treatment with anti-TNF antibody or dexamethasone. *Toxicol. Appl. Pharmacol.* **117**, 126–132.

Tryphonas, H., Hayward, S., O'Grady, L., Loo, J. C. K., Arnold, D. L., Bryce, F., and Zawidzka, Z. Z. (1989). Immunotoxicity studies of PCB (Aroclor 1254) in the adult rhesus (*Macaca mulatta*) monkey—Preliminary report. *Int. J. Immunopharmacol.* **11(2)**, 199–206.

Tubbs, R., Gephardt, G., McMohon, J., Pohl, M., Vidt, D., Barenberg, S., and Valenzuela, R. (1982). Membranous glomerulonephritis associated with industrial mercury exposure. *Am. J. Clin. Pathol.* **77**, 409–413.

Vanderberg, J., and Epstein, W. (1963). Experimental contact sensitization in man. *J. Invest. Dermatol.* **41**, 413–416.

Vorwald, A. J., Pratt, P. C., and Urban, E. J. (1955). The production of pulmonary cancer in albino rats exposed by inhalation to an aerosol of beryllium sulfate. *Acto Unio. Int. Contra. Cancrum* **11**, 735–749.

Vos, J. G., and Luster, M. I. (1989). Immune alterations. *In* "Halogenated Biphenyls, Terphenyls, Napthalenes, Dibenzodioxins, and Related Compounds" (K. Kimbrough and T. Jensen, eds.), 2d Ed., pp. 295–322. Raven Press, New York.

Vos, J. G., Kreeftenberg, J. G., Engle, H. W. B., Minderhood, A., and Van Noorle Jansen, Z. M. (1978). Studies on 2,3,7,8-tetrachlorodibenzo(*p*)dioxin induced immune suppression and decreased host resistance to infection: Endotoxin hypersensitivity, serum zinc concentrations, and effect of thymosin treatment. *Toxicology* **9**, 75.

Watzl, B., and Watson, R. (1990). Immunomodulation by cocaine: A neuroendocrine mediated response. *Life Sci.* **46**, 1319–1329.

Zeiss, C. R., Wolkonsky, P., Chacon, R., Turtland, P. A., Levitz, D., Prunzansky, J. J., and Patterson, R. (1983). Syndromes in workers exposed to trimellitic anhydrides. *Ann. Intern. Med.* **98**, 8–29.

2

The Inflammatory Process

Elizabeth J. Kovacs and Michelle R. Frazier-Jessen

I. Introduction

Inflammation, the response of the body to injury, is characterized by (1) increased blood flow to the affected area to dilute potentially toxic agents, (2) increased capillary permeability to facilitate transmission of larger molecules across the endothelium, and (3) the migration of leukocytes (primarily neutrophils and, to a lesser extent, macrophages) out of the circulatory system into the surrounding tissue to remove debris and restore normal tissue structure and activity. The duration and magnitude of the inflammatory response dictate the ultimate outcome. If the tissue is more severely damaged and the inflammatory response is prolonged, restoring normal tissue architecture and function may be more difficult.

II. Inflammatory Cells

Leukocytes, which normally constitute 1% of the circulating cells, are active in the repair process that follows tissue injury as well as in fighting infection. Histologically, the first cell type to appear at an inflammatory site is the neutrophil. The acute neutrophilic infiltration is followed by an influx of macrophages and lymphocytes. This event marks the beginning of chronic inflammation, which is of longer duration and involves several different types of cells from the blood and the connective tissue, including lymphocytes and fibroblasts.

A. Cells of Acute Inflammation

1. Neutrophils
Neutrophils are the most abundant leukocyte, constituting 55–65% of the total cell count. Their importance was first appreciated by Elie Metchni-

Xenobiotics and Inflammation
Copyright 1994 © by Academic Press, Inc. All rights of reproduction in any form reserved.

koff in the 1880s (Metchnikoff, 1907). Neutrophils share structural and developmental similarities with monocytes, eosinophils, and basophils. These cells are easily identified in peripheral blood smears by their highly characteristic nucleus consisting of two or more lobules connected by narrow strands. The variability of nuclear shape is the basis for the other name applied to these cells: polymorphonuclear leukocytes (PMNs) or polys. When correctly stained the cytoplasm of neutrophils shows the presence of small granules that have little affinity for dyes and are referred to as specific granules. In addition, larger reddish-purple azurophilic granules are present that may appear quite pale in routinely stained preparations. At the electron microscopic level, granules of human neutrophils can be detected throughout the cytoplasm, except for a thin peripheral zone thought to be involved in cell motility.

Neutrophils are the first line of defense against invasion from pathogenic bacteria. At sites of inflammation, these cells adhere to the walls of postcapillary venules and migrate between the endothelial cells into the connective tissue matrix below. Once at their target site, neutrophils exert their effects by releasing hydrolytic enzymes and reactive oxygen metabolites. In addition, neutrophils are avid phagocytic cells that are particularly effective against bacteria. The contents of their phagocytic vacuoles fuse with lysosomes containing hydrolytic enzymes to digest the contents.

2. *Mast Cells*

Mast cells, first described by Paul Ehrlich in 1879, are best distinguished by their large metachromatic-staining cytoplasmic granules containing histamine, heparin, an assortment of proteolytic and degradative enzymes, and chemotactic factors (including eosinophil chemotactic factor and neutrophil chemotactic factor), all of which are released on degranulation. Mast cells also synthesize and release a variety of factors, including prostaglandins, slow releasing factors of anaphylaxis (SRS-A), platelet activating factor (PAF), growth factors, and a wide variety of cytokines: interleukin 3 (IL-3), interleukin 4 (IL-4), interleukin 5 (IL-5), interleukin 6 (IL-6), tumor necrosis factor α (TNFα), and granulocyte–macrophage colony stimulating factor (GM-CSF; Plaut et al., 1989; Wodnar-Filipowicz et al., 1989; Gordon and Galli, 1990; for a review, see Gordon et al., 1990).

Mast cells are most commonly known for their role in Type I (immediate hypersensitivity) reactions in which the fixation of IgE and antigen to mast cells via high-affinity Fc receptors causes the mast cells to degranulate, thus releasing their chemical mediators. These mediators initiate an inflammatory event by causing an increase in the blood flow and in the permeability of capillary endothelial cells (histamine), a decrease in blood coagulability (heparin), an increase in muscle tone (SRS-A), an increase in pain perception, contraction of smooth muscle cells (prostaglandins), and chemotaxis of an assortment of cell types.

Although mast cells are mainly associated with acute inflammatory events, they have also been linked to chronic inflammatory states such as systemic sclerosis (Hawkins *et al.*, 1985) and rheumatoid arthritis (Malone *et al.*, 1987). The exact function of mast cells in such states is currently unclear, but the cells appear to be localized in fibrotic lesions and may stimulate the proliferation of fibroblasts and the production of collagen directly (Druvefors and Norrby, 1988). Mast cells also contain a host of proteolytic enzymes that may be involved in normal connective tissue repair and remodeling. Further, fibroblasts produce many mediators that play a critically important role in the development and differentiation of normal mast cells (Davidson *et al.*, 1983; Davidson, 1986).

3. Platelets

Platelets have been implicated in the pathogenesis of atherosclerosis and inflammation, among other disorders. Platelets are anuclear cytoplasmic fragments derived from megakaryocytes in the bone marrow and, at 2–4 μm in size, are the smallest blood-borne elements. In their inactive state in the circulation, platelets tend to be dispersed but, on interaction with various stimuli, they clump to initiate blood coagulation. Normally, these cell fragments arrest bleeding by activating the clotting cascade.

Platelets contain three types of granules in their cytoplasm: dense granules, α granules, and lysosomes. Dense granules, also called delta granules, contain serotonin, ATP, ADP, and calcium ions; α granules contain fibrinogen, platelet-derived growth factor (PDGF), and other factors involved in the clotting cascade. Lysosomes, also referred to as small or lambda granules, contain hydrolytic enzymes. Transforming growth factor β (TGFβ) is also found in platelets.

When the endothelium is damaged and the underlying basement membrane exposed, platelets become activated (Ginsberg *et al.*, 1988; Terkeltaub and Ginsberg, 1989). These cell fragments have high affinity for connective tissue elements including fibronectin, fibrinogen, thrombospondin, and collagen; on interaction with these proteins, platelets change shape and degranulate, thereby triggering the clotting cascade aimed at repairing the walls of damaged blood vessels to prevent blood loss.

4. Eosinophils

Paul Ehrlich was the first to describe the eosinophil subclass with its distinctive cytoplasmic granules characterized by staining with acidic dyes. Eosinophils contain bilobed or multilobed nuclei with an abundance of red–orange cytoplasmic granules. These granules contain hydrolytic enzymes and peroxidases as well as mediators that modulate allergic responses and aid in resisting parasitic infection.

Eosinophils are commonly found in the connective tissue of the digestive and respiratory systems, they are elevated in these regions and in the circulation during allergic responses (asthma and hay fever) and after parasitic infection. Under these conditions, enhanced mobilization from the bone marrow allows an increased number of eosinophils to enter the circulatory system.

In addition to their role in acute inflammatory processes, eosinophils also participate in chronic inflammation although their numbers may be quite low. These cells do not directly phagocytose bacteria or other particulate antigens, but take up antigen–antibody complexes. Further, they release pharmacologically active mediators, including histaminase, serotonin, and prostaglandins, that increase vascular permeability.

Finally, eosinophils play a critical role in the response to parasitic infection. Major basic protein (MBP) contained in their granules is released on degranulation to coat the cell surface of the parasites and facilitate antibody-dependent killing of the organisms.

5. Basophils

Basophils are rare but distinctive cells with bilobed or U-shaped nuclei and large metachromatic or basophilic granules containing glycosaminoglycans and pharmacologically active mediators. The strongly anionic sulfated mucopolysaccharide of the glycosaminoglycans accounts for the staining pattern of basophils.

Basophils resemble connective tissue mast cells in both structure and function, yet they arise from different lineages. Both are involved in increasing the permeability of the vascular system during inflammation and in binding immunoglobulin—primarily IgE. Degranulation occurs in allergic reactions after the binding, of antigen-bound immunoglobulin to the cells surface. The granules of basophils contain agents that are chemotactic for leukocytes, as well as histamine, which causes vasodilation and promotes the migration of those cells from the circulatory system to the connective tissue. This phenomenon can cause local swelling and, in extreme cases, anaphylactic shock.

B. Cells of Chronic Inflammation

If the infiltration of neutrophils is not sufficient to clear an inflamed area, additional support is provided by nongranular leukocytes: lymphocytes and macrophages.

1. Lymphocytes

Lymphocytes constitute the second most numerous class of leukocytes, comprising 20–35% of the circulating white blood cells. These cells belong to two functional classes: thymus-dependent T lymphocytes and B cells, which are derived from the Bursa of Fabricius in chickens or the bone marrow in mammals. T and B cells are distinguished from one another by their class-specific cell surface antigens. In addition, they are classified by size into the arbitrary designations of small, medium, and large; the small lymphocyte is the predominant class.

Lymphocytes perform most of their immunological functions in connective tissue and are the immune-specific effector cells in delayed-type hypersensitivity. On activation by antigen, small lymphocytes undergo blast transformation and become large lymphocytes. The large lymphocytes then replicate, giving rise to cells of small and medium size that are progeny of the original small lymphocyte.

Plasma cells, found exclusively in tissues and not in the circulatory system, represent the end stage of B cell differentiation. These cells can be distinguished readily with the electron microscope by the presence of an extensive rough endoplasmic reticulum. Mature plasma cells are the major sources of secretory immunoglobulin (Leduc, 1955) and lack the normal surface immunoglobulin of precursor B cells. T lymphocytes also play a role in chronic inflammation by producing mediators that help attract and activate macrophages.

2. Macrophages

Monocytes constitute 3–8% of the circulating leukocyte population and mature into connective tissue macrophages on migration out of the circulatory system into specific extravascular compartments. After derivation from precursors in the bone marrow, monocytes remain in the circulation for 1–2 days before they differentiate into macrophages.

Macrophages are long-lived, highly motile, phagocytic cells with large numbers of lysosomes, endocytic vacuoles, and intracellular vesicles containing undigestible material. Macrophages ingest extracellular material by phagocytosis and pinocytosis. These internalized components are digested by lysosomal enzymes to clear them from the extracellular environment. On activation, the number of lysosomes per cell increases, as does the amount of hydrolytic enzyme per lysosome, to facilitate the digestion of material taken up by phagocytosis.

Under certain conditions, such as the invasion of foreign material, macrophages can form multinucleated giant cells resulting from the fusion of several macrophages. These giant cells can remain in the tissue for extended periods of time and are thought to act as barricades that surround foreign material, thus separating it from normal tissue.

In culture as well as in vivo, macrophages adhere to surfaces of cells and to extracellular matrix elements, and are able to migrate. In addition to making directed and random movements as cellular entities, macrophages can extend pseudopods in an ameboid fashion to reach out and explore their environment.

Tissue macrophages were initially named for the specific tissues in which they were identified, for example, alveolar or pulmonary macrophages of the lung. Although the macrophages from different tissues share certain "generic" characteristics, some characteristics are tissue specific. For example, because of the high concentration of oxygen in the lung, alveolar macrophages have a higher capacity to produce reactive oxygen metabolites than do macrophages from other tissues.

In addition to being migratory and phagocytic macrophages are also highly secretory, producing variety of mediators that range from cytokines and prostaglandins to connective tissue elements, (for a review, see Nathan, 1987).

C. Nonlymphoid Cells

In addition to leukocytes, epithelial and connective tissue cells play a role in the inflammatory process. Once thought of as passive bystanders in inflammatory events, fixed mesenchymal cells including epithelial cells, endothelial cells, and fibroblasts clearly play important roles in both acute and chronic inflammation.

Embryologically, connective tissue mesenchymal cells fill the spaces between developing organs. Mature connective tissue cells provide the structure for the delicate network of fibers and other extracellular matrix proteins. Moreover, connective tissue has a great capacity to repair itself.

1. *Fibroblasts*

Fibroblasts are the most abundant of connective tissue cell types. Although they may be dormant for prolonged periods of time, these cells are capable of returning to the cell cycle on stimulation by appropriate environmental cues. Fibroblasts then replicate and produce high levels of extracellular matrix proteins, primarily type I collagen, to fill the spaces left after inflammation or traumatic injury.

2. *Epithelial Cells*

Epithelial tissues have the following functions: (1) covering and lining surfaces, (2) absorption (e.g., in the intestine), (3) secretion (e.g., in glands), and (4) contractility (e.g., in the myoepithelium). These cells are labile structures and are renewed continuously by means of mitotic activity. Their renewal capacity is variable and is highly dependent on their rate of replication and their ability to migrate. In the lung, for example, where the alveolar epithelium must be maintained as a thin barrier to permit readily the exchange of oxygen between the alveolar space and the lumen of capillaries that lie in the alveolar septum, diffuse damage to the epithelium could be lethal. The alveolar type I pneumocyte, a squamous epithelial cell that covers the alveolar surface, is an end-stage cell with no ability to replicate. For the alveoli to regenerate an epithelial cover, cuboidal type II pneumocytes that are present in the alveoli must dedifferentiate, replicate, and migrate to the appropriate sites—a slow, inefficient, and therefore life-threatening process.

3. Endothelial Cells

The barrier between the connective tissue and the vascular system is the capillary endothelial cell. Endothelial cells constitute a subclass of epithelial cells that surround the lumen of blood vessels. Derived from the same mesenchymal cell precursor as the fibroblast, endothelial cells maintain capillary structure and function as (1) a selectively permeable barrier, (2) a synthetic and metabolic system, and (3) a nonthrombogenic container for blood. Under abnormal conditions, for example, when inflammation occurs, capillary and postcapillary venular permeability is greatly increased by altering the state of the junctional complexes between adjacent endothelial cells; thus, leukocytes may leave the bloodstream by passing between endothelial cells and entering the underlying tissue, a process called diapesis. The opening of these junctions appears to be caused by local release of mediators such as histamine and bradykinin.

Capillary endothelial cells also produce cell adhesion molecules and a variety of cytokines that allow margination of neutrophils prior to their migration from the blood vessels to the site of inflammation (for a review, see Mantovani and Dejana, 1989).

III. Inflammatory Process

Inflammation is the process by which leukocytes and materials derived from the serum are directed to the site of tissue injury. In the skin, for example, inflammation is characterized by local redness and swelling. Clotting factors, as well as factors that alter vascular permeability, aid in bringing about (1) vasodilation and enhanced blood flow to the affected area, (2) enhanced permeability of the capillaries, and (3) increased migration of effector cells (leukocytes) from the circulatory system to the connective tissue.

The inflammatory response can be divided into a series of overlapping stages: acute vascular, acute cellular, chronic cellular, and resolution. This response is triggered by trauma, infection, tissue necrosis, or immune reaction, which leads to the dilation of blood vessels causing the leakage of fluid from precapillary arterioles. Acute changes in blood flow pattern lead to margination of neutrophils along the vascular surface of the endothelial cells, followed by the directed migration of neutrophils through the endothelial cell monolayer into the connective tissue below. Depending on the degree of infection or tissue damage, this process may be sufficient to remove debris and to restore normal tissue structure. However, a chronic inflammatory infiltrate of macrophages and lymphocytes is usually necessary to remove bacteria and necrotic tissue. When the damage is more extensive, normal tissue is replaced in the resolution phase by scar tissue, a result of the proliferation of fibroblasts and the depositing of connective tissue proteins.

A. Chemotaxis

Histological analysis reveals that mononuclear leukocytes and PMNs are present in inflammatory tissue (for review, see Rot, 1992). A key element in the inflammatory process is chemotaxis, the directed migration of leukocytes diverted from the vascular system to sites of tissue damage by chemotactic factors that are generated at the site of inflammation and diffuse laterally. Chemotactic factors are small molecules with short half-lives that readily permit their diffusion and the termination of their effects.

A wide variety of agents is chemotactic for leukocytes, including C5A, formyl peptides (Schiffman et al., 1975), leukotriene B_4 (Palmblad et al., 1981), thrombin (Bar-Shavit et al., 1983), TGFβ, neutrophil activating/attracting peptide (NAP-1/IL-8; Kownatzki et al., 1986; Waltz et al., 1987; Yoshimura et al., 1987; Van Damme et al., 1988), monocyte chemotactic peptide (MCP-1; Leonard and Yoshimura, 1990), PAF (Shaw et al., 1981), the connective tissue proteins, fibronectin (Norris et al., 1982), collagen (Postlethwaite and Kang, 1976), laminin (Terranova et al., 1986), and fragments of elastin (Senior et al., 1980). Thus, blood-borne agents and components of disrupted basement membranes can attract cells to the extravascular space.

B. Cell Adhesion Molecules

For cells to migrate to and through endothelial cell monolayers, adhesion must take place. Whereas endothelial cells attach to one another by junctional complexes, leukocytes use a set of cell surface proteins called cell adhesion molecules (CAMs), which play roles in the processes of cell growth, migration, and differentiation (for reviews, see Albelda and Buck, 1990; Figdor et al., 1990; Springer, 1990). CAMs are categorized into the following superfamilies:

Integrins: Representative members of the integrin family, LFA-1 and Mac-1, contain α and β subunits of about 1100 and 750 amino acids, respectively (Hynes, 1987; Kishimoto et al., 1989).

Adhesion molecules of the immunoglobulin superfamily: Members of this class of adhesion molecules have sets of immunoglobulin domains composed of 90–100 amino acids, arranged in sheets of antiparallel β strands stabilized by disulfide bridges (Alzari et al., 1988; Williams and Barclay, 1988).

Selectins: Mel-14/LAM-1, ELAM-1, and CD62 are examples of this class of adhesion molecules. These proteins have an N-terminal domain of 117–120 amino acids that is homologous to that of the Ca^{2+}-dependent animal lectins (Bevilacqua et al., 1989; Stoolman, 1989; Tedder et al., 1989).

The adhesion of leukocytes to the endothelial cell surface, and their migration out of the vascular system to the interstitial space, requires CAMs. Neutrophils, for example, express Mac-1 or LFA-1, enabling them to adhere to endothelial cells expressing ICAM-1. LFA-1 can also interact with ICAM-2. The endothelial cell adhesion molecule that binds Mel-14/LAM-1 is unknown. Lymphocytes bearing LFA-1 can also bind to ICAM-expressing cells. Cytokines and bacterial products up-regulate the expression of CAMs on the surfaces of both leukocytes and endothelial cells (Albelda and Buck, 1990). For example, IL-1 and TNFα induce the expression of ICAM on endothelial cells (Pober et al., 1986; Pohlman et al., 1986).

To initiate wound healing, platelets adhere to the extracellular matrix products that are exposed after damage to the endothelium (Ginsberg et al., 1988). The activation of the clotting cascade stimulates aggregation of additional platelets that degranulate to release thrombin and TGFβ. The expression of fibronectin receptors on keratinocytes, for example, facilitates their migration over the fibronectin molecules abundant in wounds (Toda et al., 1987). Neutrophils then adhere to the surfaces of capillary endothelial cells and pass through gaps between the cells of postcapillary venules in response to neutrophil-specific chemotactic signals. Tissue necrosis is triggered by the release of hydrolytic enzymes and reactive metabolites of oxygen from neutrophils (Varani et al., 1989).

Thrombin and TGFβ also play a role in chronic inflammation by stimulating the expression of integrins on the surfaces of macrophages and fibroblasts, facilitating their infiltration into the site of injury (Heino and Massague, 1989).

C. Actions of Effector Cells

Once leukocytes have been summoned to an injured site, they exert effects on target tissues either directly through cell contact or indirectly via secretory mediators such as cytokines and eicosanoids. A description of the various inflammatory cytokines and their actions is included in Chapter 3.

In addition to cytokines, other nonpeptide mediators, such as the products of arachidonic acid metabolism—including prostaglandins, leukotrienes, and thromboxanes—are produced by effector cells during the inflammatory process. Derived from the breakdown of membrane phospholipids, these metabolites are produced by most, if not all, of the cells that participate in inflammatory responses, including cells of immune and nonimmune origin.

Arachidonic acid metabolism can be divided into the cyclooxygenase pathway and the lipoxygenase pathway. The role of prostaglandins—products of the cyclooxygenase pathway—in the activation of macrophages, for example, has been reviewed elsewhere (Zwilling and Justement, 1988). Several laboratories have demonstrated the role of prostaglandin E_2 (PGE$_2$) in regulating production of IL-1 and TNFα (for a review, see Kovacs, 1991b). Studies have reported the coincidental production of cytokines and PGE$_2$, suggesting a possible autocrine or paracrine role for arachidonate metabolites in the control of IL-1 and TNFα gene expression (Kunkel et al., 1986a). Prostaglandins induce cytokines and cytokines induce prostaglandins, thus completing an additional autocrine loop.

Histamine is the major preformed mediator of mast cells. Formed from the amino acid histidine by an enzyme found in the cytoplasm of mast cells and basophils, its effects are mediated by two distinct classes of receptors, designated H_1 and H_2. Acute vascular inflammatory effects are transduced through H_1 receptors on the surfaces of smooth muscle cells; antiinflammatory effects involve H_2 receptors.

In addition, nitric oxide and reactive oxygen intermediates could be thought of as secretory mediators because they are made by one cell type and exhibit their effects on another. The production of reactive nitrogen intermediates by mammalian cells is a relatively recent observation (Stuehr and Marletta, 1985; Ignarro et al., 1987; Palmer et al., 1987; Amber et al., 1988), whereas the generation of reactive metabolites of oxygen has been known for some time. The oxygen intermediates include superoxide (Drath and Karnovsky, 1975), hydroxyl radical (Weiss et al., 1977), and hydrogen peroxide (Nathan and Root, 1977). Nitric oxide, synthesized from L-arginine in macrophages, appears to play a critical role in antimicrobial activity (for a review, see Marletta et al., 1989). The activity of nitric oxide synthase, the enzyme responsible for the production of the reactive intermediate, is prompted by both cytokines and microbial products (for a review, see Nathan and Hibbs, 1991). Thioglycolate-elicited peritoneal macrophages, as well as macrophage cell lines, do not have enzymatic activity prior to stimulation (Stuehr and Marletta, 1985). Exposure to interferon γ (IFNγ) alone can induce a low level of activity of the enzyme (Ding et al., 1988); however, treatment with IFNγ in the presence of lipopolysaccharide or muramyl dipeptide triggers high levels of enzymatic activity (Stuehr and Marletta, 1987; Ding et al., 1988; Drapier et al., 1988). IFNγ also acts synergistically with TNFα and TNFβ to induce nitrogen oxide (Esparza et al., 1987; Bogdan et al., 1990). Since bacterial products are good inducers of TNFα production, the role played by microorganisms in the generation of nitrogen oxide may be mediated in part by their induction of TNFα production and by the consequent macrophage response (Green et al., 1990). Finally, several cytokines have been shown to interfere with nitrogen oxide synthase activity, including macrophage deactivating factor, TGF $β_1$, $β_2$, and $β_3$ (Ding et al., 1990), and IL-10 (Gazzinelli et al., 1992).

IV. Resolution of Inflammation

The return to normal tissue structure and function following a local inflammatory event depends on the degree of damage to the tissue and the ability of cells within the tissue to regenerate (as described earlier). In the lung, for example, after the removal of the epithelium, a "competition" arises between reepitheliazation and fibrosis (Terzaghi *et al.*, 1978; Hascheck and Witschi, 1979; Hastlet and Henson, 1988). Evidence suggests that macrophages play a critical role in both processes (Leibovich and Ross, 1975) by elaborating cytokines that stimulate interstitial fibroblasts to replicate and synthesize extracellular matrix proteins, primarily type I collagen (Fulmer *et al.*, 1980; Scharffetter *et al.*, 1989; Darby *et al.*, 1990; for a review, see Kovacs, 1991b). PDGF, derived in part from macrophages, is thought to play a major role in wound healing (Pierce *et al.*, 1991) and in the pathogenesis of pulmonary fibrosis (Shaw *et al.*, 1991). In the absence of inhibitory signals, the aberrant production of these mediators sustains the connective tissue accumulation, which results in permanent alteration of tissue architecture.

The replacement of the epithelial cell layer consisting of type I pneumocytes has been studied to a lesser extent. Researchers believe that type II pneumocytes represent the precursor cells for the alveolar epithelium, and that they replicate and differentiate into the cells that cover the alveolar surface (Witschi, 1991). Mediators derived from macrophages also stimulate the replication of alveolar type II cells (Leslie *et al.*, 1985;1990), thus aiding in the reepitheliazation process.

V. Summary

Inflammation is the process by which proteins and cells accumulate at a site of tissue damage or infection. The activation of the cells at these sites leads to the removal of necrotic tissue and either regeneration of normal tissue or replacement with scar tissue. The inflammatory process is designed to provide a rapid mechanism by which the host can respond to the invasion of foreign materials and return to a homeostatic equilibrium. Excessive or inadequate activation of the system can have serious effects, as can the failure of inactivation mechanisms.

Acknowledgments

This work was sponsored by grants from the Elsa U. Pardee Foundation and the Office of Naval Research.

References

Albelda, S. M., and Buck, C. A. (1990). Integrins and other cell adhesion molecules. *FASEB J.* **4**, 2868–2880.

Alzari, P. M., Lascombe, M-B., and Poljak, R. J. (1988). Three dimensional structure of antibodies. *Ann. Rev. Immunol.* **6**, 555–580.

Amber, I. J., Hibbs, J. B., Jr., Taintor, R. R., and Vavrin, Z. (1988). The L-arginine dependent effector mechanism is induced in murine adenocarcinoma cells by supernatant from cytotoxic activated macrophages. *J. Leukocyte Biol.* **43**, 187–192.

Bar-Shavit, R., Kahn, A., Fenton, J. W., II, and Wilner, G. D. (1983). Chemotactic response of monocytes to thrombin. *J. Cell Biol.* **96**, 282–285.

Bevilacqua, M. P., Stengelin, S., Gimbrone, M. A., and Seed, B. (1989). Endothelial leukocyte adhesion molecule 1: An inducible receptor for neutrophils related to complement regulatory proteins and lectins. *Science* **243**, 1160–1165.

Bogdan, C., Moll, H., Solbach, W., and Rollinghoff, M. (1990). Tumor necrosis factor α in combination with interferon-γ, but not with interleukin-4 activates murine macrophages for elimination of *Leishmania major* amastigotes. *Eur. J. Immunol.* **20**, 1131–1135.

Darby, I., Skalli, O., and Gabbiani, G. (1990). α-Smooth muscle cell actin is transiently expressed by myofibroblasts during experimental wound healing. *Lab. Invest.* **63**, 21–29.

Davidson, S. (1986). Fibroblasts are required for mast cell granule synthesis. *In* "Mast Cell Differentiation and Heterogeneity" (A. D. Befus, J. Bienenstock, and J. A. Denburg, eds.), pp. 115–124. Raven Press, New York.

Davidson, S., Mansour, A., Gallily, R., Smolarski, M., and Ginsburg, H. (1983). Mast cell differentiation depends on T cell and granule synthesis in fibroblasts. *Immunology* **48**, 439–452.

Ding, A., Nathan, C. F., and Stuehr, D. J. (1988). Nitrogen intermediates from mouse peritoneal macrophages: Comparison of activating cytokines and evidence for independent production. *J. Immunol.* **141**, 96–103.

Ding, A., Nathan, C. F., Graycar, J., Derynck, R., Stuehr, D. J., and Srimal, S. (1990). Macrophage deactivating factor and transforming growth factors β_1, β_2 and β_3 inhibit induction of macrophage nitrogen oxide synthesis by interferon γ. *J. Immunol.* **145**, 940–944.

Drapier, J. C., Wietzerbin, J., and Hibbs, J. B., Jr. (1988). Interferon γ and tumor necrosis factor induce L-arginine dependent cytotoxic effector mechanism in murine macrophages. *Eur. J. Immunol.* **18**, 1587–1592.

Drath, D. B., and Karnovsky, M. L. (1975). Superoxide production by phagocytic leukocytes. *J. Exp. Med.* **141**, 257–262.

Druvefors, P., and Norrby, K. (1988). Molecular aspects of mast cell-mediated mitogenesis in fibroblasts and mesothelial cells in situ. *Virchow's Arch. B* **55**, 187–192.

Esparza, I., Mannel, D., Ruppel, A., Falk, W., and Krammer, P. (1987). Interferon-γ and lymphotoxin or tumor necrosis factor act synergistically to induce macrophage killing of tumor cells and schistosomula of *Schistosoma mansini*. *J. Exp. Med.* **166**, 589–594.

Figdor, C. G., van Kooyk, Y., and Keizer, G. D. (1990). On the mode of action of LFA-1. *Immunol. Today* **11**, 277–280.

Fulmer, J. D., Beinkowski, R. S., Cowan, M. J., Breul, S. D., Bradley, K. M., Ferrans, J., Roberts, W. C., and Crystal, R. G. (1980). Collagen concentration and rates of synthesis in idiopathic pulmonary fibrosis. *Am. Rev. Resp. Dis.* **122**, 289–301.

Gazzinelli, R. T., Oswald, I. P., James, S. L., and Sher, A. (1992). IL-1 inhibits parasite killing and nitrogen oxide production by IFNγ activated macrophages. *J. Immunol.* **148**, 1792–1796.

Ginsberg, M. H., Loftus, J. C., and Plow, E. F. (1988). Cytoadhesions, integrins and platelets. *Thromb. Hemostasis* **59**, 1–6.

Gordon, J. R., and Galli, S. L. (1990). Mast cells as a source of both preformed and immunologically inducible TNFα/cachectin. *Nature (London)* **339**, 274–276.

Gordon, J. R., Burd, P. R., and Galli, S. L. (1990). Mast cells as a source of multifunctional cytokines. *Immunol. Today* **11**, 458–464.

Green, S. J., Mellouk, S., Hoffman, S. L., Meltzer, M. S., and Nacy, C. A. (1990). Cellular mechanisms of nonspecific immunity to intracellular infection: Cytokine induced synthesis of toxic nitrogen oxides from L-arginine by macrophages and hepatocytes. *Immunol. Lett.* **25**, 15–20.

Haslett, C., and Henson, P. M. (1988). Resolution of inflammation. In "The Molecular and Cellular Biology of Wound Repair" (R. A. F. Clark and P. M. Henson, eds.), pp. 185–211. Plenum, New York.

Hascheck, W. M., and Witschi, P. (1979). Pulmonary fibrosis—A possible mechanism. *Toxicol. Appl. Pharmacol.* **51**, 475–487.

Hawkins, R. A., Claman, H. N., Clark, R. A. F., and Steigerwals, J. C. (1985). Increased dermal mast cell populations in progressive systemic sclerosis: A link to chronic fibrosis. *Ann. Intern. Med.* **102**, 182–186.

Heino, J., and Massague, J. (1989). Transforming growth factor β switches the pattern of integrins expressed in MG-63 human osteosarcoma cells and causes a selective loss of cell adhesion to laminin. *J. Biol. Chem.* **264**, 21806–21811.

Hynes, R. O. (1987). Integrins: A family of cell surface receptors. *Cell* **48**, 549–554.

Ignarro, L. J., Buga, G. M., Wood, K. S., Byrnes, R. E., and Chaudhuri, G. (1987). Endothelium-derived relaxing factor produced and released by artery and vein is nitric oxide. *Proc. Natl. Acad. Sci. USA* **84**, 9265–9269.

Kishimoto, T. K., Larson, R. S., Corbi, A. L., Dustin, M. L., Staunton, D. E., and Springer, T. A. (1989). The leukocyte integrins. *Adv. Immunol.* **46**, 149–182.

Kovacs, E. J. (1991a). Fibrogenic cytokines: The role of immune mediators in the development of fibrosis. *Immunol. Today* **12**, 17–23.

Kovacs, E. J. (1991b). Control of IL-1 and TNF mRNA expression by inhibitors of second messenger pathways. In "Cytokines in Inflammatory Diseases" (E. Kimball, ed.), pp. 87–105. CRC Press, Boca Raton, Florida.

Kownatzki, E., Kapp, A., and Ulrich, S. (1986). Novel neutrophil chemotactic factor derived from human peripheral blood leukocytes. *Clin. Exp. Immunol.* **64**, 214–222.

Kunkel, S. L., Chensue, S. W., and Phan, S. H. (1986a). Prostaglandins as endogenous mediators of interleukin 1 production. *J. Immunol.* **136**, 182–192.

Kunkel, S. L., Wiggins, R. C., Chensue, S. W., and Larrick, J. (1986b). Regulation of macrophage tumor necrosis factor production by prostaglandin E_2. *Biochem. Biophys. Res. Commun.* **137**, 404–412.

Leduc, E. H. (1955). Studies on antibody production. II. The primary and secondary responses in the popliteal lymph node of the rabbit. *J. Exp. Med.* **102**, 61–72.

Leibovich, S. J., and Ross, R. (1975). The role of macrophages in wound repair: A study with hydrocortisone and anti-macrophage serum. *Am. J. Physiol.* **78**, 71–91.

Leonard, E. J., and Yoshimura, T. (1990). Human monocyte chemoattractant protein-1 (MCP-1). *Immunol. Today* **11**, 97–101.

Leslie, C. C., McCormick-Shannon, K., Cook, J. L., and Mason, R. J. (1985). Macrophages stimulate DNA synthesis in rat alveolar type II cells. *Am. Rev. Resp. Dis.* **132**, 1246–1252.

Leslie, C. C., McCormick-Shannon, K., and Mason, R. J. (1990). Heparin-binding growth factors stimulate DNA synthesis in rat alveolar type II cells. *Am. J. Resp. Cell. Mol. Biol.* **2**, 99–106.

Malone, D. G., Wilder, R. L., Saaverda-Delgado, A. M., and Metcalf, D. D. (1987). Mast cell numbers in rheumatoid synovial tissues. *Arthritis Rheum.* **30**, 130–137.

Mantovani, A., and Dejana, E. (1989). Cytokines and communication signals between leukocytes and endothelial cells. *Immunol. Today* **10**, 370–375.

Marletta, M. A. (1989). Nitric oxide: Biosynthesis and biological significance. *Trends Biochem. Sci.* **14**, 488–452.

Metchnikoff, E. (1907). "Immunity in Infective Diseases" (F. A. Starling and E. H. Starling, transl.). Paul Trench, Trubner, London.

Nathan, C. F. (1987). Secretory products of macrophages. *J. Clin. Invest.* **79**, 319–326.

Nathan, C. F., and Hibbs, J. B., Jr. (1991). Role of nitric oxide synthesis in macrophage antimicrobial activity. *Curr. Opin. Immunol.* **3**, 65–70.

Nathan, C. F., and Root, R. K. (1977). Hydrogen peroxide release from mouse peritoneal macrophages: Dependence on sequential activation and triggering. *J. Exp. Med.* **146**, 1648–1662.

Norris, D. A., Clark, R. A. F., Swigart, L. M., Huff, J. C., Weston, W. L., and Howell, S. E. (1982). Fibronectin fragment(s) are chemotactic for human peripheral blood monocytes. *J. Immunol.* **129**, 1612–1618.

Palmblad, J., Malmsten, C. L., Uden, A.-M., Radmark, O., Engstedt, L., and Samuelsson, B. (1981). Leukotriene B$_4$ is a potent and stereospecific stimulator of neutrophil chemotaxis and adherence. *Blood* **58**, 658–661.

Palmer, R. M. J., Ferrige, A. G., and Moncada, S. (1987). Nitric oxide release accounts for the biological activity of endothelium-derived relaxing factor. *Nature (London)* **327**, 524–526.

Pierce, G. F., Mustoe, T. A., Altrock, B. W., Deuel, T. F., and Thomason, A. (1991). Role of platelet derived growth factor in wound healing. *J. Cell. Biochem.* **45**, 319–326.

Plaut, M., Pierce, J. H., Watson, C. J., Hanley-Hyde, J., Nordan, R. P., and Paul, W. E. (1989). Mast cell lines produce lymphokines in response to cross-linkage of Fc epsilon RI or to calcium ionophores. *Nature (London)* **339**, 64–67.

Pober, J. S., Gimbrone, M. A., Jr., Lapierre, L. A., Mendrick, D. L., Fiers, W., Rothlein, R., and Springer, T. A. (1986). Overlapping patterns of activation of human endothelial cells by interleukin 1, and tumor necrosis factor, interferon-γ. *J. Immunol.* **137**, 1893–1896.

Pohlman, T. H., Stanness, K. A., Beat, P. G., Ochs, H. D., and Harlan, J. M. (1986). An endothelial cell surface factor(s) induced in vitro by lipopolysaccharide, interleukin-1, and tumor necrosis factor α increased neutrophil adherence by a CDw18-dependent mechanism. *J. Immunol.* **136**, 4548–4553.

Postlethwaite, A. E., and Kang, A. H. (1976). Collagen- and collagen peptide-induced chemotaxis of human blood monocytes. *J. Exp. Med.* **143**, 1299–1307.

Rot, A. (1992). The role of leukocyte chemotaxis in inflammation. *In* "Biochemistry of Inflammation" (J. Whicher and S. Evans, eds.), pp. 263–296. Kluwer Publishing, Lancaster, England.

Scharffetter, K., Kulozik, M., Stolz, W., Lankat-Buttgereit, B., Hatamochi, A., Sohnchen, R., and Krieg, T. (1989). Localization of collagen α$_1$ (I) gene during wound healing by in situ hybridization. *J. Invest. Dermatol.* **93**, 405–412.

Schiffman, E., Corcoran, B. A., and Wahl, S. M. (1975). N-Formylmethionyl peptides as chemoattractants for leukocytes. *Proc. Natl. Acad. Sci. USA* **72**, 1059–1062.

Senior, R. M., Griffin, G. L., and Mecham, R. P. (1980). Chemotactic activity of elastin-derived peptides. *J. Clin. Invest.* **66**, 859–862.

Shaw, J. O., Pinckard, R. N., Ferrigni, K. S., McManus, L. M., and Hanahan, D. J. (1981). Activation of human neutrophils with 1-O-hexadecyl/octadecyl-2-acetyl-sn-glyceryl-3-phosphorylcholine (platelet-activating factor). *J. Immunol.* **127**, 1250–1255.

Shaw, R. J., Benedict, S. H., Clark, R. A. F., and King, T. E., Jr. (1991). Pathogenesis of pulmonary interstitial lung disease: Alveolar macrophage PDGF(B) gene activation and up-regulation by interferon-γ. *Am. Rev. Resp. Dis.* **143**, 167–173.

Springer, T. A. (1990). Adhesion receptors of the immune system. *Nature (London)* **346**, 425–434.

Stoolman, L. M. (1989). Adhesion molecules controlling lymphocyte migration. *Cell* **24**, 907–910.

Stuehr, D. J., and Marletta, M. A. (1985). Mammalian nitrate biosynthesis: Mouse macrophages produce nitrate and nitrite in response to *Escherichia coli* lipopolysaccharide. *Proc. Natl. Acad. Sci. USA* **82**, 7738–7742.

Stuehr, D. J., and Marletta, M. A. (1987). Induction of nitrite/nitrate synthesis in murine macrophages by BCG infection, lymphokines or interferony. *J. Immunol.* **139,** 518–525.

Tedder, T. F., Issacs, C. M., Ernst, Y. J., Demetri, G. D., Adler, D. A., and Disteche, C. M. (1989). Isolation and chromosomal localization of cDNAs encoding a novel lymphocyte cell surface molecule, LAM-1: Homology with the mouse lymphocyte homing receptor and other human adhesion proteins. *J. Exp. Med.* **170,** 123–133.

Terkeltaub, R. A., and Ginsberg, M. H. (1989). Platelets and response to injury. In "Molecular and Cell Biology of Wound Healing" (R. A. F. Clark and P. M. Henson, eds.), pp. 35–55. Plenum Press, New York.

Terranova, V. P., DiFlorio, R., Hujanen, E. S., Lyall, R. M., Liota, L. A., Thorgeirsson, U., Siegal, G. P., and Schiffmann, E. (1986). Laminin promotes rabbit neutrophil motility and attachment. *J. Clin. Invest.* **77,** 1180–1186.

Terzaghi, M., Nettesheim, P., and Williams, M. L. (1978). Population of denuded tracheal grafts with normal, preneoplastic, and neoplastic epithelial cell populations. *Cancer Res.* **38,** 4546–4553.

Toda, K.-L., Tuan, T.-L., Brown, P. J., and Grinnell, F. (1987). Fibronectin receptors of human keratinocytes and their expression during cell culture. *J. Cell. Biol.* **104,** 3097–3104.

Van Damme, J., Van Beeuman, J., Opdenakker, G., and Billiau, A. (1988). A novel NH_2-terminal sequence-characterized human monokine possessing neutrophil chemotactic, skin-reactive, and granulocyte-promoting activity. *J. Exp. Med.* **167,** 1364–1376.

Varani, J., Ginsberg, I., Schuger, L., Gibbs, D. F., Bromberg, J., Johnson, K. J., Ryan, U. S., and Ward, P. A. (1989). Endothelial cell killing by neutrophils: Synergistic interaction of oxygen products and proteases. *Am. J. Pathol.* **135,** 435–438.

Waltz, A., Peveri, P., Aschauer, H., and Baggoiolini, M. (1987). Purification and amino acid sequence of NAF, a novel neutrophil-activating factor produced by monocytes. *Biochem. Biophys. Res. Commun.* **149,** 755–761.

Weiss, S. J., King, G. W., and LoBuglio, A. F. (1977). Evidence for hydroxyl radical generation by human monocytes. *J. Clin. Invest.* **60,** 370–373.

Williams, A. F., and Barclay, A. N. (1988). The immunoglobulin superfamily—Domains for cell surface recognition. *Ann. Rev. Immunol.* **6,** 381–405.

Witschi, H. (1991). Role of the epithelium in lung repair. *Chest* **99,** 22S–25S.

Wodnar-Filipowicz, A., Heusser, C. H., and Moroni, C. (1989). Production of the hematopoietic growth factors GM-CSF and interleukin-3 by mast cells in response to IgE receptor-meditated activation. *Nature (London)* **339,** 150–152.

Yoshimura, T., Matsushima, K., Tanaka, S., Robinson, E. A., Appella, E., Oppenheim, J. J., and Leonard, E. J. (1987). Purification of a human monocyte-derived neutrophil chemotactic factor that has peptide sequence similarity to the host defence cytokines. *Proc. Natl. Acad. Sci. USA* **84,** 9233–9237.

Zwilling, B. S., and Justement, L. B. (1988). Prostaglandin regulation of macrophage function. In "Macrophages and Cancer" (G. H. Heppner and A. M. Fulton, eds.), pp. 62–78. CRC Press, Boca Raton, Florida.

3

Inflammatory Cytokines: An Overview

Mary E. Brandes and Sharon M. Wahl

I. Introduction

The inflammatory response that ensues after an insult to the body is characterized by an influx of neutrophils and monocytes. If the inciting agent is antigenic, lymphocytes are also present in the cellular infiltrate, and play a central role in the initiation and maintenance of immunologically mediated inflammation. Protein, peptide, and lipid mediators produced by these leukocytes, as well as by cells of the injured tissue, precisely control the inflammatory events (Wong and Wahl, 1990). One class of these mediators is the inflammatory cytokines, small proteins produced and secreted in response to exogenous stimulation. These signaling molecules interact with specific receptors on target cells, causing a modification in the function or behavior of those cells. Often, the effects of cytokines are confined to the local environment in which they were generated. However, some cytokines attain very significant concentrations in the serum, where they may mediate systemic manifestations after certain kinds of injury. Cytokines are instrumental in moderating every stage of the inflammatory response, from the initial recruitment of inflammatory cells to the resolution of the injury.

The terms growth factor, monokine, and lymphokine are sometimes used instead of the term cytokine to refer to a subset of the cytokines. In general, monokines are monocyte/macrophage-derived molecules and lymphokines are produced by T or B lymphocytes. Historically, the term "growth factor" has been used to identify proteins that affect the growth status of nonhematopoietic cells, whereas "cytokine" has been used to refer to molecules that alter cellular function relevant to immune and inflammatory processes. However, as our understanding of the multiple roles of these signaling molecules has grown, the distinction between cytokines and growth factors has blurred. Specific growth factors have been shown to regulate events within the inflammatory response, and some inflammatory cytokines ap-

Xenobiotics and Inflammation
Copyright 1994 © by Academic Press, Inc. All rights of reproduction in any form reserved.

pear to control a variety of noninflammatory activities including the growth state of cells under normal homeostatic conditions. In general, the term "cytokine" is currently used to refer to all polypeptide regulators of cell function. However, this chapter focuses only on those cytokines that have been shown to be important during inflammation, either immunologically mediated or otherwise: interleukins 1, 2, 4, 6 (IL-1, IL-2, IL-4, IL-6), tumor necrosis factor α (TNFα), interferon γ (IFNγ), macrophage inflammatory proteins (MIP-1, -2 families, also known as intercrines), transforming growth factor β (TBFβ), and colony stimulating factors: granulocyte, macrophage, granulocyte–macrophage, and multicolony stimulating factors (G-CSF, M-CSF, GM-CSF, multi-CSF/IL-3). Cytokines involved in repair and resolution of the injury [platelet-derived growth factor (PDGF), fibroblast growth factor (FGF), epidermal growth factor (EGF/TGFα)] and those that appear primarily to affect the humoral immune response but also may affect inflammatory events, will be considered briefly at the end of the chapter. The participation of the newly identified cytokines IL-9 (Kelleher et al., 1991), IL-10 (Thompson-Snipes et al., 1991), and IL-11 (Paul et al., 1990) in inflammation has not yet been extensively studied, and hence will not be considered here.

As mentioned earlier, the inflammatory cytokines are produced by many cell types. Cells of the inflammatory infiltrate including polymorphonuclear neutrophils (PMNS), monocytes, and lymphocytes are the major sources of cytokines during the inflammatory reaction because of their large number and persistence at the site of the injury (Table I). However, tissue macrophages, parenchymal cells, and stromal cells (fibroblasts and endothelial cells) are also important contributors to the generation of inflammatory cytokines. These resident cells may be most significant immediately after insult to the tissue and later, during the resolution of the inflammatory response. Overt injury to the tissue by certain toxic agents may result in the release of cytokines stored by parenchymal cells; for example, injury to the skin is followed by keratinocyte release of IL-1 (Kupper, 1990a; Figure 1). Platelets also contain large stores of cytokines, including TGFβ, PDGF, and EGF (Oka and Orth, 1983; Wong and Wahl, 1990). If the tissue injury results in damage to endothelial cells, platelet aggregation and release of stored platelet cytokines rapidly follows.

Many of the inflammatory cytokines do not exist as stored proteins, but are generated by stimulated cells. Some xenobiotics may cause an immediate activation of tissue macrophages, resulting in the production and release of cytokines by these cells. For instance, deposition of inhaled particulates such as asbestos fibers in the alveolar region of the lung results in the activation of the resident macrophages and the subsequent production and release of inflammatory cytokines (Brandes and Finkelstein, 1990; Kelley, 1990). Thus, the rapid release of cytokines locally by resident cells in response to xenobiotics may provide the origin for the evolution of an inflammatory response.

Table I Major Sources of the Inflammatory Cytokines

Cytokine[a]	Major source
MIP/intercrines	Monocytes/macrophages, T cells, fibroblasts, endothelial cells, platelets
TGFβ	Platelets, many cell types
IL-1	Monocytes/macrophages, T and B cells, neutrophils, fibroblasts, endothelial cells, other cell types
TNFα	Monocytes/macrophages, T and B cells, neutrophils, endothelial cells, other cell types
M-CSF	Monocytes/macrophages, fibroblasts, endothelial cells
GM-CSF	Monocytes/macrophages, T cells, fibroblasts, endothelial cells
G-CSF	Monocytes/macrophages, endothelial cells
IL-3	T cells
IL-2	T cells
IFNγ	T cells
IL-4	T cells
IL-6	Monocytes/macrophages, fibroblasts, endothelial cells, B and T cells, other cell types

[a] Abbreviations: MIP, macrophage inflammatory protein; TGFβ, transforming growth factor β; IL, interleukin; TNFα, tumor necrosis factor α; M-CSF, macrophage colony stimulating factor; GM-CSF, granulocyte–macrophage colony stimulating factor; G-CSF, granulocyte colony stimulating factor; IFNγ, interferon γ.

Cytokines generated as an immediate result of tissue injury function in multiple ways to promote the inflammatory response (Wong and Wahl, 1990). Some of these proteins are chemotactic factors for specific leukocyte populations (Table II). For instance, TGFβ is a very potent chemotactic factor for monocytes and neutrophils, stimulating their chemotaxis at femtomolar concentrations (Wahl et al., 1987a; Brandes et al., 1991a). Other chemotactic factors that are generated in the early stages of the inflammatory response, for example, the complement component C5a and leukotriene B$_4$ (LTB$_4$), are also effective, although at much higher concentrations (Goldstein, 1988). In addition to promoting leukocyte chemotaxis, cytokines can promote the infiltration of these cells by stimulating the increased expression of adhesion molecules on both leukocytes and endothelial cells (Springer, 1990). Another role cytokines play in the earliest stages of the inflammatory response is activation of the leukocytes that have just migrated into the tissue. In this regard, some of the cytokines that function as chemotactic factors at low concentrations activate the leukocytes at the higher concentrations present at the injury site (Wahl et al., 1987a). Activation of inflammatory leukocytes has multiple effects, including the production of potentially destructive reactive oxygen intermediates and the release of protease-containing granules. In addition, leukocyte activation by cytokines stimulates the synthesis and release of additional cytokines that can act in similar capacities, thus establishing autocrine and paracrine regulatory loops and maintaining the inflammatory state. As the inflammatory response wanes,

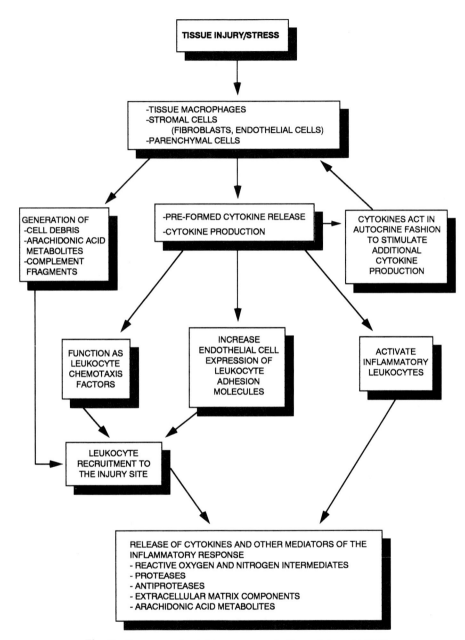

Fig. 1 Sequence of cytokine response to tissue injury or stress.

Table II   Cellular Responses Induced by Cytokines during Inflammation

Cytokine-stimulated cellular effects	Cytokines[a]
Promotion of chemotaxis	
monocytes	MIP/intercrines, TGFβ, M-CSF, G-CSF
neutrophils	MIP/intercrines, TGFβ, G-CSF
lymphocytes	MIP/intercrines
fibroblasts	MIP/intercrines, TGFβ, TNFα
endothelial cells	G-CSF, GM-CSF
Enhanced leukocyte–endothelial cell adhesion	MIP/intercrines, IL-1, TNFα, GM-CSF, TGFβ
Increased cellular cytotoxicity (phagocytosis, degranulation, generation of reactive oxygen, and nitrogen intermediates)	MIP/intercrines, TNFα, IL-1, CSF, IL-2, IFNγ
Prostaglandin synthesis	
stimulation	IL-1, TNFα, GM-CSF
inhibition	IFNγ, IL-4
Synthesis of inflammatory cytokines	
stimulation	TGFβ, IL-1, TNFα, GM-CSF, IL-2, IFNγ, IL-4
inhibition	TGFβ, IL-4
Altered expression of cytokine receptors	
increases	IL-1
decreases	TNFα, IFNγ
Protease synthesis	
stimulation	IL-1, TNFα, TGFβ
inhibition	IL-4, TGFβ
Inhibition of monocyte programmed cell death	IL-1, TNFα, M-CSF, GM-CSF
Cell proliferation and differentiation	
stimulation	
hematopoietic progenitors	IL-1, M-CSF, GM-CSF, G-CSF, IL-3, IL-6
T cells	IL-1, IL-2, IL-6
fibroblasts	MIP/intercrines, TGFβ
endothelial cells	G-CSF, GM-CSF
inhibition	TGFβ
Stimulate synthesis of matrix proteins	TGFβ, IL-1, TNFα

[a] For abbreviations, see Table I.

absence or low concentrations of appropriate activating signals may foster leukocyte programmed cell death (apoptosis) and cessation of the inflammatory response (Mangan *et al.*, 1991).

The concept that cellular interactions during inflammation are controlled by cytokine cascades or networks, rather than by the action of individual cytokines on discrete cell populations, has gained wide acceptance in recent years (Arai *et al.*, 1990; Kelley, 1990; Warren, 1990). Most cytokines are now recognized to be pleiotropic and to express multiple biological activities. The functional outcome of cytokine–cell interactions is often dependent on the type of target cell, its maturation state, target cell receptor expression, the type and density of surrounding cells, the concentration of the cytokine, and the presence or absence of other cytokines. These variables are often held constant during *in vitro* studies, yielding consistent results, but ones that do not necessarily mimic the range or magnitude of effects the cytokine might express when generated *in vivo*. In this regard, results of *in vitro* studies must be interpreted narrowly, and conclusions about parallel effects in *in vivo* systems must be drawn with caution. Therefore, studies that examine the effects of cytokine administration *in vivo*, and *in vitro* studies that use crude cytokine mixtures derived from fluids and effluents from inflamed tissues, are important adjuncts to studies that use purified or recombinant cytokine preparations in well-defined *in vitro* systems.

The successful use of *in vitro* culture systems to identify the action of cytokines also depends on a tissue culture system that closely mimics the cellular environment *in vivo*. Consideration must be given to the type and concentration of serum or serum analogs, the concentration of necessary nutrients and cofactors, the type of extracellular matrix, and the necessity of accessory cells to maintain normal cell function. In the absence of adequate culture conditions, primary cell cultures have been shown to lose receptors and, thus, responsiveness to various cytokines. Despite the inherent artificial nature of *in vitro* culture systems, these systems are necessary simplifications of the complex *in vivo* system and have yielded the bulk of our understanding of the diverse actions of cytokines.

II. Inflammatory Cytokines: Biology and Biochemistry

This section focuses on each cytokine in turn, summarizing information on its physical structure and that of its receptor(s), on the cells that synthesize the cytokine (Table I), and on those that respond to it with functional effects relevant to the inflammatory response (Table II). Most of the cytokines have been cloned from one or more species. Much current research emphasis is directed at understanding the upstream regulatory elements and the transcriptional factors that control gene expression. Space limitations preclude the detailing of these devleopments. As indicated in each section, many of the cytokine receptors have been cloned as well. Interestingly, marked structural similarities are evident among several of the cytokine receptors and many appear to fall into one of three superfamilies (Williams and Barclay, 1988; Bazan, 1990; Cosman *et al.*, 1990; C. A. Smith *et al.*, 1990). In addition, current work is showing that many of the cytokines appear to have multiple receptor types that differ in location (cell surface versus extracellular or soluble) and affinity. Much current work is directed at understanding the physical structure of the multiplicity of receptors and the functional effects of this redundancy. Knowledge of the signal transduction pathways employed by the cytokine receptors is very limited for many of the cytokines, but this area of research already promises to be one of rapid development.

A. Macrophage Inflammatory Proteins

Among the earliest events in the evolution of the inflammatory response is the necessary generation of chemotactic factors for leukocytes. Many of the various members of the superfamily of MIPs or intercrines are chemotactic for specific leukocytes (monocytes, neutrophils, T lymphocytes) and/or fibroblasts (for a review, see Wolpe and Cerami, 1989; Oppenheim et al., 1991). The superfamily name "macrophage inflammatory proteins" reflects some of the earliest work, which characterized two distinct proteins that were among the major macrophage products after endotoxin administration. The two proteins were of similar molecular mass—8 and 6 kDa (MIP-1, MIP-2), shared conserved regions including 4 half-cystines, but were separable by other physical characteristics. Both proteins were identified as inflammatory cytokines, able to activate neutrophils in vitro and to cause a localized inflammatory reaction or fever in vivo (Wolpe and Cerami, 1989). Simultaneous studies in other laboratories, many employing subtractive DNA hybridization techniques, identified additional proteins synthesized by other cell types that were structurally related to MIP-1 or MIP-2 based on amino acid sequence, especially the positioning of the cysteines, but sometimes differed slightly in estimated molecular mass (6–12 kDa) and the presence or absence of glycosylation sites. The designation of the entire superfamily as the "intercrines" reflected a desire to emphasize that cells other than macrophages also synthesized members of this cytokine family (Oppenheim et al., 1991).

The members of the MIP-1 or intercrine β subfamily and the MIP-2 or intercrine α subfamily are listed in Table III. Several of the family members have been given multiple names, reflecting their discovery by independent researchers. For example, neutrophil activating protein 1 (NAP-1), neutrophil activating factor (NAF), monocyte-derived neutrophil chemotactic factor (MDNCF), monocyte-dervied neutrophil activating peptide (MONAP), lymphocyte-derived neutrophil activating peptide (LYNAP), and granulocyte chemotactic peptide (GCP) all specify the same monocyte–derived gene product, which is now frequently referred to as interleukin 8 (IL-8). However, the use of the interleukin terminology here is confusing since it groups this single MIP-2/intercrine α family member, NAP-1/NAF, with the interleukins, making no provision for all the related MIP/intercrine proteins. Some insight into the basis for the similarity among the MIP-1 and MIP-2 family members is found at the gene level. All the members of the MIP-1/intercrine β family map to human chromosome 17 and murine chromosome 11; the MIP-2 family members all map to human chromosome

Table III   Members of the Intercrine or Macrophage Inflammatory Protein Family[a]

Protein[b]	Cell source
MIP-1 or Intercrine β Subfamily	
MIP-1α (mu)	Monocytes/macrophages, T cells
LD78/PAT464 (hu)	T cells, B cells, tumor cells
MIP-1β (mu)	Monocytes/macrophages, T cells
ACT2/PAT744 (hu)	T cells, B cells, tumor cell line
TCA3 (mu)	T cells
I309 (hu)	T cells
RANTES (hu)	T cells
JE (mu)	Monocytes/macrophages, fibroblasts, endothelial cells
MCAF/MCP-1 (hu)	Monocytes/macrophages, fibroblasts, endothelial cells, keratinocytes, smooth muscle cells
MIP-2 or Intercrine α Subfamily	
MIP-2/KC (mu)	Monocytes/macrophages, fibroblasts
GRO/MGSA (hu)	Monocytes/macrophages, endothelial cells, synovial cells, tumor cells
CRG-2 (mu)	—
IP10 (hu)	Monocytes/macrophages, fibroblasts, endothelial cells, keratinocytes
PF4 (hu)	Platelets
PBP, CTAP3, βTG, NAP-2 (hu)[c]	Platelets
IL-8/NAP-1/NAF/MDNCF/MONAP/ LYNAP/GCP (hu)	Monocytes/macrophages, T cells, neutrophils, chondrocytes, fibroblasts, endothelial cells, keratinocytes, hepatocytes

[a] Data from Wolpe and Cerami (1989) and Oppenheim et al. (1991).
[b] Multiple names for the same gene product are separated by a slash; the murine (mu) and human (hu) homologs are grouped together.
[c] CTAP3, βTG, and NAP-2 are all cleavage products of the 15-kDa PBP precursor.

4 (Oppenheim et al., 1991). This relationship suggests that the families arose through duplication and subsequent divergence (Wolpe and Cerami, 1989).

In general, all the members of the MIP/intercrine superfamily are involved in mediating the induction of acute inflammation. In nontransformed cells, the MIP/intercrine family members appear to be inducible by particulates, microorganisms or their products [e.g., lipopolysaccharide (LPS)], viruses, or inflammatory cytokines rather than being constitutively expressed (Oppenheim et al., 1991). Although the biological activities of the individual members of the MIP-1 and MIP-2 families have not been thoroughly elucidated, the chemotactic effects of many of the family members have been examined. Most of the MIP/intercrine family members have been shown in vitro to be chemoattractants (Oppenheim et al., 1991). For instance, MIP-1α, -1β, MIP-2, connective tissue activating protein (CTAP)/

β thromboglobulin (βTG)/NAP-2, platelet factor 4 (PF4). GRO/melanoma growth stimulatory activity (MGSA), and IL-8 all stimulate neutrophil chemotaxis; PF4, monocyte chemotactic and activating factor (MCAF)/MCP-1, JE, and RANTES are chemotactic for monocytes, IL-8 for lymphocytes, and PF4 and CTAP/βTG/NAP-2 for fibroblasts. *In vivo* studies have confirmed the chemotactic activity of some of these proteins. Although the chemotactic properties of the MIP/intercrine proteins have been studied most thoroughly, other cellular functions also have been shown *in vitro* to be affected by specific family members. For instance, many of MIP/intercrine proteins that function as neutrophil chemotactic factors also increase specific neutrophil activities such as degranulation and the respiratory burst. MCAF/MCP-1 stimulates monocyte cytostatic activity and superoxide anion release (Zachariae *et al.*, 1990). CTAP/βTG/NAP-2 and PF4 increase fibroblast proliferation (Senior *et al.*, 1983). Other studies have expanded our understanding of the roles these proteins play *in vivo*. PF4 has been shown to induce fibrosis (Sharpe *et al.*, 1990) and act as an immunostimulant (Katz *et al.*, 1986; Zucker *et al.*, 1989); IL-8 increases vascular permeability (Foster *et al.*, 1989); and MIP-1α and -1β are pyrogenic (Devatelis *et al.*, 1989).

Our current understanding of receptors for MIP family members is limited to studies of receptors for IL-8 and MCAF/MCP-1. Monocytes have been shown to express MCAF/MCP-1 receptors of moderately high affinity ($K_d = 2$ nM) (Yoshimura and Leonard, 1990). Neutrophils and monocytic cell lines have been shown to express glycosylated IL-8 receptors (Besemer *et al.*, 1989; Grob *et al.*, 1990; Samanta *et al.*, 1989a, b; although some discrepancy exists over whether the binding sites are of multiple affinities. The inability of other chemotactic factors and cytokines (IL-1, TNFα, GM-CSF, EGF, insulin, C5a, FMLP, LTB$_4$) to compete with IL-8 for binding suggests that IL-8 has a separate receptor (Besemer *et al.*, 1989; Grob *et al.*, 1990). Several studies have indicated that the structural similarity among subfamily members may allow sharing of receptors or receptor subunits (Oppenheim *et al.*, 1991).

B. Transforming Growth Factor β

In addition to the MIP/intercrine superfamily, TGFβ is another cytokine generated early in the inflammatory response that functions as a chemotactic factor. TGFβ has a broad spectrum of cellular targets and a wide range of functional effects, many of which directly influence the inflammatory response (for reviews, see Massague, 1990; Nilsen-Hamilton, 1990; Roberts and Sporn, 1990). TBFβ is a misnomer because this cytokine does not cause oncogenic transformation. Instead, the name reflects the assay system in which TGFβ was originally distinguished as a unique activity (De Larco and Todaro, 1978; Moses *et al.*, 1981; Roberts *et al.*, 1981). In the assay,

TGFβ was identified as the agent that caused normal rodent fibroblasts to exhibit characteristics of transformed cells.

TGFβ has multiple diverse effects on hematopoietic cells and may be considered both pro- and anti-inflammatory, as well as immunosuppressive (Wahl et al., 1989). This cytokine is released by aggregated platelets after vascular injury (Assoian et al., 1983). In this environment, TGFβ is thought to exert its pro-inflammatory effects. TBGβ is the most potent monocyte and neutrophil chemoattractant known; for both cell types, its maximal chemotactic effects are achieved at femtomolar levels (Wahl et al., 1987a; Brandes et al., 1991a). Activated monocytes (Assoian et al., 1987; McCartney-Francis et al., 1990) and neutrophils (Grotendorst et al., 1989) have both been shown to synthesize TGFβ, so the infiltrating leukocytes can release additional TGFβ, thus promoting the inflammation. Supporting this hypothesis are in vivo studies that have shown that TGFβ causes inflammatory cell recruitment when administered locally (Roberts et al., 1986; Allen et al., 1990a). This phenomenon likely occurs not only through the ability of TGFβ to induce directed migration, but also through its enhancement of monocyte integrin expression, which facilitates cell–cell and cell–matrix interaction, and its induction of type IV collagenase, which aids cell movement through the basement membrane (Wahl et al., 1993). Another important pro-inflammatory effect of TGFβ is its ability to stimulate the increased expression of FcγRIII (Welch et al., 1990), a membrane protein that is central to immunophagocytic activity. Further, TGFβ can activate monocytes to synthesize inflammatory cytokines including IL-1, TNFα, Il-6, FGF, PDGF, and TGFβ (Wahl et al., 1987a; McCartney-Francis et al., 1990; Turner et al., 1990). However, TGFβ-stimulated monocytes also demonstrate increased expression of an IL-1 receptor antagonist (IL-1ra or IRAP; S. M. Wahl et al., unpublished results), suggesting that at least the IL-1-mediated pro-inflammatory effects induced by TGFβ may be self-regulating. These activities, in conjunction with TGFβ production early in the sequence of events culminating in inflammation, make TGFβ a pivotal mediator of the inflammatory response.

The multiple effects of TGFβ on lymphocyte populations also show its importance as a negative immunoregulatory agent. In vitro studies have shown that TGFβ antagonizes specific effects of IL-1 (Wahl et al., 1988), IL-2 (Kehrl et al., 1986a, b), IL-3 (Ohta et al., 1987), TNFα (Ranges et al., 1987), and IFNγ (Czarniecki et al., 1988). TGFβ inhibits the proliferation of thymocytes (Ristow, 1986; Wahl et al., 1988, B cells (Kehrl et al., 1986a, 1989), and hematopoietic progenitor cells (Keller et al., 1988). In addition, TGFβ suppresses the activity of natural killer (NK) cells (Rook et al., 1986), inhibits the development of cytotoxic T lymphocytes (Espevik et al., 1988) and lymphokine-activated killer (LAK) cells (Mule et al., 1988), and can inhibit lymphocyte production of IFNγ, TNFα, and TNFβ (Ranges et al., 1987; Espevik et al., 1988). Additional studies have shown that systemic administration of TGFβ can suppress immune function *in vivo* as well, and thus can antagonize the development of various disease states such as experimental arthritis (Brandes *et al.*, 1991b; Kuruvilla *et al.*, 1991), multiple sclerosis (Kuruvilla *et al.*, 1991), graft rejection (Wallick *et al.*, 1990), and reperfusion injury (Lefer *et al.*, 1990). TGFβ also appears to have suppressive effects on the stimulated release of reactive oxygen (Tsunawaki *et al.*, 1988) and nitrogen (Ding *et al.*, 1990) intermediates by tissue macrophages, although a similar suppression does not occur with blood monocytes and neutrophils (Brandes *et al.*, 1991a).

In addition to its myriad effects on inflammatory and immune cells, TGFβ also profoundly affects virtually all other cell populations. This cytokine often functions as a growth inhibitor, antagonizing the actions of cell mitogens, but also has been shown to stimulate the growth of some mesenchymal cells, possibly indirectly, by influencing the expression of extracellular matrix proteins (Roberts and Sporn, 1990). This ability of TGFβ to stimulate the production of matrix proteins suggests that TGFβ is also important in wound healing. The chemotactic activity of TGFβ for fibroblasts is also indicative of a role for this protein in repair (Postlethwaite *et al.*, 1987). In a complementary fashion, TGFβ also increases the expression of cell receptors for the matrix molecules, decreases the synthesis of matrix-degrading proteolytic enzymes, and enhances the production of antiproteases by fibroblasts (Roberts and Sporn, 1990). In this fashion TGFβ aids in the resolution of inflammatory lesions and, if it persists, may promote fibrotic sequelae (Manthey *et al.*, 1990).

TGFβ actually comprises a family of closely related molecules including TGFβ1, -β2, -β3, -β4, and -β5 (Roberts and Sporn, 1990); these molecules are differentially expressed among various species, often in a tissue-specific fashion (Miller *et al.*, 1989a,b; Thompson *et al.*, 1989). Histochemical studies have shown that many tissues express specific types of TGFβ, often in a developmentally regulated fashion (Heine *et al.*, 1987; Miller *et al.*, 1989a,b; Pelton *et al.*, 1990). Conservation at the amino acid level among the TGFβ species ranges from 64 to 82%, but each TGFβ species is very highly conserved across taxonomic groups ($>$ 97%), suggesting specific roles for each of the TGFβs (Roberts and Sporn, 1990). The TGFβ molecules are 25-kDa homodimers, with the exception of TGFβ1.2, a heterodimer synthesized in small quantities by platelets and some cultured cells and composed of one TGFβ1 chain and one TGFβ2 chain (Cheifetz *et al.*, 1988; Danielpour *et al.*, 1989). Mammalian species primarily express TGFβ1, -β2, and -β3. These proteins are derived from 390-, 412-, and 412-amino-acid precursors, respectively; their 112-amino-acid chains are $\geq$ 71% identical, including the conservation of all 9 cysteine residues (Roberts and Sporn, 1990). All are released from cells in a biologically inactive form because of association with a 75-kDa noncovalently associated latency protein and are unable to bind to cell receptors (Pircher *et al.*, 1986; Miyazono *et al.*, 1988; Wakefield *et al.*, 1988). The mechanism of the activation of latent TGFβ *in vivo* is unclear, but some evidence indicates that specific proteases (Lyons *et al.*, 1988) or sialidases (Miyazono and Heldin, 1989), such as those that are found at inflammatory sites, may function in this capacity. In addition, researchers have shown that the latency protein must be bound to a cell surface mannose-6-phosphate receptor for the protease to act (Dennis and Rifkin, 1991). The release of TGFβ in a latent state is thought to be a critical regulatory step, since virtually all cells express TGFβ receptors.

At least three proteins are expressed by many cells that specifically bind TGFβ. These proteins are referred to as the type I (53 kDa), type II (70–100 kDa), and type III (200–400 kDa) TGFβ receptors (Roberts and Sporn, 1990). Although most cells express one or more of these three receptor types, some cell types have been shown to express a different panel of TGFβ binding proteins (MacKay *et al.*, 1990). Studies indicate that only the type I and type II receptors appear to be involved in signal transduction (Segarini *et al.*, 1989; Laiho *et al.*, 1990), whereas the type III receptor, a proteoglycan, has been suggested to be involved in the storage, delivery, or clearance of TGFβ (Andres, 1989). TGFβ1 and -β2 demonstrate different affinities for the type I and II TGFβ receptors (Roberts and Sporn, 1990). This difference is thought to underlie the observation that TGFβ1 and -β2 often stimulate the same functional consequences, but differ in their potencies. Although the genes for the TGFβ receptor have not yet been cloned, studies have begun to identify agents that can regulate TGFβ receptor expression. Relevant to the inflammatory response, IFNγ and LPS have been shown to down-regulate monocyte type I TGFβ receptors, an event that may be important in the resolution of the inflammatory response (Brandes *et al.*, 1991c). In addition, mitogenic agents such as phytohemagglutinin (PHA) have been shown to induce T lymphocyte expression of all three TGFβ receptor types (Ellingsworth *et al.*, 1989). Since TGFβ inhibits T cell proliferation, this up-regulation of TGFβ receptors may effectively autoregulate clonal expansion.

C. Interleukin 1

The cytokines IL-1 and TNFα (considered next) are central mediators of the inflammatory changes induced by pathogenic organisms and injury to the body. Like MIP proteins and TGFβ, both appear to be produced early in the sequence of events following tissue injury; however, instead of a primary role in promoting chemotaxis, these mediators appear to function on multiple levels to promote local and systemic inflammatory events (for reviews, see Strober and James, 1988; Mizel, 1989; Arai *et al.*, 1990; Warren, 1990). Like most of the cytokines, IL-1 is produced by hematopoietic cells (monocytes, T and B lymphocytes, neutrophils (Arai *et al.*, 1990; Marucha *et al.*, 1990). However, increasing evidence suggests that IL-1 is also made by many tissue cells including fibroblasts, endothelial cells, keratinocytes, astrocytes, microglia, mesangial cells, and Kupffer cells. Some cells such as keratinocytes (Mizutani *et al.*, 1991) and Kupffer cells (Manthey *et al.*, 1992) have also been shown to store IL-1 intracellularly, leading to the hypothesis that the release of this cytokine following direct cellular injury can serve as an initiating signal for the inflammatory response (Kupper, 1990a,b). In support of this hypothesis, IL-1 receptors have been identified on many cell types and IL-1 has been shown to stimulate directly events in the tissue that promote inflammation (Mizel, 1989). For instance, IL-1 stimulates fibroblast prostaglandin E_2 (PGE_2) production (Dejana *et al.*, 1987), and induces the expression of adhesion molecules on the surface of endothelial cells, thereby promoting increased adherence of neutrophils, monocytes, and lymphocytes (Arai *et al.*, 1990). In addition, IL-1 has been shown to stimulate tissue cells to release collagenase (Dejana *et al.*, 1987) as well as other cytokines that participate in the inflammatory cascade (Arai *et al.*, 1990; Kupper, 1990a).

The effects of IL-1 are not always confined to the locale in which it was generated; IL-1 production may also trigger a systemic response to injury (Strober and James, 1988). For example, IL-1 is an endogenous pyrogen; it mediates this response at the level of the hypothalamic thermoregulatory center, possibly indirectly by stimulating prostaglandin synthesis. IL-1 also acts on the central nervous system to increase production of certain neuro-peptides, corticotropin releasing factor, and adrenocorticotropic hormone (ACTH). ACTH and IL-1 can then act directly on the adrenal gland to bring about increased circulating steroid levels. IL-1 also plays a role in mediating the acute-phase response by promoting the synthesis of acute-phase proteins in the liver and decreasing albumin production.

The local and systemic effects of IL-1 as an inflammatory mediator are also caused by its myriad of effects on the immune system. IL-1 modulates the activation state of neutrophils, priming or directly stimulating the respiratory burst and release of granule contents (Figari *et al.*, 1987; Ferrante *et al.*, 1988; Steinback and Roth, 1989) and stimulating their tissue infiltration *in vivo* (Sayers *et al.*, 1988). IL-1 has also been shown to stimulate lymphocytes and monocytes to express various pro-inflammatory cytokines including IL-1, IL-2, and CSFs (Dinarello *et al.*, 1987; Arai *et al.*, 1990). IL-1 directly modulates the growth and differentiation of hematopoietic cells and, through its ability to induce CSFs, does so indirectly as well (Arai *et al.*, 1990). In addition, IL-1 promotes T cell proliferation. Specifically IL-1 stimulates T lymphocytes to synthesize IL-2 and express the IL-2 receptor. Then, in the presence of antigen, the combined action IL-1 and IL-2 stimulates T cell clonal expansion. IL-1 is also thought to extent the life-span, and therefore the functional activity, of monocytes at inflammatory sites by preventing programmed cell death (Mangan *et al.*, 1991).

IL-1 exists as two distinct molecules, IL-1α and IL-1β, derived from separate genes (Arai *et al.*, 1990). IL-1α and -1β are synthesized as 31-kDa precursors. Cell types appear to differ in their ability to express and translate

IL-1α and -1β mRNA, and to process the precursor proteolytically to the active 17.5-kDa form and secrete it. For example, activated monocytes produce IL-1α and -1β protein, but only IL-1β is converted to the mature form and secreted, whereas IL-1α remains cell associated. Keratinocytes, however, produce pro-IL-1α and pro-IL-1β but can only convert the α form into a mature molecule. Pro-IL-1β is only released after keratinocyte lysis; then the action of an extracellular protease is required to convert it to an active form (Mizutani et al., 1991).

Although IL-1α and -1β show only 26% homology in amino acid sequence, they share 7 highly conserved exons that confer a similarity in tertiary structure and allow the two molecules to bind to the same receptor and stimulate very similar biological activities (Arai et al., 1990). The IL-1 receptor is an 80-kDa glycoprotein belonging to the Ig-like superfamily of receptors (Williams and Barclay, 1988). This receptor has been cloned from murine fibroblasts (Sims et al., 1988) and from a helper T cell line (Sims et al., 1989) and has been shown to be very highly conserved across species. A soluble secreted form of the receptor has also been identified, consisting primarily of the extracellular Ig-like portion of the membrane-bound receptor type (Dower et al., 1989).

D. Tumor Necrosis Factor α

Like IL-1, TNFα is a pro-inflammatory cytokine with pleiotropic effects mediating many local and systemic aspects of the inflammatory response (for review, see Sherry and Cerami, 1988; Warren, 1990). TNFα is primarily a product of monocytes and macrophages that have been activated by foreign substances or by bacterial, viral, or parasitic infections. However, neutrophils, NK cells (Dubravec et al., 1990), T and B lymphocytes (Ware and Green, 1987; Sung et al., 1988), mast cells (Gordon and Galli, 1990), astrocytes (Chung and Benveniste, 1990), endothelial cells, and smooth muscle cells have also been shown to synthesize TNFα. Three convergent lines of investigation that led to the discovery of TNFα sought to identify a transferable serum protein that mediated LPS-induced shock, hemorrhagic necrosis of solid tumors, and cachexia (wasting syndrome). Thus the discovery that these systemic effects were mediated by TNFα contradicted the understanding at the time that cytokines, unlike endocrine hormones, work only on a local level. The identification of soluble cytokine binding proteins and the development of more sensitive assay systems have led to an appreciation that many other cytokines can also be found at significant levels in the serum following injury. The systemic effects of TNFα can be very toxic (Sherry and Cerami, 1988; Tracey and Cerami, 1990). When generated in large quantities during invasive infection, TNFα can lead to hemodynamic shock, diffuse tissue injury, and death. However, moderate TNFα production in the tissues defends against local infection and promotes healing and tissue remodeling after injury.

The systemic effects of TNFα are mediated by its diverse effects on many cell populations (Tracey and Cerami, 1990). For instance, the TNFα-induced cachexia (from which the alternative name for TNFα, cachectin, is derived) is caused, in part, by the suppression of adipocyte lipoprotein lipase; fever is mediated by induced prostaglandin synthesis in the brain; and the acute-phase response by the induction of acute-phase proteins by hepatocytes. The cellular effects of TNFα relevant to inflammation include stimulating endothelial cell production of procoagulant activity, IL-1, hematopoietic growth factors, arachidonic acid metabolites, and platelet activating factor (PAF) and induced endothelial cell expression of ICAMs and ELAMs (adhesion molecules), thus promoting leukocyte adherence and transmigration (Bevilacqua et al., 1986; Libby et al., 1986; Pober et al., 1986; Broudy et al., 1987; Camussi et al., 1987). Recent work by other investigators has also shown that TNFα has profound effects on neutrophils, priming or directly stimulating adherence, phagocytosis, degranulation, reactive oxygen intermediate production, and possibly migration (Broudy et al., 1986; Figari et al., 1987; Shalaby et al., 1987; Ferrante et al., 1988; Sayers et al., 1988; Livingston et al., 1989; Steinbeck and Roth, 1989). TNFα has also been shown to stimulate leukocyte synthesis of other inflammatory cytokines such as GM-CSF, TCFβ, IL-1, IL-6, PDGF, and TNFα itself (Broudy et al., 1986; Libby et al., 1986; Hajjar et al., 1987; Cicco et al., 1990; Marucha et al., 1990). Like IL-1, TNFα also acts to extend the life-span of monocytes in inflammatory lesions by delaying the onset of programmed cell death (Mangan et al., 1991). This cytokine acts on fibroblasts to promote chemotaxis and to stimulate synthesis of IL-6, PGE_2, and collagenase, and is a weak fibroblast mitogen, its effects ablated by the growth inhibitory effects of the released IL-6 and PGE_2 (Dayer et al., 1985; Kohase et al., 1986; Elias et al., 1987).

TNFα is synthesized as a prohormone that is subsequently processed to yield the mature 17.5-kDa species, containing 154–157 amino acid residues. Both the pro-region and the mature protein are highly conserved (80%) (Sherry and Cerami, 1988). Three TNFα receptors have been identified and cloned: a soluble form (Gatanaga et al., 1990; Heller et al., 1990) and two membrane-bound forms of apparent molecular sizes 60 and 80 kDa by SDS–PAGE, but 440 amino acids each (C. A. Smith et al., 1990; Loetscher et al., 1990; Schall et al., 1990). Most cells appear to express both cell surface forms. Purified TNFα has been found in noncovalently associated dimers, trimers, and pentamers, depending on the isolation procedure employed. The trimeric form has been shown to be eight times more effective at receptor binding than the monomer, possibly engaging three TNFα receptors simultaneously, and is postulated to be the active form in vivo (Smith and Baglioni, 1987). A membrane-associated form of TNFα has also been identified. This form is thought to allow a localization of the action of this potentially toxic cytokine (Perez et al., 1990). TNFα shares 30% sequence homology with lymphotoxin, also called TNFβ, a cytokine synthesized by

T lymphocytes. TNFβ binds to the TNFα receptors and often elicits similar biological activities (Gatanaga *et al.*, 1990; Loetscher *et al.*, 1990; Schall *et al.*, 1990). Only recently has evidence been found to suggest that TNFα and β do modulate certain bioactivities very differently, including endothelial cell promotion of neutrophil adherence and production of CSFs (Broudy *et al.*, 1987).

E. Colony Stimulating Factors

The CSFs are similar to IL-1 and TNFα because they also function to activate endothelial cells and infiltrating leukocytes, thereby promoting the inflammatory response on a local level. As their name implies, the CSFs are a family of cytokines involved in the growth and differentiation of hematopoietic precursor cells; this function is manifested as colony formation in cultures of bone marrow precursor cells (for review, see Strober and James, 1988; Arai *et al.*, 1990; Monroy *et al.*, 1990). The predominant lineage of the colony cells is determined by the type of CSF to which cells are exposed. The family members follow. (1) M-CSF (also referred to as CSF-1) is a heavily glycosylated protein of 47–76 kDa that stimulates the growth and differentiation of monocytes and macrophages (Arai *et al.*, 1990). This cytokine is synthesized by monocytes, fibroblasts, and endothelial cells. M-CSF is a disulfide-linked dimer that exists in multiple forms because of alternative RNA processing of the single gene transcript. (2) GM-CSF induces colonies that contain granulocytes, monocytes/macrophages, and eosinophils (Arai *et al.*, 1990; Monroy *et al.*, 1990). GM-CSF is a product of multiple cell types: fibroblasts, macrophages, endothelial cells, and activated T lymphocytes. A single gene encodes the 141- or 144- (murine or human) amino-acid protein, which displays a range of molecular mass (14–35 kDa) because of variable glycosylation. (3) G-CSF, a macrophage and endothelial cell product, predominantly supports granulocyte colony formation (Arai *et al.*, 1990). This cytokine is a 204- or 208- (human or murine) amino-acid, 19- to 20-kDa glycoprotein. G-CSF is also encoded by a single gene, but through alternative splicing many forms of the molecule are produced. (4) Multi-CSF or IL-3 promotes the growth of virtually all types of hematopoietic progenitors, especially at early stages of their development (Mizel, 1989; Arai *et al.*, 1990). As are the other CSFs, IL-3 is a glycoprotein (20–25 kDa) of 166 amino acids (murine). This cytokine is produced by activated T lymphocytes. IL-3 and GM-CSF will also promote erythroid cell differentiation when used in conjunction with erythropoietin. The actions of the CSFs are often species specific because of poor conservation of the genes and/or variable glycosylation.

Through their ability to promote the proliferation and differentiation of precursor cells into inflammatory leukocytes, the CSFs may be considered to play an indirect role as mediators of inflammation. However, the CSFs also directly influence inflammatory events through their effects on mature cell populations. For instance, numerous *in vitro* and *in vivo* studies have shown that GM-CSF modulates neutrophil function and phenotype, often serving as a priming stimulus (Steinbeck and Roth, 1989; Monroy *et al.*, 1990). GM-CSF has been shown to induce TNFα, G-CSF, and M-CSF production (Lindemann *et al.*, 1989), to alter the number and affinity of neutrophil FMLP receptors (Weisbart *et al.*, 1986) and/or affect the FMLP signal transduction pathway (McColl *et al.*, 1990), to increase the expression of a neutrophil cell adhesion protein (CD11b, Mo1; Griffin *et al.*, 1990), to up-regulate complement receptors types 1 and 3 (Neuman *et al.*, 1990), and to enhance phagocytosis (Fleischmann *et al.*, 1986; Lopez *et al.*, 1986) and the release of reactive oxygen intermediates in response to a second stimulus (Weisbart *et al.*, 1987). In addition, monocytes treated with GM-CSF demonstrate increased cytotoxicity, enhanced production of IL-1 (P. D. Smith *et al.*, 1990), IL-6 (Janoff *et al.*, 1991), and PGE$_2$, and increased expression of the cell adhesion protein Mo1 (CD11b; Griffin *et al.*, 1990) and the surface protein HLA-DR, important in T lymphocyte–monocyte interactions (P. D. Smith *et al.*, 1990). Both G-CSF and M-CSF have been shown to act as chemotactic factors: M-CSF for monocytes (Pierce *et al.*, 1990) and G-CSF for neutrophils and monocytes (Wang *et al.*, 1988b). In addition, new evidence suggests that nonhematopoietic cells can also express CSF receptors and respond to CSFs with augmented function. G-CSF and GM-CSF have both been shown to induce endothelial cell migration and proliferation and, thus, support angiogenesis at a wound site (Bussolino *et al.*, 1991).

The CSF receptors are expressed to a varying extent on undifferentiated and mature cells of different lineages. Distinct receptors for each of the CSFs have been identified and cloned: GM-CSF (Gearing *et al.*, 1989); G-CSF (Fukunaga *et al.*, 1990); M-CSF (Sherr *et al.*, 1985); and IL-3 (Itoh *et al.*, 1990). Despite the separate receptors, some evidence exists that the CSFs cross-compete for receptor binding (Walker *et al.*, 1985). Some new evidence suggests that this competition may be the result of shared receptor subunits. The receptors for GM-CSF and IL-3 each consist of an α and β chain, which together form the respective high affinity receptors. Interestingly, the human GM-CSF and IL-3 receptors share the same β chain (p120); thus, high affinity binding of one ligand can block the binding of the other (Miyajima *et al.*, 1991). The α chains of the GM-CSF and IL-3 receptors, as well as the G-CSF receptor, belong to an emerging hematopoietin receptor superfamily that also includes receptors for IL-2, -4, -6, -7, and erythropoietin (Bazan, 1990; Cosman *et al.*, 1990). The M-CSF receptor (*c-fms* gene product) appears to be distinct. Unlike the hematopoietin receptor superfamily members, which appear to associate with separate tyrosine kinases, the M-CSF receptor has intrinsic tyrosine kinase activity (Yarden and Ullrich, 1988).

F. Interleukin 2

The presence of T lymphocytes in the inflammatory infiltrate, as seen in beryllium disease of the lung (Kriebel *et al.*, 1988) and streptococcal cell wall-induced arthritis in rats (Allen *et al.*, 1985), characterizes the inflammation triggered by specific antigenic xenobiotics. IL-2 and IFNγ (considered next) are T lymphocyte-derived cytokines that play a role in inflammation with T cell involvement (for review, see Smith, 1988; Mizel, 1989; Arai *et al.*, 1990). When T lymphocytes are stimulated by engagement of the T cell receptor and by IL-1 released by the antigen-presenting cell, IL-2 synthesis is stimulated. Resting T lymphocytes do not express the high affinity IL-2 receptor, but the IL-1 that stimulates the production of IL-2 also induces the T lymphocytes to express the IL-2 receptor. The secreted IL-2 primarily functions within this milieu by stimulating T lymphocytes to proliferate and by increasing their synthesis of other cytokines that contribute to the recruitment and activation of additional inflammatory cells. Although much of our understanding of the biological activities of IL-2 deals with its effects on the growth and activation of T lymphocytes, IL-2 has also been shown to modulate the function of activated monocytes (Wahl *et al.*, 1987b), activated B cells (Kishi *et al.*, 1985; Mond *et al.*, 1985), NK cells, and LAK cells (Ortaldo *et al.*, 1984). For instance, IFNγ- and LPS-activated monocytes are induced to express IL-2 receptors and respond to IL-2 with an augmented generation of reactive oxygen intermediates and an increase in cytotoxic activity (Wahl *et al.*, 1987b).

IL-2 is a 133-amino-acid protein with a 20-residue signal sequence. This cytokine is a glycoprotein containing a variable number of O-linked saccharides. Its membrane receptor has at least two components: an α chain (p55) and a β chain (p70). The α chain binds IL-2 with low affinity and the β chain with intermediate affinity; the noncovalent association of the α and β chains forms the high affinity IL-2 receptor (Leonard *et al.*, 1984; Waldmann, 1986; Dukivich *et al.*, 1987). The binding of IL-2 to the β chain by itself, but not the α chain, is sufficient to generate a stimulatory signal for T lymphocytes. The β chain of the IL-2 receptor has been cloned (Hatakeyama *et al.*, 1989) and has been shown to belong to the hematopoietin receptor superfamily, by virtue of sequence and structural homology over a 200-amino-acid stretch (Bazan, 1990; Cosman *et al.*, 1990). The members of this family are postulated to interact with accessory proteins, such as the IL-2 receptor α chain, which facilitate the receptor–ligand interaction. A soluble form of the IL-2 receptor has also been identified, and has been shown to be released by activated lymphocytes (Rubin *et al.*, 1985) and monocytes (Allen *et al.*, 1990b).

G. Interferon γ

As mentioned earlier, IFNγ is an important inflammatory mediator when T lymphocytes are present in the cellular infiltrate. Interferon refers to a group of molecules—α, β, and γ—all of which were originally discovered because of their ability to "interfere" with virus replication in cells (for review, see Billiau, 1988; Nathan and Yoshida, 1988; Heremans and Billiau, 1989). IFNα and β (also known as type I IFNs) are encoded by the same gene cluster and act through the same cellular receptor. These cytokines are typically synthesized concurrently and are produced by a wide variety of cells. IFNγ, also known as "immune interferon" or "type II interferon," is derived from a different gene and acts through a separate receptor. The IFNγ receptor is the product of a single gene (Aguet et al., 1988) and is a 90-kDa variably glycosylated protein that binds IFNγ with high affinity. The molecular mass of monomeric IFNγ is approximately 17 kDa, but variable glycosylation yields proteins in the 20- to 25-kDa range. The sequence of IFNγ is poorly conserved across species (as little as 40% amino acid sequence homology) and often displays little activity outside the species of origin (Arai et al., 1990).

IFNγ is primarily a product of T lymphocytes activated by exposure to antigen or mitogen. This protein is a potent stimulator of monocytes/macrophages, neutrophils, and endothelial cells, often acting to promote a more vigorous response to another stimulus (Nathan and Yoshida, 1988). For instance, IFNγ synergizes with TNFα, TNFβ, and IL-1, enhancing their actions (Lee et al., 1984; Stone-Wolff et al., 1984; Ding et al., 1988) and their further production. IFNγ also amplifies the LPS-induced response of monocytes and macrophages, which consists of increased production of inflammatory cytokines (Donnelly et al., 1990) and increased release of reactive oxygen and nitrogen intermediates (Ding et al., 1988), phagocytosis, and cytotoxicity (Schultz et al., 1983). IFNγ also acts directly on cells to alter their phenotypic characteristics. In this regard, IFNγ has been shown to induce the expression of class II major histocompatibility complex (MHC) molecules on monocytic cells and epithelial, endothelial, and connective tissue cells, thus allowing these cells to become active in antigen presentation (Arai et al., 1990).

Although IFNγ often has marked pro-inflammatory effects, under appropriate conditions it may also have anti-inflammatory effects. For instance, systemic administration of IFNγ has been shown to cause suppression of the local Schwartzman reaction (Heremans et al., 1987) and a particulate-induced arthritis in rats (Wahl et al., 1991a). The mechanism of these anti-inflammatory effects is unclear; this phenomenon may be, in part, an indirect effect mediated through endocrine and neuroendocrine changes. IFNγ may also have direct anti-inflammatory effects. For instance, IFNγ has been shown to inhibit phospholipase A_2 and, thus, decrease monocyte production of the inflammatory mediators PGE_2 and collagenase (L. M. Wahl et al., 1990). Other in vitro evidence suggests that some of the anti-inflammatory effects of IFNγ may be mediated by alterations in the expression of receptors for other inflammatory mediators. For instance, IFNγ has been shown to modulate the expression of TGFβ (Brandes et al., 1991c),

TNFα (Drapier and Wietzerbin, 1991), and C5a (Katona *et al.*, 1991; Wahl *et al.*, 1991) receptors on monocytes and macrophages, thus altering their responsiveness to these agents.

H. Interleukin 4

Like IFNγ, IL-4 is a product of activated T lymphocytes and exhibits both pro- and anti-inflammatory activities (for review, see Paul and O-Hara, 1987; Mizel, 1989; Arai *et al.*, 1990). The single IL-4 gene encodes a 140- (murine) or 153- (human) amino-acid protein with a 20- or 24-amino-acid signal sequence. After processing, the IL-4 protein has a molecular mass of 15 kDa, with additional mass added by posttranslational glycosylation. Human and murine IL-4 share approximately 50% sequence homology but are poorly cross-reactive. In addition, they appear to have some species-specific effects. The IL-4 receptor (140 kDa) is expressed as a membrane-bound and a secreted soluble form. This receptor is a member of the hemato-poietin receptor superfamily and, as such, has no intrinsic tyrosine kinase activity (Bazan, 1990; Cosman *et al.*, 1990). Cloning of the IL-4 receptor showed that the secreted form of the receptor is encoded by a gene that is separate from that encoding of the membrane-bound form, and is not generated by proteolytic processing of the membrane-bound form, as are many of the other soluble receptors (Mosley *et al.*, 1989).

The effects of IL-4 on the inflammatory state appear to be dependent on the maturational state and the species of origin of the target cell. For instance, IL-4 induces the production of IL-1 and TNFα by murine macrophages (Wolpe *et al.*, 1987), but functions in an anti-inflammatory capacity in human monocytes by inhibiting the stimulated production of these cytokines (Essner *et al.*, 1989; Hart *et al.*, 1989; Donnelly *et al.*, 1990; Wong *et al.*, 1991). Other pro-inflammatory effects of IL-4 include its ability to stimulate tumoricidal activity in cultured macrophages (Crawford *et al.*, 1987) and enhance antigen-presenting ability (Zlotnik *et al.*, 1987; Aiello *et al.*, 1990). In addition, IL-4 promotes the proliferation of T lymphocytes and mast cells and can act synergistically with CSFs to support the growth of various hematopoietic cells (Arai *et al.*, 1990). Other anti-inflammatory effects of IL-4 on human monocytes are its ability to inhibit the induced production of specific prostaglandins (Hart *et al.*, 1989), block TGFβ-induced CD16 expression (Wong *et al.*, 1991), inhibit active collagenase production (Corcoran *et al.*, 1992), and promote programmed cell death of stimulated cells (Mangan *et al.*, 1992). In addition, IL-4 stimulates human monocytes to synthesize IRAP (H. Wong, personal communication), a soluble IL-1 receptor antagonist (considered in the last section). Studies have also shown that IL-4, possibly through these anti-inflammatory mechanisms, can inhibit an induced arthritic condition in rats (Allen *et al.*, 1991). However, the actions of IL-4 are not limited strictly to monocytes and T lymphocytes. IL-4 also has multiple effects on B cells, acting as a co-stimulator to promote the proliferation of quiescent and activated B cells and influencing isotype differentiation by promoting class switching, inducing expression of class II MHC, and augmenting expression of Fcε receptor II (Arai *et al.*, 1990).

I. Interleukin 6

IL-6, like TNFα, IL-1, and TGFβ, is a cytokine that mediates a broad range of host responses affecting multiple cell types (for review, see Arai *et al.*, 1990; Sehgal, 1990a,b; Warren, 1990). IFNγ and IL-4, IL-6 has anti-inflammatory activity, activating local and systemic host defense mechanisms that limit the tissue damage brought about by injury and, potentially, by the ensuing inflammatory response (Sehgal, 1990a,b). As was TNFα, IL-6 was characterized independently by several lines of investigation (Warren, 1990). This cytokine was simultaneously defined as a B cell differentiation factor (BGF2), a hybridoma/plasmacytoma growth factor (HGF), a hepatocyte stimulatory factor (HSF), a monocyte/granulocyte inducer (MGI$_2$), and a second type of IFNβ released by fibroblasts (IFNβ2). IL-6 is synthesized by a wide variety of cells including fibroblasts, endothelial cells, keratinocytes, monocytes/macrophages, mast cells, and B and T cell lines (Sehgal, 1990a). Production of IL-6 is induced by many types of agents, each effective in only certain cell types, including certain inflammatory cytokines such as IL-1, IL-2, IL-4, TNFα, IFNγ, and PDGF, as well as LPS, viruses, PGE$_1$, substance P, and substance K (Sehgal, 1990a). In addition, direct trauma to the tissue, such as thermal or surgical injury, also induces IL-6 production. In fact, IL-6 synthesis is preferentially enhanced when cellular synthesis of other proteins is compromised by cellular injury, thus allowing IL-6 to be secreted even by a dying cell (Kohase *et al.*, 1986; May *et al.*, 1988).

Many of the actions of IL-6 to limit tissue injury are encompassed in the hepatic acute-phase response, the metabolic reaction of the liver to tissue injury (Sehgal, 1990a). IL-6 stimulates hepatocytes to increase the production of specific plasma proteins, while decreasing the synthesis of others. These acute-phase proteins all function to neutralize the harmful products of injury and inflammation. For example, specific proteins act to opsonize particulate matter, promote clotting, inhibit proteases, neutralize reactive oxygen intermediates, modulate the activity of the immune system, and provide substrates for tissue repair (Sehgal, 1990a). In addition to the induction of acute-phase reactants, IL-6 also directly modulates the inflammatory and immune response to injury by augmenting B cell immunoglobulin production (Baumann *et al.*, 1987) and, when acting with other cytokines, by stimulating the growth and differentiation of specific thymocyte populations and hematopoietic stem cells (Arai *et al.*, 1990).

IL-6 is encoded by a single gene and is synthesized as a 212-amino-acid precursor, then processed to a 184- to 186-amino-acid protein (Sehgal, 1990b). The molecular mass of the secreted IL-6 varies from cell to cell in the range of 21–70 kDa, because of variable N- and O-linked glycosylation and phosphorylation (May *et al.*, 1989). At least two IL-6 receptors exist: a soluble form (Novick *et al.*, 1989) and a high affinity transmembrane receptor (80 kDa) (Yamasaki *et al.*, 1988). The IL-6 receptor is a member of the hematopoietic receptor superfamily (Bazan, 1990; Cosman *et al.*, 1990) and, like other family members, is thought to associate with a membrane accessory protein (130 kDa) to form the high affinity signal-transducing receptor (Taga *et al.*, 1989). The relative ability of the differentially modified forms of IL-6 to interact with these receptors has not yet been characterized.

J. Cytokines Involved in Repair

Cytokines such as PDGF, TGFα, EGF, and the members of the FGF family may not be involved in the acute inflammatory response, but instead mediate its resolution—tissue repair or fibrosis.

As its name indicates, PDGF is released by platelets during adherence or aggregation, as occurs during clot formation initiated by injury to the vasculature (Wong and Wahl, 1990). PDGF is also synthesized by smooth muscle cells, fibroblasts, and endothelial and epithelial cells, as well as by activated monocytes and macrophages. PDGF is a potent mesenchymal cell mitogen promoting the growth of fibroblasts, smooth muscle cells, chondrocytes, and glial cells. In addition, PDGF is a fibroblast and smooth muscle cell chemotaxis factor and therefore promotes the formation of granulation tissue during wound repair (Ross *et al.*, 1986). Some investigations have also shown that PDGF is a monocyte and neutrophil chemotaxis factor (Deuel *et al.*, 1982; Williams *et al.*, 1983); however, more recent studies have not supported this concept (Graves *et al.*, 1989).

PDGF is a cationic heat stable glycoprotein composed of two subunits to form a 27- to 31-kDa protein. Separate genes encode the two subunit chains, A and B which combine by disulfide bridges to form the homodimers AA and BB and the heterodimer AB (Ross *et al.*, 1986). The type of PDGF dimer expressed varies with species and cell type. PDGF receptors also consist of a combination of two chains, designated α and β chains; each is the product of a separate gene and belongs to the Ig-like superfamily of receptors that are characterized by a split tyrosine kinase domain and amino acid spans homologous to immunoglobulin (Williams and Barclay, 1988). The three possible PDGF receptors—αα, ββ, and αβ—have been found on various cells. Careful analysis has shown that these receptors bind only select PDGF isoforms: ββ binds only BB, αβ binds AB and BB, and αα binds BB, AB, and AA (Hart *et al.*, 1988). The receptors are expressed differentially by cells and are thought to mediate specific biological actions of PDGF (Bowen-Pope *et al.*, 1989).

The acidic and basic FGFs constitute a multimember family of structurally related proteins that stimulate mesenchymal cell chemotaxis and proliferation (for review, see Gospodarowicz, 1988; Rifkin and Moscatelli, 1989). The members of this family have been divided into two groups according to their affinity for heparin; the prototypes for these groups are acidic FGF (aFGF, 140 amino acids) and basic FGF (bFGF, 146 amino acids), polypeptides that are 55% homologous but are encoded by separate genes found on different chromosomes. The acidic FGFs are anionic polypeptides (15–18 kDa) (Lobb et al., 1986). The members of this family have been given a variety of names, often referring to the tissue of origin (Gospodarowicz, 1988). Many of these proteins have been shown to represent different molecular weight forms of the same gene product. The basic FGFs are cationic polypeptides (16–18.5 kDa). Like the acidic FGFs, the multiple members of this family derived from various tissues probably represent different molecular weight forms of the same gene product (Gospodarowicz, 1988).

A wide variety of cell types express bFGF, including most mesenchymal cells and activated monocytes, probably an important source during resolution of inflammation. The manner in which bFGF is released from cells remains unclear since the molecule lacks the classical signal sequence that directs secretion. Researchers propose that significant bFGF release may only occur through cell death (Rifkin and Moscatelli, 1989). Acidic FGF expression appears to be limited to cells of the brain, retina, bone, and kidney. Acidic and basic FGF interact with a common cell surface receptor (Rifkin and Moscatelli, 1989), a member of the Ig-like receptor superfamily (Williams and Barclay, 1988), and thus can elicit similar biological effects over a wide range of tissues.

The FGFs are mitogens for virtually all mesenchymal cells including fibroblasts, endothelial cells, and smooth muscle cells. These proteins are also endothelial cell chemotaxis factors and, as such, promote angiogenesis, a critical event in the formation of granulation tissue (Folkman and Klagsbrun, 1987). Interestingly, bFGF has been found to be stored in the basement membrane in association with heparin, a molecule that aids the binding of bFGF to its receptor (Vlodavsky et al., 1991). Heparinase derived from degranulating platelets, neutrophils, and mast cells has been shown to release bFGF from the matrix in which it is sequestered.

EGF and TGFα are polypeptides that bind with similar affinity to the same receptor (170 kD) and share similar biological activity—mitogenic for epithelial cells, keratinocytes, endothelial cells, and fibroblasts (for review, see Carpenter and Cohen, 1990; Massague, 1990). When fully processed, TGFα and EGF are 5.6 and 6.0 kDa, respectively. Both are sometimes synthesized as glycosylated membrane-anchored precursors (Bringman et al., 1987; Wong et al., 1989; Massague, 1990) and can be found as larger molecules if released from the membrane before full processing (Linsley et al., 1985; Bringman et al., 1987). Although EGF and TGFα share only 40% sequence homology, they have considerable structural homology including the conservation of all 3 disulfide bridges (Stoschek and King, 1986). TGFα is unrelated to TGFβ and, despite its name, exhibits no transforming activity. This cytokine is synthesized by activated macrophages, keratinocytes, epithelial cells, brain, pituitary, and various tissues in embryonic development. EGF production appears to take place in a wide variety of tissues; this protein is found in nearly all body fluids (Carpenter, 1985). Relevant to the inflammatory response, platelets contain large quantities of EGF. Recently, a heparin-binding form of EGF has been identified. Unlike TGFα and (non-heparin-binding) EGF, this novel form can be stored in the extracellular matrix and is also mitogenic for smooth muscle cells (Higashiyama et al., 1991). Heparin-binding EGF is produced by activated macrophages and is found in wound fluids. This form of EGF, as well as platelet-derived EGF and TGFα, undoubtedly plays an important role in the resolution of inflammation and wound repair.

K. Cytokine Mediators of Humoral Immunity

The cytokines discussed in the preceding sections each mediate some aspect of the inflammatory response. Some of the cytokines, including IL-4, IL-6, and TGFβ, were also noted to be important mediators of B cell function. Other characterized cytokines, IL-5 and IL-7, function primarily as modulators of the humoral immune response, that is, B cell-mediated immunity. In addition, these cytokines may also indirectly affect the inflammatory response.

IL-5, a product of activated T lymphocytes, is a 133- or 134-amino-acid protein (murine, human) with a 21- or 22-amino-acid signal sequence and multiple glycosylation sites (Strober and James, 1988; Arai et al., 1990). The molecular mass of mature IL-5 is 18 kDa, with 12.8 kDa contributed by the polypeptide core. Like IL-4, IL-5 promotes the growth of B cells; however, its effects are restricted to activated cells. IL-5 also appears to modulate B cell isotype differentiation, and has been shown to augment T cell cytotoxic capacity and promote eosinophil growth (colony formation) in culture.

IL-7, a 25-kDa protein, is produced by bone marrow and thymus stromal cells and appears to be a lymphoid-specific growth regulator (Mizel, 1989; Arai et al., 1990). IL-7 promotes proliferation of primitive B cells at the pro- and pre-B cell stages, but is inactive with mature B cells. In addition, IL-7 supports the growth of thymocytes and mature T lymphocytes, the latter possibly through the induction of IL-2 and the IL-2 receptor. Additional investigation is necessary to determine whether IL-7 is involved in the activation of T lymphocytes during the inflammatory response.

III. Additional Considerations

As the preceding overview has indicated, the various inflammatory cytokines that can contribute to the inflammatory response often appear to have overlapping or synergistic functional effects, thus raising the following question. What control mechanisms mediate the effects of these molecules? Increasing evidence suggests that the regulatory mechanisms are as complex and multifaceted as the cytokine cascade being regulated.

The first level of control is the production of active cytokines. Evidence for the exertion of control of this process by the cell is seen in the very defined temporal order of cytokine synthesis, and its transient nature even in the presence of a persistent stimulus. Regulation of cytokine production can occur at the level of transcription or translation, depending on the cytokine; alternatively, the cytokine may be synthesized constitutively with regulation at the level of cellular release. Some cytokines are not immediately released from the cell, but are tethered to the cell surface (e.g., M-CSF, TNFα, TGFα, EGF); thus, their activity is limited to adjacent cells expressing the appropriate receptor unless the cytokines are released from the cell surface by the action of a specific enzyme (Massague, 1990). Other cytokines (TGFβ, IL-1β) can be released from the cell in a latent form, requiring activation by extracellular enzymes before they achieve biological activity (Roberts and Sporn, 1990; Mizutani et al., 1991).

A second level of regulation of cytokine activity is supplied by extracellular proteins and structures that limit the activity of the secreted cytokines. Tight junctions between cells, the basement membrane, and extracellular matrix can all limit the diffusion of a released cytokine. However, injury often compromises the integrity of these structures. In addition to these physical barriers, proteins found within the extracellular milieu can bind the cytokine, thus neutralizing its activity. For example, the serum protein α_2-macroglobulin, when converted to an active form by the action of a protease such as plasmin, is able to bind TGFβ, PDGF, IL-1β, and IL-6 (Sottrup-Jensen, 1989). In addition, soluble receptors for specific cytokines (IL-1, TNFα, IFNγ, IL-2, IL-6, EGF, TGFα) can be found extracellularly (Novick et al., 1989; Gatanaga et al., 1990; Giri et al., 1990; Gunther et al., 1990); these receptors can scavenge released cytokine and thus effectively and specifically eliminate the cell-mediated biological activity. However, as shown for the soluble IL-6 receptor, soluble receptor peptides need not act as ligand antagonists and may, instead, exert stimulatory effects (Taga et al., 1989). Heparin sulfate found within the basement membrane also binds certain cytokines (aFGF, bFGF, heparin-binding EGF), thus temporarily inhibiting their biological activity (Rifkin and Moscatelli, 1989). Since the actions of all cytokines are concentration dependent, limitation in the access of cytokines to target cells may prevent the necessary concentration of cytokine from being achieved, thereby eliminating its biological effects.

A third level of control of the activities of cytokines released during the inflammatory response is at the level of the effector cell. The cell must first express the receptor for the cytokine. In some cases, receptor expression must be induced by an activating stimulus or other cytokines. For example, expression of the IL-2 receptor is induced in monocytes when they are activated by LPS or IFNγ (Wahl *et al.*, 1987b) and in T lymphocytes when they are activated by IL-1. Many cytokines have multiple receptors of differing affinity for the various isoforms. Selective expression of receptor subtypes could also be important in modulating the cellular response. Once expressed, receptors can be down-regulated by inflammatory stimuli or cytokines. For instance, monocyte TGFβ receptors are down-regulated by LPS, IFNγ (Brandes *et al.*, 1991c), and streptococcal cell wall (M. E. Brandes and S. M. Wahl, unpublished results); LPS and IFNγ down-regulate macrophage TNFα receptors (Ding *et al.*, 1989; Drapier and Wietzerbin, 1991); and TNFα decreases macrophage M-CSF receptors (Shieh *et al.*, 1989). Another means by which a receptor may become unavailable for cytokine binding is through the action of a receptor antagonist. An IL-1 receptor antagonist, referred to as IL-1ra or IRAP, binds to the IL-1 receptor, preventing IL-1 from binding, but has no discernable IL-1 agonist effects (Arend *et al.*, 1990). The receptor antagonist is released by activated monocytes and is thought to be present at inflammatory sites. In addition to modulation of receptor expression and availability, cytokines can antagonize each others' effects. The best example of antagonistic activity is that of TGFβ which inhibits the action of several cytokines and consequently interferes with the proliferation and functional activity of several types of leukocytes (Roberts and Sporn, 1990).

Despite the enormous complexity of the cytokine network, it is efficiently regulated. The inflammatory response that ensues after injury typically restricts the damage and removes or neutralizes the injurious agent. These processes are mediated to a large extent by the inflammatory cytokines released by cells of the tissue involved and by circulating leukocytes. Our understanding of the intricacies of the inflammatory response is far from complete, but the identification of cytokines as controllers of the various stages of inflammation provides a solid foundation for characterizing these cellular and molecular events.

References

Aguet, M., Dembic, Z., and Merlin, G. (1988). Molecular cloning and expression of the human interferon-γ receptor. *Cell* **55**, 273–280.

Aiello, F. B., Longo, D. L., Overton, R., Takacs, L., and Durum, S. K. (1990). A role for cytokines in antigen presentation: IL-1 and IL-4 induce accessory cell functions of antigen-presenting cells. *J. Immunol.* **144**, 2572–2581.

Allen, J. B., Malone, D. G., Wahl, S. M., Calandra, G. B., and Wilder, R. L. (1985). Role of the thymus in streptococcal cell-wall induced arthritis and hepatic granuloma formation. *J. Clin. Invest.* **76**, 1042–1056.

Allen, J. B., Manthey, C. L., Hand, A. R., Ohura, K., Ellingsworth, L., and Wahl, S. M. (1990a). Rapid onset synovial inflammation and hyperplasia induced by transforming growth factor β. *J. Exp. Med.* **171**, 231–247.

Allen, J. B., McCartney-Francis, N., Smith, P. D., Simon, G., Gartner, S., Wahl, L. M., Popovic, M., and Wahl, S. M. (1990b). Expression of interleukin 2 receptors by monocytes from patients with acquired immunodeficiency syndrome and induction of monocyte interleukin 2 receptors by human immunodeficiency virus in vitro. *J. Clin. Invest.* **85,** 192–199.

Allen, J. B., Wong, H., Costa, G., Bienkowski, M. J., and Wahl, S. M. (1993). Suppression of monocyte function and differential regulation of IL-1 and IL-1ra by IL-4 contribute to resolution of experimental arthritis. *J. Immunol.* **151,** 4344–4351.

Andres, J. L., Stanley, K., Cheifetz, S., and Massague, J. (1989). Membrane-anchored and soluble forms of betaglycan, a polymorphic proteoglycan that binds transforming growth factor-β. *J. Cell Biol.* **109,** 3137–3145.

Arai, K., Lee, F., Miyajima, A., Shoichiro, M., Arai, N., and Yokota, T. (1990). Cytokines: Coordinators of immune and inflammatory responses. *Annu. Rev. Biochem.* **59,** 783–836.

Arend, W. P., Welgus, H. G., Thompson, R. C., and Eisenberg, S. P. (1990). Biological properties of recombinant human monocyte-derived interleukin-1 receptor antagonist. *J. Clin. Invest.* **85,** 1694–1697.

Assoian, R. K., Komoriya, A., Meyers, C. A., Miller, D. M., and Sporn, M. B. (1983). Transforming growth factor-beta in human platelets. *J. Biol. Chem.* **258,** 7155–7160.

Assoian, R. K., Fleurdelys, B. E., Stevens, H. C., Miller, P. J., Madtes, D. K., Raines, E. W., Ross, R., and Sporn, M. B. (1987). Expression and secretion of type β transforming growth factor by activated human macrophages. *Proc. Natl. Acad. Sci. USA* **84,** 6020–6024.

Baumann, H., Richards, C., and Gauldie, J. (1987). Interaction among hepatocyte-stimulating factors, interleukin 1, and glucocorticoids for regulation of acute phase plasma proteins in human hepatoma (HepG2) cells. *J. Immunol.* **139,** 4122–4128.

Bazan, J. F. (1990). Structural design and molecular evolution of a cytokine receptor superfamily. *Proc. Natl. Acad. Sci. USA* **87,** 6934–6938.

Besemer, J., Hujber, A., and Kuhn, B. (1989). Specific binding, internalization, and degradation of human neutrophil activating factor by human polymorphonuclear leukocytes. *J. Biol. Chem.* **264,** 17409–17415.

Bevilacqua, M. P., Pober, J. S., Majeau, G. R., Fiers, W., Cotran, R. S., and Gimbrone, M. A. (1986). Recombinant tumor necrosis factor induces procoagulant activity in cultured human vascular endothelium. *Proc. Natl. Acad. Sci. USA* **83,** 4533–4537.

Billiau, A. (1988). Gamma-interferon: The match that lights the fire? *Immunol. Today* **9,** 37–40.

Borish, L., Rosenbaum, R., Albury, L., and Clark, S. (1989). Activation of neutrophils by recombinant interleukin 6. *Cell. Immunol.* **121,** 280–289.

Bowen-Pope, D. F., Hart, C. E., and Seifert, R. A. (1989). Sera and conditioned media contain different isoforms of platelet-derived growth factor (PDGF) which bind to different classes of PDGF receptor. *J. Biol. Chem.* **264,** 2504–2508.

Brandes, M. E., and Finkelstein, J. N. (1990). The production of alveolar macrophage-derived growth-regulating proteins in response to lung injury. *Toxicol. Lett.* **54,** 3–22.

Brandes, M. E., Mai, U. E. H., Ohura, K., and Wahl, S. M. (1991a). Type I TGFβ receptors on neutrophils mediate chemotaxis to TGFβ. *J. Immunol.* **147,** 1600–1606.

Brandes, M. E., Allen, J. B., Yasushi, O., and Wahl, S. M. (1991b). Transforming growth factor β1 suppresses acute and chronic arthritis in experimental animals. *J. Clin. Invest.* **87,** 1108–1113.

Brandes, M. E., Wakefield, L. M., and Wahl, S. M. (1991c). Modulation of monocyte type I transforming growth factor beta (TGFβ) receptors by inflammatory stimuli. *J. Biol. Chem.* **266,** 19697–19703.

Bringman, T. S., Lindquist, P. B., and Derynck, R. (1987). Different transforming growth factor-α species are derived from a glycosylated and palmitoylated transmembrane precursor. *Cell* **48,** 429–440.

Broudy, V. C., Kaushansky, K., Segal, G. M., Harlan, J. M., and Adamson, J. W. (1986). Tumor necrosis factor-α stimulates human endothelial cells to produce granulocyte/macrophage colony stimulating factor. *Proc. Natl. Acad. Sci. USA* **83**, 7467–7474.

Broudy, V. C., Harlan, J. M., and Adamson, J. W. (1987). Disparate effects of tumor necrosis factor-α/cachectin and tumor necrosis factor β/lymphotoxin on hematopoietic growth factor production and neutrophil adhesion molecule expression by cultured human endothelial cells. *J. Immunol.* **138**, 4298–4306.

Bussolino, F., Ziche, M., Wang, J., Alessi, D., Morbidelli, L., Cremona, O., Bosia, A., Marchisio, P. C., and Mantovani, A. (1991). *In vitro* and *in vivo* activation of endothelial cells by colony-stimulating factors. *J. Clin. Invest.* **87**, 986–995.

Camussi, G., Bussolino, F., Salvidio, G., and Baglioni, C. (1987). Tumor necrosis factor/cachectin stimulates peritoneal macrophages, polymorphonuclear leukocytes, and vascular endothelial cells to synthesize and release platelet activating factor. *J. Exp. Med.* **166**, 1390–1404.

Carpenter, G. (1985). Epidermal growth factor: Biology and reception metabolism. *J. Cell Sci. Suppl.* **3**, 1–9.

Carpenter, G., and Cohen, S. (1990). Epidermal growth factor. *J. Biol. Chem.* **265**, 7709–7712.

Cheifetz, S., Bassols, A., Stanley, K., Ohta, M., Greenberger, J., and Massague, J. (1988). Heterodimeric transforming growth factor-β. Biological properties and interaction with three types of cell surface receptors. *J. Biol. Chem.* **263**, 10783–10789.

Chung, I. Y., and Benveniste, E. N. (1990). Tumor necrosis factor-α production by astrocytes. Induction by lipopolysaccharide, IFN-γ, and IL-1β. *J. Immunol.* **144**, 2999–3007.

Cicco, N. A., Lindenmann, A., Content, J., Vandenbussche, P., Lubbert, M., Gauss, J., Mertelsmann, R., and Herrmann, F. (1990). Inducible production of interleukin-6 by human polymorphonuclear neutrophils: Role of granulocyte-macrophage colony-stimulating factor and tumor necrosis factor-alpha. *Blood* **75**, 2049–2052.

Corcoran, M. L., Stetler-Stevenson, W. G., Brown, P. D., and Wahl, L. M. (1992). Interleukin 4 inhibition of prostaglandin E2 synthesis blocks interstitial collagenase and 92-kDa type IV collagenase/gelatinase production by human monocytes. *J. Biol. Chem.* **267**, 515–519.

Cosman, D., Lyman, S. D., Idzerda, R. L., Beckmann, M. P., Park, L. S., Goodwin, R. G., and March, C. J. (1990). A new cytokine receptor superfamily. *Trends Biochem. Sci.* **15**, 265–270.

Crawford, R. M., Finbloom, D. S., Ohara, J., Paul, W. E., and Meltzer, M. S. (1987). B cell stimulatory factor-1 (interleukin 4) activates macrophages for increased tumoricidal activity and expression of Ia antigens. *J. Immunol.* **139**, 135–141.

Czarniecki, C. W., Chiu, H. H., Wong, G. H. W., McCabe, S. M., Palladino, M. A. (1988). Transforming growth factor-β1 modulates the expression of class II histocompatability antigens on human cells. *J. Immunol.* **140**, 4217–4223.

Danielpour, D., Dart, L. L., Flanders, K. C., Roberts, A. B., and Sporn, M. B. (1989). Immuno-detection and quantitation of the two forms of transforming growth factor-beta (TGF-beta 1 and TGF-beta 2) secreted by cells in culture. *J. Cell. Physiol.* **138**, 79–86.

Dayer, J. M., Beutler, B., and Cerami, A. (1985). Cachectin/tumor necrosis factor stimulates collagenase and prostaglandin E2 production by human synovial cells and dermal fibroblasts. *J. Exp. Med.* **162**, 2163–2168.

Dejana, E., Breviario, F., Erroi, A., Bussolino, F., Mussoni, L., Gramse, M., Pintucci, G., Casali, B., Dinarello, C. A., Van Damme, J., and Mantovani, A. (1987). Modulation of endothelial cell functions by different molecular species of interleukin 1. *Blood* **69**, 695–699.

De Larco, J. E., and Todaro, G. J. (1978). Growth factors from murine sarcoma virus-transformed cells. *Proc. Natl. Acad. Sci. USA* **75**, 4001–4005.

Dennis, P. A., and Rifkin, D. B. (1991). Cellular activation of latent transforming growth factor β requires binding to the cation-independent mannose 6-phosphate/insulin-like growth factor type II receptor. *Proc. Natl. Acad. Sci. USA* **88**, 580–584.

Deuel, T. F., Senior, R. M., Huang, J. S., and Griffin, G. L. (1982). Chemotaxis of monocytes and neutrophils to platelet-derived growth factor. *J. Clin. Invest.* **69**, 1046–1049.

Devatelis, G., Wolpe, S. D., Sherry, B., Dayer, J.-M., Chicheportiche, R., and Cerami, A. (1989). Macrophage inflammatory protein 1: A prostaglandin-independent endogenous pyrogen. *Science* **243**, 1066–68.

Dinarello, C. A., Ikejima, T., Warner, S. J. C., Orencole, S. F., Lonnemann, G., Cannon, J. G., and Libby, P. (1987). Interleukin-1 induces interleukin-1. Induction of circulating interleukin-1 in rabbits *in vivo* and in human mononuclear cells *in vitro*. *J. Immunol.* **139**, 1902–1910.

Ding, A., Nathan, C. F., and Stuehr, D. J. (1988). Release of reactive nitrogen intermediates and reactive oxygen intermediates from mouse peritoneal macrophages: Comparison of activating cytokines and evidence for independent production. *J. Immunol.* **141**, 2407–2412.

Ding, A. H., Sanchez, E., Srimal, S., and Nathan, C. F. (1989). Macrophages rapidly internalize their tumor necrosis factor receptors to bacterial lipopolysaccharide. *J. Biol. Chem.* **264**, 3924–3929.

Ding, A., Nathan, C. F., Graycar, J., Derynck, R., Stuehr, D. J., and Srimal, D. (1990). Macrophage deactivating factor and transforming growth factors-β1, -β2 and -β3 inhibit induction of macrophage nitrogen oxide synthesis by IFN-γ. *J. Immunol.* **145**, 940–944.

Donnelly, R. P., Fenton, M. J., Finbloom, D. S., and Gerrard, T. L. (1990). Differential regulation of IL-1 production in human monocytes by IFN-γ and IL-4. *J. Immunol.* **145**, 569–575.

Dower, S. K., Wignall, J., Schooley, K., McMahan, C. J., Jackson, J., Prickett, K. S., Lupton, S., Cosman, D., and Sims, J. E. (1989). Retention of ligand binding activity by the extracellular domain of the IL-1 receptor. *J. Immunol.* **142**, 4314–4320.

Drapier, J. C., and Wietzerbin, J. (1991). IFN-γ reduces specific binding of tumor necrosis factor on murine macrophages. *J. Immunol.* **146**, 1198–1203.

Dubravec, D. B., Spriggs, D. R., Mannick, J. A., and Rodrick, M. L. (1990). Circulating human peripheral blood granulocytes synthesize and secrete tumor necrosis factor α. *Proc. Natl. Acad. Sci. USA* **87**, 6758–6761.

Dukovich, M., Wano, Y., Thuy, L. T. B., Katz, P., Cullen, B. R., Kehrl, J. H., and Greene, W. C. (1987). A second human interleukin-2 binding protein that may be a component of high affinity interleukin-2 receptors. *Nature (London)* **327**, 518–522.

Elias, J. A., Gustilo, K., Baeder, W., and Freundlich, B. (1987). Synergistic stimulation of fibroblast prostaglandin production by recombinant interleukin 1 and tumor necrosis factor. *J. Immunol.* **138**, 3812–3816.

Ellingsworth, L., Nakayama, D., Dasch, J., Segarini, P., Carrillo, P., and Waegell, W. (1989). Transforming growth factor beta 1 (TGF-β_1) receptor expression on resting and mitogen-activated T cells. *J. Cell. Biochem.* **39**, 489–500.

Espevik, T., Figari, I. S., Ranges, G. E., and Palladino, M. A. (1988). Transforming growth factor-β1 (TGF-β1) and recombinant human tumor necrosis factor-alpha reciprocally regulate the generation of lymphokine-activated killer cell activity. *J. Immunol.* **140**, 2312–2316.

Essner, R., Phoades, K., McBride, W. H., Morton, D. L., and Economou, J. S. (1989). IL-4 down-regulates IL-1 and TNF gene expression in human monocytes. *J. Immunol.* **142**, 3857–3861.

Ferrante, A., Nandoskar, M., Walz, A., Goh, D. H. B., and Kowanko, I. C. (1988). Effects of tumor necrosis factor alpha and interleukin- alpha and beta on human neutrophil migration, respiratory burst and degranulation. *Int. Arch. Allergy Appl. Immunol.* **86**, 82–91.

Figari, I. S., Mori, N. A., and Palladino, M. A. (1987). Regulation of neutrophil migration and superoxide production by recombinant tumor necrosis factors-α and -β: Comparison to recombinant interferon-γ and interleukin-1α. *Blood* **70**, 979–984.

Fleischmann, J., Golde, D., Wiesbart, R., and Gasson, J. C. (1986). Granulocyte-macrophage colony-stimulating factor enhances phagocytosis of bacteria by human neutrophils. *Blood* **68**, 708–711.

Folkman, J., and Klagsbrun, M. (1987). Angiogenic factors. *Science* **235**, 442–447.

Foster, S. J., Aked, D. M., Schroder, J.-M., and Christophers, E. (1989). Acute inflammatory effects of a monocyte-derived neutrophil-activating peptide in rabbit skin. *Immunology* **67,** 181–83.

Fukunaga, R., Ishizaka-Ikeda, E., Seto, Y., and Nagata, S., (1990). Expression cloning of a receptor for murine granulocyte colony-stimulating factor. *Cell* **61,** 341–350.

Gatanaga, T., Hwang, C., Kohr, W., Cappuccini, F., Lucci, J. A., Jeffes, E. W. B., Lentz, R., Tomich, J., Yamamoto, R. S., and Granger, G. A. (1990). Purification and characterization of an inhibitor (soluble tumor necrosis factor receptor) for tumor necrosis factor and lymphotoxin obtained from the serum ultrafiltrates of human cancer patients. *Proc. Natl. Acad. Sci. USA* **87,** 8781–8784.

Gearing, D. P., King, J. A., Gough, N. M., and Nicola, N. A. (1989). Expression cloning of a receptor for human granulocyte-macrophage colony-stimulating factor. *EMBO J.* **8,** 3667–3676.

Giri, J. G., Newton, R. C., and Horuk, R. (1990). Identification of soluble interleukin-1 binding protein in cell-free supernatants. *J. Biol. Chem.* **265,** 17416–17419.

Goldstein, I. M. (1988). Complement: Biologically active products. *In* "Inflammation: Basic Principles and Clinical Correlates" (J. I. Gallin, I. M. Goldstein, and R. Snyderman, eds.), pp. 55–74. Raven Press, New York.

Gordon, J. R., and Galli, S. J. (1990). Mast cells as a source of both preformed and immunologically inducible TNF-α/cachectin. *Nature (London)* **346,** 274–276.

Gospodarowicz, D. (1988). Fibroblast growth factor. *In* "ISI Atlas of Science: Biochemistry," pp. 101–108. Institute for Scientific Information, Philadelphia.

Graves, D. T., Grontendorst, G. R., Antoniades, H. N., Schwartz, C. J., and Valente, H. A. (1989). Platelet-derived growth factor is not chemotactic for human peripheral blood monocytes. *Exp. Cell Res.* **180,** 497–503.

Griffin, J. D., Spertini, O., Ernst, T. J., Belvin, M. P., Levine, H. B., Kanakura, Y., and Tedder, T. F. (1990). Granulocyte-macrophage colony-stimulating factor and other cytokines regulate surface expression of the leukocyte adhesion molecule-1 on human neutrophis, monocytes, and their precursors. *J. Immunol.* **145,** 576–584.

Grob, P. M., David, E., Warren, T. C., DeLeon, R. P., Farina, P. R., and Homon, C. A. (1990). Characterization of a receptor for human monocyte-derived neutrophil chemotactic factor/interleukin-8. *J. Biol. Chem.* **265,** 8311–8316.

Grotendorst, G. R., Smale, G., and Pencev, D. (1989). Production of transforming growth factor beta by human peripheral blood monocytes and neutrophils. *J. Cell. Immunol.* **140,** 396–402.

Gunther, N., Betzel, C., and Weber, W. (1990). The secreted form of the epidermal growth factor receptor. *J. Biol. Chem.* **265,** 22082–22085.

Hajjar, K. A., Hajjar, D. P., Silverstein, R. L., and Nackman, R. L. (1987). Tumor necrosis factor-mediated release of platelet-derived growth factor from cultured endothelial cells. *J. Exp. Med.* **166,** 235–245.

Hart, C. E., Forstrom, J. W., Kelley, J. D., Seifert, R. A., Smith, R. A., Ross, R., Murray, M. J., and Bowen-Pope, D. F. (1988). Two classes of PDGF receptors recognize different isoforms of PDGF. *Science* **240,** 1529–1531.

Hart, P. H., Vitti, G. F., Burgess, D. R., Whitty, G. A., Piccoli, D. S., and Hamilton, J. A. (1989). Potential anti-inflammatory effects of interleukin 4: Suppression of human monocyte tumor necrosis factor alpha, interleukin 1, and prostaglandin E2. *Proc. Natl. Acad. Sci. USA* **86,** 3803–3807.

Hatakeyama, M., Tsudo, M., Minamoto, S., Kono, T., Doi, T., Miyata, T., Miyasaka, M., and Taniguchi, T. (1989). Interleukin-2 receptor β chain gene: Generation of three receptor forms by cloned human α and β chain cDNAs. *Science* **244,** 551–556.

Heller, R. A., Song, K., Onasch, M. A., Fischer, W. H., Chang, D., and Ringold, G. M. (1990). *Proc. Natl. Acad. Sci. USA* **87,** 6151–6155.

Heine, U. I., Flanders, K., Roberts, A. B., Munoz, E. F., and Sporn, M. B. (1987). Role of transforming growth factor-β in the development of the mouse embryo. *J. Cell Biol.* **105,** 2861–2876.

Heremans, H., and Billiau, A. (1989). The potential role of interferons and antagonists in inflammatory disease. *Drugs* **38,** 957–972.

Heremans, H., Dijkmans, R., Sobis, H., Vandekerckhove, F., and Billiau, A. (1987). Regulation by interferons of the local inflammatory response to bacterial lipopolysaccharide. *J. Immunol.* **138,** 4175–4179.

Higashiyama, S., Abraham, J. A., Miller, J., Fiddes, J. C., and Klagsbrun, M. (1991). A heparin-binding growth factor secreted by macrophage-like cells that is related to EGF. *Science* **251,** 936–939.

Itoh, N., Yonehara, S., Schreurs, J., Gorman, D. M., Maruyama, K., Ishii, A., Yahara, I., Arai, K., and Miyajima, A. (1990). Cloning of an interleukin-3 receptor gene: A member of a distinct receptor gene family. *Science* **247,** 324–327.

Janoff, E. N., Smith, P. D., Wahl, L. M., Thomas, K., and Wahl, S. M. (1991). Human recombinant GM-CSF enhances monocyte-dependent lymphocyte proliferation and immunoglobulin production. Submitted.

Katona, I. M., Ohura, K., Allen, J. B., Wahl, L. M., Chenoweth, D. E., and Wahl, S. M. (1991). Modulation of monocyte chemotactic function in inflammatory lesions. *J. Immunol.* **146,** 708–714.

Katz, I. R., Thorbecke, G. J., Bell, M. K., Yin, J. Z., Clarke, D., Zucker, M. B. (1986). Protease-induced regulatory activity of platelet factor 4. *Proc. Natl. Acad. Sci. USA* **83,** 3491–3495.

Kehrl, J. H., Roberts, A. B., Wakefield, L. M., Jakowlew, S., Sporn, M. B., and Fauci, A. S. (1986a). Transforming growth factor β is an important immunomodulatory protein for human B lymphocytes. *J. Immunol.* **137,** 3855–3860.

Kehrl, J. H., Wakefield, L. M., Roberts, A. B., Jakowlew, S., Alvarez-mon, M., Derynck, R., Sporn, M. B., and Fauci, A. S. (1986b). Production of transforming growth factor β by human T lymphocytes and its potential role in the regulation of T cell growth. *J. Exp. Med.* **163,** 1037–1050.

Kehrl, J. H., Taylor, A. S., Delsing, G. A., Roberts, A. B., Sporn, M. B., and Fauci, A. S. (1989). Further studies of the role of TGF-β in human cell function. *J. Immunol.* **143,** 1868–1874.

Kelleher, K., Bean K., Clark, S. C., Leung, W. Y., Yang-Feng, T. L., Chen, J. W., Lin, P. F., Luo, W., and Yang, Y. C. (1991). Human interleukin-9: Genomic sequence, chromosomal location, and sequences essential for its expression in human T-cell leukemia virus (HTVL)-I-transformed human T cells. *Blood.* **77,** 1436–1441.

Keller, J. R., Mantel, C., Sing, G. K., Ellingsworth, L. R., Ruscetti, S. K., and Ruscetti, F. W. (1988). Transforming growth factor-$\beta1$ selectively regulates early murine hematopoietic progenitors and inhibits the growth of IL-3 dependent myeloid leukemia cell lines. *J. Exp. Med.* **168,** 737–750.

Kelley, J. (1990). Cytokines of the lung. *Am. Rev. Resp. Dis.* **141,** 765–788.

Kishi, H., Inui, S., Muraguchi, A., Hirano, T., Yamamura, Y., and Kishimoto, T. (1985). Induction of IgG secretion in a human B cell clone with recombinant IL 2. *J. Immunol.* **134,** 3104–3107.

Kohase, M., Heneriksen-DiStefano, D., May, L. T., Vilcek, J., and Sehgal, P. B. (1986). Induction of β_2-interferon by tumor necrosis factor: A homeostatic mechanism in the control of cell proliferation. *Cell* **45,** 659–666.

Kriebel, D., Brain, J. D., Sprince, N. L., and Kazemi, H. (1988). The pulmonary toxicity of beryllium. *Am. Rev. Resp. Dis.* **137,** 464–473.

Kupper, T. S. (1990a). Immune and inflammatory processes in cutaneous tissues. *J. Clin. Invest.* **86,** 1783–1789.

Kupper, T. S. (1990b). The activated keratinocyte: A model for inducible cytokine production by non-bone marrow-derived cells in cutaneous inflammatory and immune responses. *Invest. Dermatol.* **94**, 146S–150S.

Kuruvilla, A. P., Shah, R., Hockwald, G. M., Liggitt, H. D., Palladino, M. A., and Thorbecke, G. J. (1991). Protective effect of transforming growth factor β_1 on experimental autoimmune diseases in mice. *Proc. Natl. Acad. Sci. USA* **88**, 2918–2921.

Laiho, M., Weis, F. M. B., and Massague, J. (1990). Concomitant loss of transforming growth factor (TGF) -β receptor types I and II in TGF-β-resistant cell mutants implicates both receptor types in signal transduction. *J. Biol. Chem.* **265**, 18518–18524.

Lee, S. H., Aggarwal, B. B., Rinderknecht, E., Assisi, F., and Chiu, H. (1984). The synergistic anti-proliferative effect of γ-interferon and human lymphotoxin. *J. Immunol.* **133**, 1083–1086.

Lefer, A. M., Tsao, P., Aoki, N., and Palladino, M. A., Jr. (1990). Mediation of cardioprotection by transforming growth factor-β. *Science* **249**, 61–64.

Leonard, W. J., Depper, J. M., Crabtree, G. R., Rudikoff, S., Pumphrey, J., Robb, R. J., Kronke, M., Svetlik, P. B., Peffer, N. J., Waldmann, T. A., and Greene, W. C. (1984). Moleculare cloning and expression of cDNAs for the human interleukin-2 receptor. *Nature (London)* **311**, 626–635.

Libby, P., Ordovas, J. M., Auger, K. R., Robbins, A. H., Biringi, L. K., and Dinarello, C. A. (1986). Endotoxin and tumor necrosis factor induce interleukin-1 gene expression in adult human vascular enodthelial cells. *Am. J. Pathol.* **124**, 179–185.

Lindemann, A., Riedel, D., Oster, W., Ziegler-Heitbrock, H. W. L., Mertelsmann, R., and Herrmann, F. (1989). Granulocyte-macrophage colony-stimulating factor induces cytokine secretion by human polymorphonuclear leukocytes. *J. Clin. Invest.* **83**, 1308–1312.

Linsley, P. S., Hargreaves, W. R., Twardzik, D. R., and Todaro, G. J. (1985). Detection of larger polypeptides structurally and functionally related to type I transforming growth factor. *Proc. Natl. Acad. Sci. USA* **82**, 356–360.

Livingston, D. H., Appel, S. H., Sonnenfeld, G., and Malangoni, M. A. (1989). The effect of tumor necrosis factor-α and interferon-γ on neutrophil function. *J. Surg. Res.* **46**, 322–326.

Lobb, R. R., Harper, J. W., and Fett, J. W. (1986). Purification of heparin-binding growth factors. *Anal. Biochem.* **154**, 1–14.

Loetscher, H., Pan, Y. C. E., Lahm, H. W., Gentz, R., Brockhaus, M., Tabuchi, H., and Lesslauer, W. (1990). Molecular cloning and expression of the human 55kd tumor necrosis factor receptor. *Cell* **61**, 351–359.

Lopez, A. F., Williamson, D. J., Begley, J. R., Harlan, J. M., Klebanoff, S. J., Waltersdorpf, A., Wong, G., Clark, S. C., and Vadas, M. A. (1986). Recombinant human granulocyte-macrophage colony-stimulating factor stimulates *in vitro* mature human neutrophil and eosinophil function, surface receptor expression and survival. *J. Clin. Invest.* **78**, 1220–1228.

Lyons, R. M., Keski-Oja, J., and Moses, H. L. (1988). Proteolytic activation of latent transforming growth factor-β from fibroblast-conditioned medium. *J. Cell. Biol.* **106**, 1659–1665.

MacKay, K., Robbins, A. R., Bruce, M. D., and Danielpour, D. (1990). Identification of disulfide-linked transforming growth factor-β1-specific binding proteins in rat glomeruli. *J. Biol. Chem.* **265**, 9351–9356.

Mangan, D., Welch, G. R., and Wahl, S. M. (1991). Lipopolysaccharide, tumor necrosis factor-α, and IL-1β prevent programmed cell death (apoptosis) in human peripheral blood monocytes. *J. Immunol.* **146**, 1541–1546.

Mangan, D. F., Robertson, B., and Wahl, S. M. (1992). Interleukin-4 enhances programmed cell death in stimulated human monocytes. *J. Immunol.* **148**, 1812–1816.

Manthey, C. L., Allen, J. B., Ellingsworth, L. R., and Wahl, S. M. (1990). *In situ* expression of transforming growth factor beta in streptococcal cell wall-induced granulomatous inflammation and hepatic fibrosis. *Growth Factors* **4**, 17–26.

Manthey, C. L., Kossmann, T., Corcoran, M. L., Brandes, M. E., Allen J. B., and Wahl, S. M. (1992). Role of Kupffer cells in streptococcal cell wall (SCW) granulomas: SCW induction of inflammatory cytokines and mediators. *Growth Factors* **7**, 73–83.

Marucha, P. T., Zeff, R. A., and Kreutzer, D. L. (1990). Cytokine regulation of IL-1β gene expression in the human polymorphonuclear leukocyte. *J. Immunol.* **145**, 2932–2937.

Massague, J. (1990). Transforming growth factor-α. *J. Biol. Chem.* **265**, 21393–21396.

May, L. T., Ghrayeb, J., Santhanam, U., Tatter, S. B., Sthoeger, Z., Helfgott, D. C., Chiorazzi, N., Grieninger, G., and Sehgal, P. B. (1988). Synthesis and secretion of multiple forms of "β_2-interferon/B cell differentiation factor 2/hepatocyte stimulating factor" by human fibroblasts and monocytes. *J. Biol. Chem.* **262**, 7760–7766.

May, L. T., Santhanam, U., Tatter, S. B., Ghrayeb, J., and Sehgal, P. B. (1989). Multiple forms human interleukin-6. *Ann. N.Y. Acad. Sci.* **557**, 353–362.

McCartney-Francis, N., Mizel, D., Wong, H., Wahl, L. M., Roberts, A. B., Sporn, M. B., and Wahl, S. M. (1990). TGF-β regulates production of growth factors and TGF-β by human peripheral blood monocytes. *Growth Factors* **4**, 27–35.

McColl, S. R., Beauseigle, D., Gilbert, C., and Naccache, P. H. (1990). Priming of the human neutrophil respiratory burst by granulocyte-macrophage colony-stimulating factor and tumor necrosis factor-α involves regulation at a post-cell surface receptor level. *J. Immunol.* **145**, 3047–3053.

Miller, D. A., Lee, A., Matsui, Y., Chen, E. Y., Moses, H. L., and Derynck, R. (1989a). Complementary DNA cloning of the murine transforming growth factor-$\beta 3$ (TGF-$\beta 3$) precursor and the comparative expression of TGF-$\beta 3$ and TGF-$\beta 1$ messenger RNA in murine embryos and adult tissues. *Mol. Endocrinol.* **3**, 1926–1934.

Miller, D. A., Lee, A., Pelton, R. W., Chen. E. Y., Moses, H. L., and Derynck, R. (1989b). Murine transforming growth factor-$\beta 2$ cDNA sequence an expression in adult tissues and embryos. *Mol. Endocrinol.* **3**, 1108–1114.

Miyajima, A., Kitamura, T., Hayashida, K., Itoh, N., Schreurs, J., Gorman, D., Wang, H.-M., Ogorochi, T., Yonehara, S., Yahara, I., Yokota, T., and Arai, K. (1991). Molecular analysis of the IL-3 and GM-CSF receptors. *J. Cell. Biochem.* **15F**, 37. (Abstract)

Miyazono, K., and Heldin, C.-H. (1989) Interaction between TGF-$\beta 1$ and carbohydrate structures in its precursor renders TGF-β_1 latent. *Nature (London)* **388**, 158–160.

Miyazono, K., Hellman, U., Wernstedt, C., and Heldin, C-H. (1988). Latent high molecular weight complex of transforming growth factor β_1. *J. Biol. Chem.* **263**, 6407–6415.

Mizel, S. B. (1989). The interleukins. *FASEB J.* **3**, 2379–2387.

Mizutani, H., Black, R., and Kupper, T. S. (1991). Human keratinocytes produce but do not process pro-interleukin-1 (IL-1) beta. *J. Clin. Invest.* **87**, 1066–1071.

Mond, J. J., Thompson, C., Finkelman, F. D., Farrar, J., Schaefer, M., and Robb, R. J. (1985). Affinity-purified interleukin 2 induces proliferation of large but not small B cells. *Proc. Natl. Acad. Sci. USA* **82**, 1518–1521.

Monroy, R. L., Davis, T. A., and MacVittie, T. J. (1990). Granulocyte-macrophage colony-stimulating factor: More than a hemopoietin. *Clin. Immunol. Immunopathal.* **54**, 333–346.

Moses, H. L., Branum, E. L., Proper, J. A., and Robinson, R. A. (1981). Transforming growth factor production by chemically transformed cells. *Cancer Res.* **41**, 2842–2848.

Mosley, B., Beckmann, M. P., March, C. J., Idzerda, R. L., Gimpel, S. D., VandenBos, T., Friend, D., Alpert, A., Anderson, D., Jackson, J., Wignall, J. M., Smith, C., Gallis, B., Sims, J. E., Urdal, D., Widmer, M. B., Cosman, D., and Park, L. S. (1989). The murine interleukin-4 receptor: Molecular cloning and characterization of secreted and membrane bound forms. *Cell* **59**, 335–348.

Mule, J. J., Schwarz, S. L. Roberts, A. B., Sporn, M. B., Rosenberg, S. A. (1988). Transforming growth factor-beta inhibits the in vitro generation of lymphokine-activated killer cells and cytotoxic T cells. *Cancer Immunol. Immunother.* **26**, 95–100.

Nathan, C., and Yoshida, R. (1988). Cytokines: Interferon-γ. *In* "Inflammation: Basic Principles and Clinical Correlates" (J. I., Gallin, I. M. Goldstein, and R. Synderman, eds.), pp. 229–251. Raven Press, New York.

Neuman, E., Huleatt, J. W., and Jack, R. M. (1990). Granulocyte-macrophage colony-stimulating factor increases synthesis and expression of CR1 and CR3 by human peripheral blood neutrophils. *J. Immunol.* **145**, 3325–3332.

Nilsen-Hamilton, M. (1990). Transforming growth factor-β and its actions on cellular growth and differentiation. *Curr. Topics Dev. Biol.* **24**, 95–136.

Novick, D., Engelmann, H., Wallach, D., and Rubinstein, M. (1989). Soluble cytokine receptors are present in normal human urine. *J. Exp. Med.* **170**, 1409–1414.

Ohta, M., Greenberger, J. S., Anklesaria, P., Bassols, A., and Massague, J. (1987). Two forms of transforming growth factor-β distinguished by multipotential hematopoietic progenitor cells. *Nature (London)* **329**, 539–541.

Koa, Y., and Orth, D. N. (1983). Human plasma epidermal growth factor/β-urogastrone is associated with blood platelets. *J. Clin. Invest.* **72**, 249–259.

Oppenheim, J. J., Zachariae, C. O. C., Mukaida, N., and Matsushima, K. (1991). Properties of the novel proinflammatory supergene "intercrine" cytokine family. *Annu. Rev. Immunol.* **9**, 617–648.

Ortaldo, J. R., Mason, A. T., Gerard, J. P., Henderson, L. E., Farrar, W., Hopkins, R. F., Herberman, R. B., and Rabin, H. (1984). Effects of natural and recombinant IL2 on regulation of IFNγ production and natural killer activity: Lack of involvement of the Tac antigen for these immunoregulatory effects. *J. Immunol.* **133**, 779–783.

Paul, S. R., Bennett, F., Calvetti, J. A., Kelleher, K., Wood, C. R., O'Hara, R. M., Jr., Leary, A. C., Sibley, B., Clark, S. C., Williams, D. A., and Yang, Y. C. (1990). Molecular cloning of a cDNA encoding interleukin-11, a stromal cell-derived lymphopoietic and hematopoietic cytokine. *Proc. Natl. Acad. Sci. USA* **87**, 7512–7516.

Paul, W. E., and Ohara, J. (1987). B-cell stimulatory factor-1/interleukin 4. *Ann. Rev. Immunol.* **5**, 429–459.

Pelton, R. W., Dickinson, M. E., Moses, H. L., and Hogan, B. L. M. (1990). *In situ* hybridization analysis of TGF-β3 RNA expression during mouse development: Comparative studies with TGF-β1 and β2. *Development* **110**, 609–620.

Perez, C., Albert I., DeFay, K., Zachariades, N., Gooding, L., and Kriegler, M. (1990). A nonsecretable cell surface mutant of tumor necrosis factor (TNF) kills by cell-to-cell contact. *Cell* **63**, 251–258.

Pierce, J. H., Di Marco, E., Cox, G. W., Lombardi, D., Ruggiero, M., Varesio, L., Wang, L. M., Choudhury, G., Sakaguchi, A. Y., Di Fiore, P. P., and Aaronson, S. A. (1990). Macrophage-colony-stimulating factor (CSF-1) induces proliferation, chemotaxis and reversible monocytic differentiation in myeloid progenitor cells transfected with the human c-*fms*/CSF-1 receptor cDNA. *Proc. Natl. Acad. Sci. USA* **87**, 5613–5617.

Pircher, R., Jullien, P., and Lawrence, D. A. (1986) β-Transforming growth factor is stored in human blood platelets as a latent high molecular weight complex. *Biochem. Biophys. Res. Commun.* **136**, 30–37.

Pober, J. S., Gimbrone, M. A., Lapierre, L. A., Mendrick, D. L., Fiers, W., Rothelein, R., and Springer, T. A. (1986). Overlapping patterns of activation of human endothelial cells by interleukin-1, tumor necrosis factor, and immune interferon. *J. Immunol.* **137**, 1893–1896.

Postlethwaite, A. E., Keski-Ola, J., Moses, H. L., and Kang, A. H. (1987). Stimulation of the chemotactic migration of human fibroblasts by transforming growth factor beta. *J. Exp. Med.* **165**, 251–256.

Ranges, G. E., Figari, I. S., Espevik, T., and Palladino, M. A. (1987). Inhibition of cytotoxic T cell development by transforming growth factor β and reversal by recombinant tumor necrosis factor alpha. *J. Exp. Med.* **166**, 991–998.

Rifkin, D. B., and Moscatelli, D. (1989). Recent developments in the cell biology of basic fibroblast growth factor. *J. Cell Biol.* **109**, 1–6.

Ristow, H. J. (1986). BSC-1 growth inhibitor/type β transforming growth factor is a strong inhibitor of thymocyte proliferation. *Proc. Natl. Acad. Sci. USA* **83**, 5531–5533.

Roberts, A. B., and Sporn, M. B. (1990). The transforming growth factor-betas. *In* "Handbook of Experimental Pharmacology" (M. B. Sporn and A. B. Roberts, eds.), pp. 419–472. Springer-Verlag, New York.

Roberts, A. B., Anzano, M. A., Lamb, L. C., Smith, J. M., and Sporn, M. B. (1981). New class of transforming growth factors potentiated by epidermal growth factor. *Proc. Natl. Acad. Sci. USA* **78**, 5339–5343.

Roberts, A. B., Sporn, M. B., Assoian, R. K., Smith, J. M., Roche, N. S., Wakefield, L. M., Heine, U. I., Liotta, L. A., Falanga, V., Kehrl, J. H., and Fauci, A. S. (1986). Transforming growth factor type β: Rapid induction of fibrosis and angiogenesis *in vivo* and stimulation of collagen formation *in vitro*. *Proc. Natl. Acad. Sci. USA* **83**, 4167–4171.

Rook, A. H., Kehrl, J. H., Wakefield, L. M., Roberts, A. B., Sporn, M. B., Burlinton, D. B., Lane, H. C., and Fauci, A. S. (1986). Effects of transforming growth factor β on the functions of natural killer cells: Depressed cytolytic activity and blunting of interferon responsiveness. *J. Immunol.* **136**, 3916–3920.

Ross, R., Raines, E. W., and Bowen-Pope, D. F. (1986). The biology of platelet-derived growth factor. *Cell* **46**, 155–169.

Rubin, L. A., Kurman, C. C., Fritz, M. E., Biddison, W. E., Boutin, B., Yarchoan, R., and Nelson, D. L. (1985). Soluble interleukin-2 receptors are released from activated human lymphoid cell *in vitro*. *J. Immunol.* **135**, 3172–3177.

Samanta, A. K., Oppenheim, J. J., and Matsushima, K. (1989a). Identification and characterization of a specific receptor for monocyte-derived neutrophil chemotactic factor (MDNCF) on human neutrophils. *J. Exp. Med.* **169**, 1185–1189.

Samanta, A. K., Oppenheim, J. J., and Matsushima, K. (1989b). Interleukin 8 (MDNCF) dynamically regulates its own receptor expression on human neutrophils. *J. Biol. Chem.* **265**, 183–189.

Sayers, T. J., Wiltrout, T. A., Bull, C. A., Denn, A. C., Pilaro, A. M., and Lokesh, B. (1988). Effect of cytokines on polymorphonuclear neutrophil infiltration in the mouse. *J. Immunol.* **141**, 1670–1677.

Schall, T. J., Lewis, M., Koller, K. J., Lee, A., Rice, G. C., Wong, G. H. W., Gatanaga, T., Granger, G. A., Lentz, R., Raab, H., Kohr, W. J., and Goeddel, D. V. (1990). Molecular cloning and expression of a receptor for human tumor necrosis factor. *Cell* **61**, 361–370.

Schultz, R. M., and Kleinschmidt, W. J. (1983). Functional identity between murine γ interferon and macrophage activating factor. *Nature (London)* **305**, 239–240.

Segarini, P. R., Rosen, D. M., and Seyedin, S. M. (1989). Binding of transforming growth factor-β to cell surface proteins varies with cell type. *Mol. Endocrinol.* **3**, 261–272.

Sehgal, P. B. (1990a). Interleukin-6: A regulator of plasma gene expression in hepatic and non-hepatic tissues. *Mol. Biol. Med.* **7**, 117–130.

Sehgal, P. B. (1990b). Interleukin-6: Molecular pathophysiology. *J. Invest. Dermatol.* **94**, 2S–6S.

Senior, R. M., Griffin, G. L., Huang, J. S., Walz, D. A., and Deuel, T. F. (1983). Chemotactic activity of a platelet alpha granule protein for fibroblasts. *J. Cell Biol.* **96**, 382–385.

Shalaby, M. R., Palladino, M. A., Hirabayashi, S. E., Eessalu, T. E., Lewis, G. D., Shepard, H. M., and Aggarwal, B. B. (1987). Receptor binding and activation of polymorphonuclear neutrophils by tumor necrosis factor-alpha. *J. Leuk. Biol.* **41**, 196–204.

Sharpe, R. J., Murphy, G. F., Whitaker, D., and Maione, T. E. (1990). Recombinant platelet factor 4 (PF-4) recuits neutrophils and mononuculear cells *in vivo*. *J. Invest. Dermatol.* **94**, 577. (Abstract)

Sherr, C. J., Rettenmier, C. W., Sacca, R., Roussel, M. F., Look, A. T., and Stanley, E. R. (1985). The c-*fms* proto-oncogene product is related to the receptor for the mononuclear phagocyte growth factor, CSF-1. *Cell* **41**, 665–676.

Sherry, B., and Cerami, A. (1988). Cachectin/tumor necrosis factor exerts endocrine, paracrine, and autocrine control of inflammatory responses. *J. Cell Biol.* **107**, 1269–1277.

Shieh, J. H., Peterson, R. H. F., Warren, D. J., and Moore, M. A. S. (1989). Modulation of colony-stimulating factor-1 receptors on macrophages by tumor necrosis factor. *J. Immunol.* **143**, 2534–2539.

Sims, J. E., March, C. J., Cosman, D., Widmer, M. B., MacDonald, H. R., McMahan, C. J., Grubin, C. E., Wignall, J. M., Call, S. M., Friend, D., Alpert, A. R., Gillis, S. R., Urdal, D. L., and Dower, S. K. (1988). cDNA expression cloning of the IL-1 receptor, a member of the immunoglobulin superfamily. *Science* **241**, 585–589.

Sims, J. E., Acres, R. B., Grubin, C. E., McMahan, C. J., Wignall, J. M., March, C. J., and Dower, S. K. (1989). Cloning of the interleukin-1 receptor from human T-cells. *Proc. Natl. Acad. Sci. USA* **86**, 8946–8950.

Smith, C. A., Davis, T., Anderson, D., Solam, L., Beckmann, M. P., Jerzy, R., Dower, S. K., Cosman, D., and Goodwin, R. G. (1990). A receptor for tumor necrosis factor defines an unusual family of cellular and viral proteins. *Science* **248**, 1019–1023.

Smith, K. A. (1988). Interleukin-2: Inception, impact, and implications. *Science* **240**, 1169–1176.

Smith, P. D., Lamerson, C. L., Wong, H. L., Wahl, L. M., and Wahl, S. M. (1990). Granulocyte-macrophage colony-stimulating factor stimulates human monocyte accessory cell function. *J. Immunol.* **144**, 3829–3834.

Smith, R. A., and Baglioni, C. (1987). The active form of tumor necrosis factor is a trimer. *J. Biol. Chem.* **262**, 6951–6954.

Sottrup-Jensen, L. (1989). α-Macroglobulins: Structure, shape, and mechanism of proteinase complex formation. *J. Biol. Chem.* **264**, 11539–11542.

Springer, T. A. (1990). Adhesion receptors of the immune system. *Nature (London)* **346**, 425–434.

Steinback, M. J., and Roth, J. A. (1989). Neutrophil activation by recombinant cytokines. *Rev. Infect. Dis.* **11**, 549–568.

Stone-Wolff, D. S., Yip, Y. K., Kelker, H. C., Le, J., Henriksen-Destefano, D., Rubin, B. Y., Rinderknecht, E., Aggarwal, B. B., and Vilcek, J. (1984). Interrelationships of human interferon-gamma with lymphotoxin and monocyte cytotoxin. *J. Exp. Med.* **159**, 828–843.

Stoschek, C. M., and King, L. E. (1986). Functional and structural characteristics of EGF and its receptor and their relationship to transforming proteins. *J. Cell. Biochm.* **31**, 135–152.

Strober, W., and James. S. P. (1988). The interleukins. *Pediatr. Res.* **24**, 549–557.

Sung, S. S. J., Bjorndahl, J. M., Wang, C. Y., Kao, H. T., and Fu, S. M. (1988). Production of tumor necrosis factor/cachectin by human T cell lines and peripheral blood T lymphocytes stimulated by phorbol myristate acetate and anti-CD3 antibody. *J. Exp. Med.* **167**, 937–953.

Taga, T., Hibi, M., Hirata, Y., Tamasaki, K., Yasukawa, K., Matsuda, T., Hirano, T., and Kishimoto, T. (1989). Interleukin-6 triggers the association of its receptor with a possible signal transducer, gp130. *Cell* **58**, 573–581.

Thompson, N. L., Flanders, K. C., Smith, J. M., Ellingsworth, L. R., Roberts, A. B., and Sporn, M. B. (1989). Expression of transforming growth factor-β1 in specific cells and tissues of adult and neonatal mice. *J. Cell. Biol.* **108**, 661–669.

Thompson-Snipes, L., Dhar, V., Bond, M. W., Mosmann, T. R., Moore, K. W., and Rennick, D. M. (1991). Interleukin 10: A novel stimulatory factor for mast cells and their progenitors. *J. Exp. Med.* **173**, 507–510.

Tracey, K. J., and Cerami, A. (1990). Metabolic responses to cachectin/TNF. *Ann. N.Y. Acad. Sci.* **587**, 325–331.

Tsunawaki, S., Sporn, M., Ding, A., and Nathan, C. (1988). Deactivation of macrophages by transforming growth factor-β. *Nature (London)* **334**, 260–262.

Turner, M., Chantry, D., and Feldmann, M. (1990). Transforming growth factor β induces the production of interleukin 6 by human peripheral blood mononuclear cells. *Cytokine* **2**, 211–216.

Vlodavsky, I., Ishai-Michaeli, R., Bashkin, P., Friedman, A., and Fuks, Z. (1991). Sequestration and release of basic fibroblast growth factor. *J. Cell. Biochem.* **15F**, 214.

Wahl, L. M., Corcoran, M. E., Mergenhagen, S. E., and Finbloom, D. S. (1990). Inhibition of phospholipase activity in human monocytes by IFN-γ blocks endogenous prostaglandin E_2-dependent collagenase production. *J. Immunol.* **144**, 3518–3522.

Wahl, S. M., Hunt, D. A., Wakefield, L. M., McCartney-Francis, N., Wahl, L. M., Roberts, A. B., and Sporn, M. B. (1987a). Transforming growth-factor beta (TGF-beta) induces monocyte chemotaxis and growth factor production. *Proc. Natl. Acad. Sci. USA* **84,** 5788–5792.

Wahl, S. M., McCartney-Francis, N., Hunt, D. A., Smith, P. D., Wahl, L. M., and Katona, I. M. (1987b). Monocyte interleukin 2 receptor gene expression and interleukin 2 augmentation of microbicidal activity. *J. Immunol.* **139,** 1342–1347.

Wahl, S. M., Hunt, D. A., Wong, H. L., Dougherty, S., McCartney-Francis, N., Wahl, L. M., Ellingsworth, L., Schmidt, J. A., Hall, G., Roberts, A. B., and Sporn, M. B. (1988). Transforming growth factor-β is a potent immunosuppressive agent that inhibits IL-1 dependent lymphocyte proliferation. *J. Immunol.* **140,** 3026–3032.

Wahl, S. M., McCartney-Francis, N., and Mergenhagen, S. E. (1989). Inflammatory and immunomodulatory role of TGF-β. *Immunol. Today* **10,** 258–261.

Wahl, S. M., Allen, J. B., Ohura, K., Chenoweth, D. E., and Hand, A. R. (1991a). IFN-γ inhibits inflammatory cell recruitment and the evolution of bacterial cell wall-induced arthritis. *J. Immunol.* **146,** 95–100.

Wahl, S. M., Allen, J. B., Weeks, B. S. Wong, H. L., and Klotman, P. E. (1993). Transforming growth factor beta enhances integrin expression and type IV collagenase secretion in human monocytes. *Proc. Natl. Acad. Sci. U.S.A.* **90,** 4577–4581.

Wakefield, L. M., Smith, D. M., Masui, T., Harris, C., and Sporn, M. B. (1988). Latent transforming growth factor-β from human platelets. *J. Biol. Chem.* **263,** 7646–7654.

Waldmann, T. A. (1986). The structure, function, and expression of interleukin 2 receptors on normal and malignant lymophocytes. *Science* **232,** 727–732.

Wallick, S. C., Figari, I. S., Morris, R. E., Levinson, A. D., and Palladino, M. A. (1990). Immunoregulatory role of transforming growth factor β (TGF-β) in development of killer cells: Comparison of active and latent TGF-β$_1$. *J. Exp. Med.* **172,** 1777–1784.

Walker, F., Nicola, N. A., Metcalf, D., and Burgess, A. W. (1985). Hierarchical downmodulation of hemopoietic growth factor receptor. *Cell* **43,** 269–276.

Wang, J. M., Griffin, J. D., Rambaldi, A., Chen, Z. G., and Mantovani, A. (1988a). Induction of monocyte migration by recombinant macrophage colony-stimulating factor. *J. Immunol.* **141,** 575–579.

Wang, J. M., Chen, Z. G., Colella, S., Bonilla, M. A., Welte, K., Bordignon, C., and Mantovani, A. (1988b). Chemotactic activity of recombinant human granulocyte colony-stimulating factor. *Blood* **72,** 1456–1460.

Ware, C. F., and Green, L. M. (1987). The cytotoxic lymphokines elaborated by effector T cells. *Lymphokines* **14,** 307–334.

Warren, J. S. (1990). Interleukins and tumor necrosis factor in inflammation. *Crit. Rev. Clin. Lab. Sci.* **28,** 37–59.

Weisbart, R. H., Golde, D. W., and Gasson, J. C. (1986). Biosynthetic human GM-CSF modulates the number and affinity of neutrophil fMet–Leu–Phe receptors. *J. Immunol.* **137,** 3584–3587.

Weisbart, R. H., Kwan, L., Golde, D. W., and Gasson, J. C. (1987). Human GM-CSF primes neutrophils for enhanced oxidative metabolism in response to the major physiologic chemoattractants. *Blood* **69,** 18–21.

Welch, G. R., Wong, H. L., and Wahl, S. M. (1990). Selective induction of FcγRIII on human monocytes by transforming growth factor-β. *J. Immunol.* **144,** 344–3448.

Williams, A. F., and Barclay, A. N. (1988). The immunoglobulin superfamily—Domains for cell surface recognition. *Annu. Rev. Immunol.* **6,** 381–405.

Williams, L. T., Antoniades, H. N., and Goetzl, E. J. (1983). Platelet-derived growth factor stimulates mouse 3T3 cell mitogenesis and leukocyte chemotaxis through different structural determinants. *J. Clin. Invest.* **72,** 1759–1763.

Wolpe, S. D., and Cerami, A. (1989). Macrophage inflammatory proteins 1 and 2: Members of a novel superfamily of cytokines. *FASEB J.* **3,** 2565–2573.

Wolpe, S. D., Davatelis, G., Luedke, C., and Cerami, A. (1987). Differential regulation of cachectin/TNF and IL-1 by IL-4 (BSF-1). *J. Leukocyte Biol.* **42,** 359. (Abstract)

Wong, H. L., and Wahl, S. M. (1990). Inflammation and repair. *In* "Handbook of Experimental Pharmacology" (M. B. Sporn and A. B. Roberts, ed.) Vol. 95/II, pp. 509–548. Springer-Verlag, New York.

Wong, H. L., Welch, G. R., Brandes, M. E., and Wahl, S. M. (1991). Interleukin-4 (IL-4) antagonized induction of FcγRIII (CD16) expression by TGFβ on human monocytes. *J. Immunol.* **147,** 1843–1848.

Wong, S. T., Winchell, L. F., McCune, B. K., Earp, H. S., Teixido, J., Massague, J., Herman, B., and Lee, D. C. (1989). The TGF-α precursor expressed on the cell surface binds to the EGF receptor in adjacent cells, leading to signal transduction. *Cell* **56,** 495–506.

Yamasaki, K., Taga, T., Hirata, Y., Yawata, H., Kawanishi, Y., Seed, B., Taniguchi, T., Hirano, T., and Kishimoto, T. (1988). Cloning and expression of the human interleukin-6 (BSF-2/IFNβ2) receptor. *Science* **241,** 825–828.

Yarden, Y., and Ullrich, A. (1988). Growth factor receptor tyrosine kinases. *Annu. Rev. Biochem.* **57,** 443–478.

Yoshimura, T., and Leonard, E. J. (1990). Identification of high affinity receptors for human monocyte chemoattractant protein-1 (MCP-1) on human monocytes. *J. Immunol.* **145,** 292–297.

Zachariae, C. O. C., Anderson, A. O., Thompson, H. L., Appella, E., Manntovani, A., Oppenheim, J. J., and Matsushima, K. (1990). Properties of monocyte chemotactic and activating factor (MCAF) purified from a human fibrosarcoma cell line. *J. Exp. Med.* **171,** 2177–2182.

Zlotnik, A., Fisher, M., Roehm, N., and Zipori, D. (1987). Evidence for effects of interleukin 4 (B cell stimulatory factor 1) on macrophages: Enhancement of antigen presenting ability of bone marrow-derived macrophages. *J. Immunol.* **138,** 4275–4279.

Zucker, M. B., Katz, I. R., Thorbecke, G. J., Milot, D. C., and Holt, J. (1989). Immunoregulatory activity of peptides related to platelet factor 4. *Proc. Natl. Acad. Sci. USA* **86,** 7571–7574.

4

Induction of Inflammation: Cytokines and Acute-Phase Proteins

C. D. Richards and J. Gauldie

I. Introduction

Tissue damage elicited by trauma, infection, burns, tumors, and other destructive agents results, in mammalian species, in initiation of a reaction called the inflammatory response. This term generally describes a complex phenomenon that involves a number of integrated immediate components at both the local and the systemic level, usually described as the acute-phase response. Local components include changes in vascular permeability, blood flow, and release of potent low molecular weight mediators such as prostaglandins, leukotrienes, and vasoactive amines (Gauldie, 1991). Systemic events include fever, leukocytosis, and alteration of plasma levels of corticosteroid and heavy metal ions such as Fe^{2+} and Zn^{2+}. Further, a striking alteration in plasma concentrations of a series of liver-derived proteins, commonly termed acute-phase proteins, is a marked characteristic of the acute inflammatory response (Koj, 1974; Kushner, 1982; Koj and Gordon, 1985). Both local and systemic phases occur independent of the type of inflammatory stimulus and act to buffer further injury and to initiate repair mechanisms. The process of acute inflammation may be thought of as homeostatic in nature, shutting off the destructive processes and facilitating return to normal function. The production of acute-phase proteins by liver is firmly conserved through evolution of vertebrates and, thus, must play an important role in host survival. As seen with other aspects of the acute-phase response, the hepatic synthesis of acute-phase proteins is rapid and relatively nonspecific. Since the induction of the hepatic response may occur in response to inflammation at distal sites, the production of systemic or blood-borne liver-specific signals caused by cell activation and tissue destruction is a logical prediction. Homburger (1945) showed that a soluble product extracted from suppurative exudate was, on injection, able to induce plasma fibrinogen levels in dogs; other investigators in the 1970s characterized a natural substance (termed leukocyte endogenous mediator, LEM) that elevated temperature and the plasma levels of fibrinogen in rats (Kampschmidt and Upchurch, 1974; Kampschmidt et al., 1982). Koj (1974) first suggested that mediators responsible for this action were released by leukocytes at sites of inflammation; these mediators circulated through bloodstream or lymph and acted specifically on hepatic tissues to induce acute-phase protein synthesis (Koj, 1974). Through the 1980s investigators recognized a small group of polypeptide hormone-like mediators or cytokines to be responsible for initiating the hepatocyte response. These cytokines are able to act on liver cells *in vitro* and *in vivo* to produce a rapid induction of the spectrum of acute-phase proteins.

In the search for hepatocyte-stimulating cytokines, researchers have defined them as molecules that interact with specific receptors on hepatocytes and induce protein expression similar to that evident in inflammatory states *in vivo*. Various advances in techniques and approaches have led to a better understanding of this phenomenon. These methods include identification, cloning, and expression of numerous cytokines and development of *in vitro* hepatocyte and hepatoma cell culture systems in which to assay for hepatocyte stimulating activities. In addition, molecular analysis of acute-phase protein genes and their regulation has provided information on gene expression by hepatocytes, while the recognition of multiple pleiotropic activities of several cytokines has brought various disciplines together to examine common lines of investigation.

II. Acute-Phase Proteins

A. Characteristics

Acute-phase proteins are predominantly liver derived and represent a diversity of functional and structural properties (Table I). These proteins collectively share the acute-phase nature of responses in inflammation, rising to maximal levels by 24 hr and returning to normal by 48–72 hr, but show individual characteristics of kinetics and magnitude of change (Schreiber, 1987; Schreiber et al., 1989). In general, the extent of tissue destruction determines the magnitude of response. Although differences among species are noted, the spectrum of acute-phase proteins as a whole appears to serve common functions (Pepys and Baltz, 1983).

Peak plasma protein levels occur 1–2 days after the onset of inflammation, declining thereafter at various rates depending on the protein examined. This increase is preceded by the accumulation in the liver of mRNA specific for acute-phase protein genes, and appears to be caused primarily by transcriptional modulation (Koj and Gordon, 1985; Birch and Schreiber, 1986;

Table I   Acute Phase Proteins

Protein	Range of change	Species	Function
Major changes			
C-reactive protein	100–1000x	Human, rabbit	Opsonin
Serum amyloid A protein	100–1000x	Human, rat, mouse	(?)
Cysteine proteinase inhibitor (thiostatin)	10–20x	Rat	Antiproteinase
α_2-Macroglobulin	10–20x	Rat	Antiproteinase, cytokine transport
α_1-Acid glycoprotein	5–20x	Most species	Transport
Medium or minor changes			
α_1-Proteinase inhibitor (α_1-antitrypsin)	3–10x	Human, rat	Antiproteinase
α_1-Antichymotrypsin (contrapsin)	5–10x	Most species	Antiproteinase
Fibrinogen	2–6x	Most species	Coagulation
Haptoglobin	2–6x	Most species	Bind and remove hemoglobin
Hemopexin	2–5x	Most species	Bind heme
Ceruloplasmin	2–3x	Most species	O_2 scavenging, transport
Complement C3	2–4x	Mouse	Opsonin
Serum amyloid P	2–5x	Human, mouse	(?)
α_2-Plasmin inhibitor	2–3x	Human	Fibrinolysis
Negative changes	30–60% decrease		
Albumin		Most species	
Transferrin		Most species	Transport
α_1-Inhibitor III		Rat	Antiproteinase

Morrone *et al.*, 1988; Schreiber *et al.*, 1989), although posttranscriptional control processes have not been studied in detail. Differences in kinetics of mRNA levels may reflect different turnover rates of separate genes. Posttranslational events such as altered glycosylation may also influence accumulation in plasma of some acute-phase proteins (Mackiewicz *et al.*, 1987; Mackiewicz and Kushner, 1989), as would utilization and turnover of the mature protein. *In vitro*, hepatocyte-stimulating cytokines induce an immediate rise in mRNA of acute-phase genes in isolated hepatocytes, where steady-state levels peak within 12–24 hr.

Evidence suggests extrahepatic synthesis of some proteins such as α_1-antichymotrypsin (α_1-ACH), α_1-protease inhibitor (α_1-PI), and complement components in monocytes/macrophages. However, the amount synthesized is low compared with that produced by hepatocytes and thus will not contribute significantly to plasma levels. Whether this production is important in the microenvironment, particularly in areas of profound monocyte/macrophage infiltration, is yet to be resolved.

Documentation of acute-phase protein responses is evident for humans undergoing surgery or suffering from clinically evident bacterial infections; for animals undergoing surgery, experimental bacterial infections, or parasite infections; or for sterile irritant treatment in rodents. Some proteins such as C-reactive protein (CRP; in human), α_2-macroglobulin (α_2-MAC; in rats), and serum amyloid A protein (SAA; in human and mouse) increase dramatically (100 to 1000-fold) in serum concentration. Others, such as α_1-ACh, fibrinogen, haptoglobin, α_1-acid glycoprotein (α_1-AGP; in most species); and α_1-cysteine protease inhibitor (α_1-CPI; in rat), increase markedly (5- to 10-fold). Ceruloplasmin and C_3 show smaller increases whereas albumin, transferrin (most species), and α_2-HS glycoprotein (in humans) show a decrease in serum concentrations (Koj, 1974; Koj and Gordon, 1985; Kushner and Mackiewicz, 1987). These decreases are evident at the mRNA level and may reflect a mechanism by which hepatocytes divert cell metabolism to the production of acute-phase proteins. Levels of serum CRP and measurement of erythrocyte sedimentation rate (ESR; a function of serum concentration of acute-phase proteins, particularly fibrinogen) are often used clinically to detect inflammation and infer the presence of infection.

B. Role in Homeostasis

Binding or opsonizing foreign particles or toxic substances facilitates activation of the complement pathway and/or removal by the reticuloendothelial system. CRP is a pentamer of 105 kDa that binds to bacterial membrane components. CRP is found deposited at local sites of inflammation and has also been shown to bind specifically to phagocytes. C_3 is an acute-phase protein, the role of which is well established to be that of an opsonin in the presence of specific antibody.

Transection of blood vessels results in rapid utilization of fibrinogen in the formation of blood clots; thus, increased output by liver in the acute-phase response replaces circulating fibrinogen levels. α_2-Plasmin inhibitor, a positive acute-phase protein in humans, also aids in coagulation. Increased levels of fibrinogen and α_2-plasmin inhibitor assist in repair from trauma and help demarcate affected tissue, thus restoring homeostasis.

Destruction of tissue and cell death results in release of neutral proteinases such as collagenase, elastase, and cathepsin G, as well as superoxide anion, from phagocytic cells that function in digestion and removal of necrotic tissue. Excessive action of these molecules could lead to damage of healthy tissue. These actions can be modulated by serum protease inhibitors, many of which are acute-phase proteins. α_2-MAC, a major acute-phase protein in rat that is constitutively expressed at high levels in human; α_1-ACH, and α_1-PI, acute-phase proteins in both human and rat; and α_1-CPI, another major acute-phase protein in rat, all have multiple antiproteinase action. Specificities range from broad (α_2-MAC inhibits all serine proteinases, some cysteine- and metallo-proteinases) to narrow (α_1-PI affects leuko-cyte elastase whereas α_1-ACH inhibits cathepsin G and chymotrypsin *in vitro*, Travis and Salvesen, 1983). The size of α_2-MAC (M_r 725 kDa) limits its penetration into tissues relative to α_1-PI (54 kDa) and α_1-ACH (68 kDa). Ceruloplasmin has been shown to inhibit superoxide anion-dependent reactions *in vitro* and, thus, may play a role in neutralizing oxygen-derived reactive metabolites. This group of acute-phase proteins constitutes a broad spectrum of antiproteinase action that presumably eliminates excess proteolytic and oxidative activities associated with inflammation.

Further, several acute-phase proteins exhibit immunomodulating effects. Endotoxin shock (Hoffman *et al.*, 1983; Van Vugt *et al.*, 1986), natural killer (NK) cell activity, and cytotoxic cell function (Hooper *et al.*, 1981; Hudig *et al.*, 1981; Ades *et al.*, 1982) have been reported to be affected by purified antiproteinases. Although these *in vitro* effects may not reflect exact events *in vivo*, they do suggest a damping of local inflammatory events as well as a contribution to control of specific immunity. In concert, enhanced levels of acute-phase proteins lead to decreased destruction at tissue sites, clearance of pathogenic substances, facilitation of wound healing, and modulation of immune responses.

III. Regulation of Hepatic Responses

A. Cytokines

As a result of initial observations that the liver responds to inflammation at distant sites, and that soluble substances from inflamed animals could elicit responses on injection into naive animals, several investigations have revealed the role of a number of cloned specific cytokines as dominant regulators of the hepatic response. These cytokines include interleukin 6 (IL-6) and corticosteroid, as well as interleukin 1 (IL-1) and tumor necrosis factor (TNF). More recently, researchers recognized the potent IL-6-like activities of leukemia inhibitory factor (LIF, Baumann and Wong, 1989) and interleukin 11 (IL-11) (Baumann and Schendel, 1991). A fourth molecule, oncostatin M (O-M), also has been identified to have similar function in inducing liver acute-phase protein synthesis (Richards *et al.*, 1992). Additional factors may remain undefined.

1. *IL-1/TNF*

The molecule LEM described by Kampschmidt and colleagues (Kampschmidt and Upchurch, 1974; Kampschmidt *et al.*, 1982) and later identified as IL-1 (Bornstein, 1982; Dinarello, 1988) is a 17-kDa nonglycosylated product of monocytes/macrophages with both α and β forms. Since IL-1 induced SAA and fibrinogen in mouse or rat *in vivo* (Kampschmidt and Mesecher,

1985), it was thought to be a major regulating cytokine of the hepatic acute-phase response. TNFα, also a 17-kDa product of macrophages (Beutler and Cerami, 1986), showed a similar action when administered to rodents. IL-1 and TNF have many common activities (Le and Vilcek, 1987); thus, researchers assumed that these two factors, released by monocytes/macrophages at sites of inflammation, mediate the overall acute-phase response.

However, detailed analysis of isolated hepatocyte cultures and hepatoma cell lines revealed that IL-1 or TNF induces only a limited set of acute-phase proteins *in vitro*. These proteins include complement components C_3 and factor B, and serum amyloid P protein (SAP) in human and mouse cells (Le and Mortensen, 1984; Ramadori *et al.*, 1985; Perlmutter *et al.*, 1986), as well as $α_1$-AGP in most systems (Baumann *et al.*, 1987a,b; Gauldie *et al.*, 1987b; Koj *et al.*, 1987; Geiger *et al.*, 1988a). Apparently, membrane-bound IL-1α was also capable of inducing C_3 in hepatoma cells (Beuscher *et al.*, 1987). Both IL-1 and TNF administered *in vivo* induced a full acute-phase protein serum response.

2. Interleukin 6

These observations regarding discrepancies between *in vitro* and *in vivo* activites led to the characterization and identification of a hepatocyte stimulating factor (HSF) from monocytes/macrophages that is distinct from IL-1/TNF. This cytokine, initially identified by Ritchie and Fuller (1983), induced the full spectrum of acute-phase proteins in isolated rat hepatocytes and hepatoma cell lines (Bauer *et al.*, 1984; Koj *et al.*, 1984; Woloski and Fuller, 1985; Darlington *et al.*, 1986; Baumann *et al.*, 1987a,b; Goldman and Liu, 1987), and is now referred to as IL-6 (Gauldie *et al.*, 1987a; Poupart *et al.*, 1987; Sehgal *et al.*, 1989). IL-6 is a 23- to 30-kDa protein of pI 5.1 with variability in glycosylation, and acts directly on hepatocytes through specific membrane receptors (Yamasaki *et al.*, 1988; Hirano *et al.*, 1989). Recombinant-derived IL-6 induces all positive acute-phase proteins and reduces albumin and transferrin in all species tested, particularly in the presence of corticosteroid (Andus *et al.*, 1987, 1988; Morrone *et al.*, 1988; Castell *et al.*, 1989). IL-6 molecules from human, pig, rat, and mouse have been cloned (Hirano *et al.*, 1986, 1989; Van Snick *et al.*, 1988; Fuller and Grenett, 1989; Northemann *et al.*, 1990a; Richards and Saklatvala, 1991); all act on the hepatocyte, with some minor effects of species differences. Murine or rat IL-6 does not stimulate human cells very well, whereas the reverse is not true. Assays of IL-6 activity in serum of animals undergoing inflammation or of burn patients show a peak of IL-6 levels 6–12 hr prior to the peak of acute-phase protein serum levels (Nijsten *et al.*, 1987). Further, IL-6 treatment *in vivo* results in liver acute-phase responses similar to those induced by inflammation (Geiger *et al.*, 1988b).

3. *Leukemia Inhibitory Factor and Interleukin 11*

Although IL-6 is the most potent inducer of the full spectrum of acute-phase proteins, other cytokines also induce a qualitatively similar response. These cytokines include a factor produced by human keratinocytes (Baumann *et al.*, 1987b; Baumann and Gauldie, 1990) that has been identified as LIF (Baumann and Wong, 1989; Baumann *et al.*, 1989b). LIF is released by T cells, Buffalo rat liver cells, and various cell lines (Fey *et al.*, 1989; Northemann *et al.*, 1990b). Recombinant LIF causes induction of a protein profile similar to that induced by IL-6 *in vitro*, although some differences may occur in the extent of stimulation. LIF acts through its own separate receptor(s) (Gearing and Bruce, 1991).

IL-11 is a novel cytokine that has been cloned from bone marrow stromal cells (Paul *et al.*, 1990) and represents a 17-kDa molecule that potently induces the same spectrum of hepatic acute-phase protein synthesis as IL-6 (Baumann and Schendel, 1991). IL-11 appears to share other activities with IL-6, such as growth of hemopoietic stem cells and megakaryocyte maturation (Kishimoto, 1989; Paul *et al.*, 1990), but works through a separate receptor. Although serum IL-6 is evident and detectable in inflammatory states, the extent to which LIF or IL-11 is found in serum, and therefore might contribute to site-derived inflammatory signals that act on liver, is not known. All three factors induce similar responses in the hepatocyte, but do so through separate receptors.

4. *Oncostatin M*

O-M is a cytokine expressed in activated human T lymphocytes (Brown *et al.*, 1987) and monocytes (Malik *et al.*, 1989). This protein was originally characterized as a growth regulator for certain tumor- and non-tumor-derived cell lines. O-M is produced as a 28-kDa single chain polypeptide with a unique primary structure (Zarling *et al.*, 1986). Specific cell surface receptors have been partially characterized (Linsley *et al.*, 1989). Brown *et al.* (1991) have shown that, similar to IL-1 and TNF, O-M induces IL-6 expression in cultured human endothelial cells. Clones for cDNA and the gene for O-M have been isolated and sequenced (Malik *et al.*, 1989). Structure-based comparisons predict similar functional properties for O-M and LIF (Bazan, 1991; Rose and Bruce, 1991). *In vitro* this molecule has been shown to stimulate human and rat hepatocytes in a fashion similar to IL-6, IL-11, and LIF (Richards *et al.*, 1992). The action of O-M is at least as potent as IL-6 in HepG2 cells but less so in rat hepatocyte cell lines and primary hepatocytes. Figure 1 shows a comparison of O-M, IL-6, and LIF, all at maximal concentrations, in their capacity to induce several acute-phase proteins *in vitro* in HepG2 cells. Similar to IL-6 and LIF, O-M acts synergistically with corticosteroid or IL-1 in the synthesis of α_1-AGP and, in addition, is able to potently enhance expression of chloramphenicol

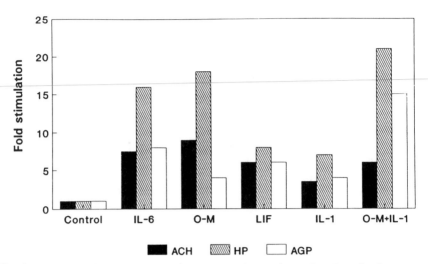

Fig. 1 Induction of acute phase protein synthesis by cytokines. HepG2 cell cultures were stimulated with optimal concentrations of interleukin 6 (IL-6; 50 ng/ml), oncostatin M (O–M; 50 ng/ml), leukemia inhibitory factor (LIF; 10,000 U/ml), and IL-1 (5 ng/ml) as previously described (Richards *et al.*, 1992). Supernatant contents of α_1-antichymotrypsin (ACH; solid), haptoglobin (HP; hatched), and α_1-acid glycoprotein (AGP; open) were measured by rocket electrophoresis (Gauldie *et al.*, 1987a,b). Results represent the average of two separate cultures and measurements of acute phase proteins.

acetyltransferase (CAT) constructs containing IL-6-specific promoter region sequences of acute-phase proteins in transfected HepG2 cells (Richards *et al.*, 1992). Since these cytokines induce CAT expression from CAT constructs containing the putative IL-6RE, IL-6, IL-11, LIF, and O-M may use (at least in part) similar mechanisms in enhancing transcription of acute-phase genes (see Section III,E).

5. *Corticosteroid*

Glucocorticoids participate in the regulation of acute-phase proteins in a permissive and synergistic fashion. The ability of cytokines such as IL-6 to induce a full acute-phase response *in vivo* and *in vitro* (particularly in rat primary hepatocyte culture) is dependent on adequate glucocorticoid levels (Koj *et al.*, 1984; Baumann, 1989). Thus, IL-6 or LIF induction of fibrinogen α_1-ACH, α_1-AGP, α_2-MAC, and other proteins is enhanced synergistically with dexamethasone in tissue culture. Some hepatoma cell lines respond to glucocorticoid addition alone (Baumann *et al.*, 1983; Gross *et al.*, 1984), possibly because of the autocrine presence of cytokines. Plasma α_1-AGP levels may be enhanced *in vivo* by dexamethasone injection alone (Baumann *et al.*, 1983). However, these responses are low in comparison with those to simultaneous cytokine/glucocorticoid induction.

Acute inflammation is also characterized by a peak of blood glucocorticoid levels (3–10 hr in rat models), which act to enhance the liver response. Both IL-1 and IL-6 have been shown to enhance adrenal corticotropic hormone (ACTH) production by At-20 pituitary cells *in vitro* (Woloski *et al.*, 1985). IL-6 has been shown to induce ACTH production *in vivo* in the rat (Naitoh *et al.*, 1988). These cytokines (and possibly others) would lead to increased adrenal output of glucocorticoids, which then act at the liver to enhance acute-phase gene regulation in an orchestrated and temporal manner (see Figure 4).

6. *Other Modulating Factors*
Analysis of the activity of many cytokines has shown that minor roles may be played by transforming growth factor β (TGFβ), epidermal growth factor (EGF), and interferon γ (IFNγ) in modifying hepatocyte responses to IL-6. TGFβ will induce α_1-ACH, α_1-PI, and fibrinogen in hepatoma cells, but to a much lower extent than IL-6 (Rokita *et al.*, 1990). IFNγ somewhat inhibits the IL-6-induced increases in α_1-ACH, haptoglobin, and fibrinogen (Magielska-Zero *et al.*, 1988). EGF also has inhibitory action on IL-6-induced alteration in albumin synthesis (Rokita *et al.*, 1990). These *in vitro* modulatory activities of IFNγ, TGFβ, and EGF may have relevance *in vivo*, contributing to the overall output of acute-phase proteins by hepatocytes. Although IL-6 and IL-1/TNF appear to be the most prominent acute-phase regulators at present, varying combinations of these and other mediators (such as oncostatin M, LIF, and others not yet identified) could account for the quantitative and temporal variation seen in acute-phase protein levels that are characteristic of different disease states (Gauldie *et al.*, 1985; Kushner and Mackiewicz, 1987).

B. Interaction of Cytokines

Examination of the effects of IL-1, TNF, IL-6, and glucocorticoids on hepatocytes *in vitro* reveals that combinations of cytokines resulted in different regulation patterns than individual cytokines alone. Additive, synergistic, and inhibitory actions of cytokine combinations on inducing specific acute-phase genes are evident. Glucocorticoids act synergistically to enhance expression of most proteins by hepatocytes; however, cytokine interaction is more complex. Acute-phase proteins can be divided into two groups: one that is stimulated by a combination of IL-1 and IL-6 with corticosteroid, the other by IL-6 and corticosteroid only (Table II). LIF, IL-11, or O-M can replace IL-6 in these induction activities, but may not stimulate production to the same extent, particularly when treated in the presence of glucocorticoid. O-M acts as an IL-6-like activity that is additive with IL-6 or LIF and synergistic with glucocorticoid or IL-1 in regulation of haptoglobin or α_1-AGP (Richards *et al.*, 1992). Additive or synergistic actions of IL-1 and IL-6 (or LIF or IL-11 or O-M) are seen in group I genes, and

Table II   Induction of Acute Phase Proteins[a]

Protein[b]	IL-1/TNF[c]	IL-6/IL-11/LIF/O-M[d]	Comment
Group One			
Haptoglobin	+ + (rat)	+ + + (human)	
Synergy (in rat)			
α_1-Acid glycoprotein	+ +	+ +	Synergy
C_3	+ +	+ +	Synergy
Factor B	+ +	+ +	
SAA	+ + +	+ + +	
SAP	+ +	+ +	
CRP	+ + +	+ + +	
Group Two			
α_1-Antichymotrypsin		+ + + +	
α_1-Protease inhibitor		+ +	
α_2-Macroglobulin (rat)		+ + + + ⎫	
Fibrinogen		+ + + + ⎬	Inhibition by
Thiostatin (rat)		+ + + + ⎭	IL-1
T1-kininogen (rat)		+ + + +	
Ceruloplasmin		+	

[a] Response of acute phase protein synthesis to cytokines *in vitro* is designated (+) weak, (+ +) medium, (+ + +) strong, and (+ + + +) very strong. Data are modified from (Gauldie (1989) and Baumann and Gauldie (1990).
[b] Abbreviations: SAA, serum amyloid A; SAP, serum amyloid P; CRP, C-reactive protein.
[c] IL-1, Interleukin 1; TNF, tumor necrosis factor.
[d] IL-6, IL-11, Interleukin 6, 11; LIF, leukemia inhibitory factor; O-M, oncostatin M.

are most pronounced in expression of α_1-AGP (Figure 1). On the other hand, inhibitory actions of IL-1 or TNF are seen on IL-6 induction of fibrinogen (most species), α_1-CPI, and α_2-MAC (in rat) *in vitro*. Since IL-1 injection *in vivo* causes enhanced plasma fibrinogen levels in rodents, the *in vitro* results suggest that the enhancement is not the result of direct action of IL-1 on hepatocytes. In examining the promoter of α_1-CPI, also known as rat T1 kininogen, Chen and colleagues (1991) found that promoter-containing CAT constructs, when transfected into Hep3B cells, responded to IL-6, showed synergy with IL-6 and glucocorticoid, and showed inhibition with IL-1 and IL-6. These experiments support the concept that different cytokine regulation involves interaction of factors that are dependent on promoting regions in acute phase genes.

IL-6 acts as a major inducer of the antiproteinases and fibrinogen (group II proteins) with modulation by IL-1/TNF. TGFβ, EGF, and IFNγ may modify the inductions by IL-6 or other mediators and thus may contribute to the complex set of cytokine/hormone concentrations available to the hepatocyte. Variations in plasma concentrations of acute-phase proteins undoubtedly reflect hepatocyte responses to these different combinations of cytokines that change over time in acute inflammation or during different disease states.

C. Receptors

Cell surface receptors for IL-6 (IL-6R) on hepatocytes are evident in relatively low numbers (400–600/cell) (Baumann *et al.*, 1988; Yamasaki *et al.*, 1988; Hirano *et al.*, 1989). Such numbers are also suggested for LIFR (Gearing and Bruce, 1991). The IL-6R cloned from B cells possesses an 80-kDa IL-6-binding domain ($K_d = 3.4 \times 10^{-10} M$) that apparently, once it has bound the IL-6 ligand, must interact with a membrane glycoprotein gp130 for signal transduction to occur (Taga *et al.*, 1989; Hibi *et al.*, 1990). Both species are present in HepG2 hepatoma cells.

Further studies have shown that Oncostatin M, LIF, IL-11, and ciliary neurtropic factor (CNTF) interact with receptor complexes that also include gp130, and that gp130 is necessary for signal transduction (Taga and Kishimoto, 1992). Unique subunits have thus been identified for IL-6 and LIF receptors (Gearing and Bruce, 1991) and it is presumed that OM and IL-11 receptors also possess unique subunits that are complexed with gp130 upon ligand interaction. Differences in tissue expression of the various receptor components may govern cell responses to these cytokines. IL-1 receptors found on T cells and fibroblasts also possess an 80-kDa binding domain (Type I; Sims *et al.*, 1988) whereas those on B cells are 65 kDa in size (Type II). The species present on hepatocytes, and whether additional membrane proteins are associated with the IL-1 binding receptor, remains unknown.

The expression of IL-6 receptor mRNA has been shown to be up-modulated *in vitro* in hepatoma cells by IL-1, IL-6, and glucocorticoid (Bauer *et al.*, 1989; Rose-John *et al.*, 1990; Gauldie *et al.*, 1992) whereas monocytes do not show this regulation. Levels of mRNA for gp130 can also be modified *in vitro* and *in vivo* (Schooltink *et al.*, 1992; Saito *et al.*, 1992). Using a homologous rat IL-6R probe (M. Baumann *et al.*, 1990), evidence also has been found of transient modulations of IL-6R mRNA expression in acute-phase inflammation in rats (Geisterfer *et al.*, 1993). Injections of corticosteroid and of IL-6 alone also up-regulate the expression of IL-6R (Gauldie *et al.*, 1992). The concomitant effects of increased cytokines and altered receptor expression may play an important part in the regulation of inflammatory models *in vivo*.

D. Signal Transduction

Events that follow receptor–ligand interaction in hepatocytes that mediate acute-phase gene expression are not clear. gp130, a membrane protein shown to mediate IL-6 biological responses in B cell lines (Hirano *et al.*, 1989; Taga *et al.*, 1989), has been cloned and possesses GTP-binding motifs in an intracytoplasmic region of the cDNA sequence (Hibi *et al.*, 1990). This structure suggests that binding of GTP is induced in some fashion in signal transduction. The gp130 protein is found on HepG2 cell surface membranes and complexes with receptor on IL-6 binding. IL-6 has been found to enhance radiolabeled GTP binding to HepG2 cell membranes *in vitro* (C. Richards, O'Neill, and J. Saklatvala, unpublished results), an observation that is consistent with this proposal.

Furthermore, it has been shown that gp130 is rapidly phosphorylated at various residues in its cytoplasmic domain upon ligand binding (Taga and Kishimoto, 1992). The receptor complexes do not have intrinsic kinase activity; however, the nature of the kinases involved or subsequent signaling events are not known at present. IL-1 has been shown to induce phosphorylation of the 27-kDa heat shock protein in fibroblasts (Kaur and Saklatvala, 1988) and HepG2 cells (Kaur *et al.*, 1989); however, IL-6 does not (C. Richards, unpublished data).

More data are available from studies of IL-6 signal transduction in B cell lines. Goldstein *et al.* (1990) provide evidence that IL-6 stimulation of IgM secretion by SKW6.4 cells is inhibited by H7 (an inhibitor of protein kinase C activity) as well as by elevated levels of cAMP. The effect of cAMP is blocked by H8 (an inhibitor of protein kinase A). However, IL-6 does not stimulate production of diacylglycerol (DAG) or induce translocation of protein kinase C. Further, IL-6 acts additively with phorbol ester (PMA) to induce IgM secretion (Goldstein *et al.*, 1990). These results suggest that, in SKW6.4 cells, IL-6 acts through an H7-inhibitable protein kinase that is distinct from protein kinase C and is inhibited by a protein kinase A-dependent pathway. PMA pretreatment does not alter IL-6 induction of acute-phase proteins in hepatoma cells (Baumann *et al.*, 1988), further suggesting a protein kinase C-independent mechanism for IL-6. PMA alone does have some effects on acute-phase protein induction (Evans *et al.*, 1987; Baumann *et al.*, 1988); thus, protein kinase C may have a minor influence on expression of some acute-phase genes.

In an IL-6-dependent B cell hybridoma system, Nakajima and Wall (1991) showed that, after IL-6 deprivation, IL-6 causes a rapid and transient increase in tyrosine phosphorylation (also H7 inhibitable) of a 160-kDa protein. This phenomenon is followed by impressive induction of mRNA for *jun*B/AP-1 and TIS11 nuclear transcription factors. *jun*B and TIS11 activation are not affected by cycloheximide, suggesting that posttranslational modifications result in their induction. Whether this H7-inhibitable kinase is identical to that in SKW6.4 cells or whether such a kinase will be found in hepatocytes is unknown.

E. Gene Regulation

Molecular cloning and sequencing of 5' promoter regions of various acute-phase protein genes has been completed and has allowed the examination of control elements responsible for tissue specificity and inducibility. Glucocorticoid response elements (GRE) are present in α_1-AGP, haptoglobin, and fibrinogen genes (Baumann and Maguat, 1986; Baumann et al., 1989a; Prowse and Baumann, 1990), and apparently account for synergistic activity of glucocorticoids in enhanced expression. Putative cytokine-specific response elements (RE) have been mapped in promoters of several acute-phase protein genes. Further, a number of DNA-binding proteins bind to cis-acting elements in these promoters, including proteins in the CCAAT element binding protein (C/EBP) nuclear factor family, all of which show high homology in their DNA-binding domains. To date, these proteins include C/EBP itself (a nuclear factor from rat liver), AGP element binding protein in mouse (AGP/EBP; Chang et al., 1990), and IL-6-dependent binding protein in rat (IL-6 DBP; Poli et al., 1990), as well as nuclear factor for IL-6 (NF-IL-6; Akira et al., 1990). NF-IL-6 is the same as C/EBPβ and binds to a putative IL-1 RE [ACATTGCACAATCT] (Akira et al., 1990; Isshiki et al., 1990) that is present in the IL-6 promoter, and also may play a role in modulating certain acute-phase proteins, such as C_3, induced by IL-1 (group 1 acute phase proteins) (Wilson et al., 1990). A consensus sequence termed IL-6 RE [(T/A)T(C/G)TGGGA(A/C)] present in rat α_2-MAC, α_1-AGP, haptoglobin, and α_1-CPI genes (Prowse and Baumann, 1988; Baumann et al., 1989a; H. Baumann et al., 1990; Hattori et al., 1990; Won and Baumann, 1990), as well as in human CRP and haptoglobin genes (Fowlkes et al., 1984; Castell et al., 1989; Fey et al., 1989; Tsuchiya et al., 1987) has been proposed to mediate IL-6-dependent transcription. The nature of factors that bind this IL-6 RE is not clear at present. Another unrelated factor, nuclear factor kappa β (NFKB), may also modulate the expression of acute-phase proteins such as SAA (Edbrooke et al., 1989). Thus, multiple transcription factors may be involved in modulating promoter activities of acute-phase genes. Interactions of different binding proteins and response elements will likely be found to regulate transcription in response to cytokines and glucocorticoid.

IV. Production of Cytokines at Tissue Sites

A. Cell Sources

Alterations in plasma levels of acute-phase proteins in vivo occur after an initial lag period from the time of tissue injury, which presumably reflects the time required to synthesize and release sufficient amounts of hepatocyte-stimulating mediators into the systemic circulation. Thus, liver mRNA for acute-phase proteins increases slightly later after subcutaneous turpentine injection than after recombinant IL-6 injection in rodents (Geiger et al., 1988b; Stadnyk et al., 1990). Enhanced serum IL-6 and TNF levels reach stimulatory concentrations shortly after inflammatory challenge; these peak levels precede those of acute-phase proteins (Nijsten et al., 1987; Jablons et al., 1989; Gauldie et al., 1992). IL-1 and IFNγ levels, in contrast, have been difficult to detect in circulation, although this difficulty may be result of technical problems in assaying these cytokines in serum.

Monocytes/macrophages are major sources of IL-1, TNF, and IL-6 on activation. Additionally, IL-1 and TNF are potent inducers of IL-6 release from stromal cells such as fibroblasts of lung, dermal, or synovial origin (May et al., 1988, 1989; Richards and Saklatvala, 1991), as well as from endothelial cells (Sironi et al., 1989). Thus, activation of monocytes/macrophages by tissue damage or infection results in cytokine release from these cells as well as from activated and recruited adjacent stromal cell populations (see Figure 4), all of which potentially contribute to the rapid rise in circulating IL-6. Some studies have suggested that hepatocytes express IL-6 under certain conditions in vitro (Northemann et al., 1990b); however, in a rat model of inflammation, hepatocytes undergoing acute-phase responses have been shown not to make their own IL-6 (Gauldie et al., 1990), so in vitro situations may not accurately reflect all in vivo conditions. Thus, IL-6 appears to act as an exocrine mediator in this context although, since Kupffer cells and endothelial cells also release IL-6 (Bauer et al., 1984), these cells could act on adjacent hepatocytes in a paracrine fashion.

B. Modulation of IL-6

The IL-6 gene has been cloned from mouse and human, and possesses 5′ flanking promoting regions with multiple potential response elements (Tanabe et al., 1989). Lipopolysaccharide (LPS) is a potent inducer of IL-6 in monocytes/macrophages, but the nature of transcriptional activation by this agent remains elusive. Two nuclear proteins, NFIL-6 (Akira et al., 1990) and NFKβ (Liberman and Baltimore, 1990), have been reported to bind to specific elements in the IL-6 promoter (NFIL-6 to IL-1RE and NFKβ to the Kβ site) and are functional in transfection assays. In addition, increases in cAMP appear to enhance IL-6 expression (Zhang et al., 1988). Prostaglandins of the E series (PGE_1 and PGE_2) have been found to up-regulate IL-6 production in vitro in fibroblasts derived from lung tissue or synovial tissue (Figure 2). This induction is seen at both the mRNA and the secreted protein level. Additional evidence suggests that other cAMP-inducing agents may not function entirely through the cAMP-responsive region in the IL-6 promoter (Ray et al., 1990). PGE was also shown to augment the LPS-induced IL-6 expression in peripheral blood monocytes and to decrease TNF expression (Scales et al., 1989; Bailly et al., 1990). Thus, the IL-6 gene appears to respond to multiple extracellular signals through different (but not mutually

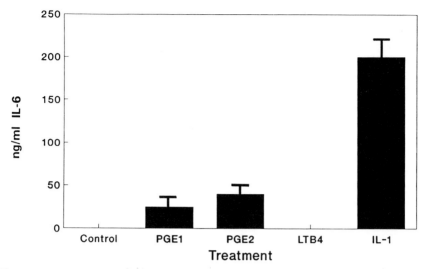

Fig. 2 Induction of interleukin 6 (IL-6) release by prostaglandin E (PGE). PGE$_1$ and PGE$_2$ (10^{-6} M) and IL-1 (0.5 ng/ml) were added to fibroblast cultures derived from human synovial biopsy specimens. Content of IL-6 in the supernatant after 6 hr was measured by the IL-6-specific B9 hybridoma proliferation assay using recombinant human IL-6 as a standard. Error bars are shown as the maximum coefficient of variation found within an assay and between assays.

exclusive) intracellular mechanisms. This multiple response system may function to insure IL-6 expression under a broad range of inflammatory stimuli.

As already stated, actions of glucocorticoid on macrophages/monocytes and stromal cells include down-regulation of expression of IL-6 as well as other cytokines. Since IL-1 and IL-6 have been implicated in stimulation of the hypothalamus/pituitary/adrenal (HPA) axis that enhances circulating levels of glucocorticoids (Woloski *et al.*, 1985; Besedovsky *et al.*, 1986; Naitoh *et al.*, 1988), this glucocorticoid action may provide a mechanism by which cytokine release from inflamed sites and recruited tissue is eventually down-regulated in a coordinated manner. Rats with deficiency in the HPA axis, or rats treated with the glucocorticoid receptor antagonist RU 486, are more susceptible to inflammatory sequelae such as arthritis (Sternberg *et al.*, 1989a,b).

TGFβ is another pleiotropic cytokine with many activities that appear to suppress lymphocyte cell functions and induce extracellular matrix formation in connective tissue through actions on collagen, matrix metalloproteinase, and tissue inhibitor of metalloproteinase (TIMP) expression (Sporn *et al.*, 1986; Edwards *et al.*, 1987; Overall *et al.*, 1989). Musso *et al.* (1990)

have found that TGFβ potently inhibits IL-1-induced expression of IL-6 in human monocytes *in vitro*. Researchers have shown that TGFβ partially down-regulates IL-6 expression in synovial cells induced by IL-1 and TNF *in vitro* (Richards and Saklatvala, 1991). Thus, TGFβ, glucocorticoid, and possibly other cytokines may modify the release of hepatocyte-stimulating cytokines from tissue sites *in vivo*, and therefore modulate the actual IL-6 concentration that affects liver responses.

C. Action of Xenobiotics

Interest has heightened in determining the role of xenobiotics in inflammation with respect to modulation of release of hepatocyte-stimulating cytokines. In earlier studies using a bleomycin-induced model of lung fibrosis in rats, intratracheal administration of bleomycin was found to cause alveolar macrophages to release IL-1 and IL-6 and bleomycin concentrations as low as $10^{-8}M$ were found to induce cytokine release *in vitro* by normal alveolar macrophages (Jordana et al., 1988). Other drugs such as benzodiazepines have been shown to modify IL-1, TNF, and IL-6 production by human monocytes *in vitro* (Taupin et al., 1991). Diazepan-binding inhibitor also modifies IL-6 production *in vitro* by monocytes (Stepien et al., 1993). These cells produce cytokines under various "stress" conditions and, since drugs or environmental pollutants in various forms are stressful to cells, the production of hepatocyte-stimulating cytokines may be significantly modulated. Further, IL-6 has been shown to induce metallothionein expression in liver (Schroeder and Cousins, 1990) and thus may play a role in clearance of heavy metals systemically.

The induction of pulmonary fibrosis by intralobar instillation of cadmium chloride in rats (Frankel et al., 1991) produces a liver acute-phase response that was proposed to be caused by local lung tissue elaboration of cytokines. Exposure of alveolar macrophages to coal dust *in vitro* caused significant release of IL-6 and TNF (Gosset et al., 1991), both of which have roles in the liver response. Examination of cytokine release from blood monocytes exposed to heavy metal salts showed a dose-dependent enhancement of TNF production by Cu^{2+} and Zn^{2+} ions *in vitro* (Scuderi, 1990), but not of IL-6. Nickel and cobalt cations at 10 μM, although without marked effect in the absence of LPS, were found to enhance LPS-induced IL-6 release from human peripheral blood monocytes in culture significantly (Figure 3). These lines of investigation suggest that various xenobiotic agents are potentially involved in modulating the production of hepatocyte-stimulating mediators and may be clinically relevant in situations of exposure to heavy metals in lungs or to prosthesis-wear particles in synovial tissues of joint replacement patients.

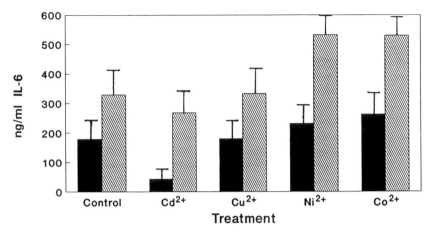

Fig. 3 Modulation of interleukin 6 (IL-6) release from monocytes by heavy metals. Adherent human peripheral blood mononuclear cells incubated in the absence (solid) or presence (hatched) of 1 μg/ml lipopolysaccharide (LPS) and 10 μM CdCl$_2$ (Cd^{2+}), CaCl$_2$ (Cu^{2+}), NiCl$_2$ (Ni^{2+}), or CoCl$_2$ (Co^{2+}). After 18 hr, supernatants were tested for IL-6 content in the B9 IL-6 assay. Error bars are shown as the maximum coefficient of variation found within an assay and between assays.

V. Summary

The induction of acute-phase protein levels in serum is mediated primarily by cytokines that act at specific receptors on hepatocytes. Ligand–receptor interactions result in transcriptional activation of acute-phase protein expression through regulatory factors that interact with 5′ flanking promoter regions in liver genes. The production of cytokines at tissue sites of inflammation, and at other sites such as the pituitary gland and adrenal cortex or liver Kupffer cells, contributes to the final milieu of mediator concentrations to which hepatocytes respond. Figure 4 summarizes the network of cytokines involved in acute-phase liver responses. The acute-phase proteins in turn circulate and may accumulate at sites of tissue damage, and function to modulate inflammation and help return the body to homeostasis. The control of cytokine release may be altered by various agents which then could alter acute-phase responses. Thus, the role of xenobiotics in modulating inflammatory responses merits further investigation.

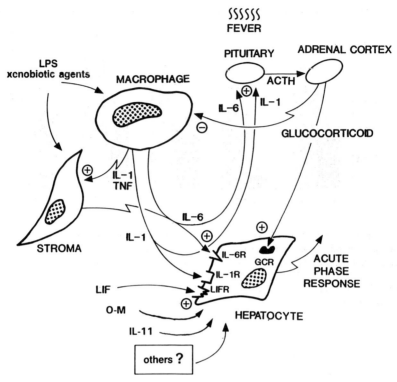

Fig. 4 Cytokine interactions in the acute phase response. Schematic representation of interactions and cytokines involved in the control of acute phase protein output by hepatocytes. Abbreviations: ACTH, adrenocorticotropic hormone; IL-6R, IL-6 receptor; IL-1R, IL-1 receptor; LIFR, LIF receptor; GCR, glucocorticoid receptor; LPS, lipopolysaccharide.

References

Ades, E. W., Hinson, A., Chapius-Cellier, C., and Arnaud, P. (1982). Modulation of the immune response by plasma protease inhibitors. I. Alpha$_2$-macroglobulin and alpha$_1$-antitrypsin inhibit natural killing and antibody-dependent cell-mediated cytotoxicity. *Scand. J. Immunol.* **15**, 109–113.

Akira, S., Isshiki, H., Sugita, T., Tanabe, O., Kinoshita, S., Nishio, Y., Nakajima, T., Hirano, T., and Kishimoto, T. (1990). A nuclear factor for IL-6 expression (NF-IL6) is a member of a C/EBP family. *EMBO J.* **9**, 1897–1906.

Andus, T., Geiger, T., Hirano, T., Northoff, H., Ganter, U., Bauer, J., Kishimoto, T., and Heinrich, P. C. (1987). Recombinant human B cell stimulatory factor 2 (BSF-2/IFN-beta2) regulates beta-fibrinogen and albumin mRNA levels in Fao-9 cells. *FEBS. Lett.* **221**, 18–22.

Andus, T., Geiger, T., Hirano, T., Kishimoto, T., Tran-Thi, T. A., Kecker, K., and Heinrich, P. C. (1988). Regulation of synthesis and secretion of major rat acute-phase proteins by recombinant human interleukin-6 (BSF-2/IL-6) in hepatocyte primary cultures. *Eur. J. Biochem.* **173**, 287–293.

Bailly, S., Ferrua, B., Fay, M., and Gougerot-Pocidalo, M. A. (1990). Differential regulation of IL 6, IL 1 A, IL 1beta and TNFalpha production in LPS-stimulated human monocytes: Role of cyclic AMP. *Cytokine* **2**, 205–210.

Bauer, J., Birmelin, M., Northoff, G. H., Northemann, W., Tran-Thi, T. A., Ueberberg, H., Decker, K., and Heinrich, P. C. (1984). Induction of rat alpha-2-macroglobulin *in vivo* and in hepatocyte primary cultures: Synergistic action of glucocorticoids and a Kupffer cell derived factor. *FEBS Lett.* **177**, 89–94.

Bauer, J., Lengyel, G., Bauer, T. M., Acs, G., and Gerok, W. (1989). Regulation of interleukin-6 receptor expression in human monocytes and hepatocytes. *FEBS Lett.* **249**, 27–30.

Baumann, H. (1989). Hepatic acute phase reaction *in vivo* and *in vitro*. *In Vitro Cell. Dev. Biol.* **25**, 115–126.

Baumann, H., and Gauldie, J. (1990). Regulation of hepatic acute phase plasma protein genes by hepatocyte stimulating factors and other mediators of inflammation. *Mol. Biol. Med.* **7**, 147–159.

Baumann, H., and Maquat, L. E. (1986). Localization of DNA sequences involved in dexamethasone-dependent expression of the rat alpha$_1$-acid glycoprotein gene. *Mol. Cell. Biol.* **6**, 2551–2561.

Baumann, H., and Schendel, P. (1991). Interleukin-11 regulates the hepatic expression of the same plasma protein genes as interleukin-6. *J. Biol. Chem.* **266**, 1–4.

Baumann, H., and Wong, G. G. (1989). Hepatocyte-stimulating Factor III shares structural and function identity with leukemia inhibitory factor. *J. Immunol.* **143**, 1163–1167.

Baumann, H., Firestone, G. L., Burgess, T. L., Gross, K. W., Yamamoto, K. R., and Held, W. A. (1983). Dexamethasone regulation of alpha-1-acid glycoprotein and other acute phase reactants in rat liver and hepatoma cells. *J. Biol. Chem.* **258**, 563–570.

Baumann, H., Richards, C., and Gauldie, J. (1987a). Interaction between hepatocyte-stimulating factors, interleukin-1 and glucocorticoids for regulation of acute phase proteins in human hepatoma (Hep-G2) cells. *J. Immunol.* **139**, 4122–4128.

Baumann, H., Onorato, V., Gauldie, J., and Jahreis, G. P. (1987b). Distinct sets of acute phase plasma proteins are stimulated by separate human hepatocyte-stimulating factors and monokines in rat hepatoma cells. *J. Biol. Chem.* **262**, 9756–9768.

Baumann, H., Isseroff, H., Latimer, J., and Jahreis, G. (1988). Phorbol ester modulates interleukin 6- and interleukin 1-regulated expression of acute phase plasma proteins in hepatoma cells. *J. Biol. Chem.* **263**, 17390–17396.

Baumann, H., Prowse, K. R., Marinkovic, S., Won, K.-A., and Jahreis, G. P. (1989a). Stimulation of hepatic acute phase response by cytokines and glucocorticoids. *Ann. N.Y. Acad. Sci.* **557**, 280–296.

Baumann, H., Won, K.-A., and Jahreis, G. P. (1989b). Human hepatocyte-stimulating factor-III and interleukin-6 are structurally and immunologically distinct but regulate the production of the same acute phase plasma proteins. *J. Biol. Chem.* **264**, 8046–8051.

Baumann, H., Morella, K. K., Jahreis, G. P., and Marinkovic, S. (1990). Distinct regulation of the interleukin-1 and interleukin-6 response elements of the rat haptoglobin gene in rat and human hepatoma cells. *Mol. Cell. Biol.* **10**, 5967–5976.

Baumann, M., Baumann, H., and Fey, G. H. (1990). Molecular cloning, characterization and functional expression of the rat liver interleukin 6 receptor. *J. Biol. Chem.* **265**, 19853–19862.

Bazan, F. (1991). Neuropeptide cytokines in the hematopoietic fold. *Neuron* **7**, 197–208.

Besedovsky, H., Del Rey, A., Sorkin, E., and Dinarello, C. A. (1986). Immunoregulatory feedback between interleukin-1 and glucocorticoid hormones. *Science* **238**, 652–654.

Beuscher, H. U., Fallon, R. J., and Colten, H. R. (1987). Macrophage membrane interleukin-1 regulates the expression of acute phase proteins in human hepatoma Hep 3B cells. *J. Immunol.* **139**, 1896–1901.

Beutler, B., and Cerami, A. (1986). Cachectin and tumour necrosis factor are two sides of the same biological coin. *Nature (London)* **320**, 584–588.

Birch, H., and Schreiber, G. (1986). Transcriptional regulation of plasma protein synthesis during inflammation. *J. Biol. Chem.* **261**, 8077–8080.

Bornstein, D. L. (1982). Leukocytic pyrogen: A major mediator of the acute phase reaction. *Ann. N.Y. Acad. Sci.* **389**, 323–337.

Brown, T. J., Lioubin, M. N., and Marquardt, H. (1987). Purification and characterization of cytostatic lymphokines produced by activated human T lymphocytes. *J. Immunol.* **139**, 2977–2983.

Brown, T. J., Rowe, J. M., and Shojab, M. (1991). Regulation of interleukin-6 expression by oncostatin M. *J. Immunol.* **147**, 2175–2180.

Castell, J. V., Andus, T., Kunz, D., and Heinrich, P. C. (1989). Interleukin-6: The major regulator of acute-phase protein synthesis in man and rat. *Ann. N.Y. Acad. Sci.* **557**, 86–101.

Chang, C.-J., Chen, T.-T., Lei, H.-Y., Chen, D.-S., and Lee, S.-C. (1990). Molecular cloning of a transcription factor, AGP/EBP, that belongs to members of the C/EBP family. *Mol. Cell. Biol.* **10**, 6642–6653.

Chen, H.-M., Considine, K. B., and Liao, W. S. L. (1991). Interleukin-6 responsiveness and cell-specific expression of the rat kininogen gene. *J. Biol. Chem.* **266**, 2946–2952.

Darlington, G. J., Wilson, D. R., and Lachman, L. B. (1986). Monocyte-conditioned medium, interleukin-1, and tumour necrosis factor stimulate the acute phase response in human hepatoma cells in vitro. *J. Cell. Biol.* **103**, 787–793.

Dinarello, C. A. (1988). Biology of interleukin-1. *FASEB. J.* **2**, 108–115.

Edbrooke, M., Burt, M. R., Cheshire, J. R., and Woo, P. (1989). Identification of cis-acting sequences responsible for phorbol ester induction of human serum amyloid A gene expression via a nuclear factor kappa B-like transcription factor. *Mol. Cell. Biol.* **9**, 1908–1912.

Edwards, D. R., Murphy, G., Reynolds, J. J., Whitham, S. E., Docherty, A. J. P., Angel, P., and Heath, J. K. (1987). Transforming growth factor beta modulates the expression of collagenase and metalloproteinase inhibitor. *EMBO J.* **6**, 1899–1904.

Evans, E., Courtois, G. M., Kilian, P. L., Fuller, G. M., and Crabtree, G. R. (1987). Induction of fibrinogen and a subset of acute phase response genes involves a novel monokine which is mimicked by phorbol esters. *J. Biol. Chem.* **262**, 10850–10854.

Fey, G. H., Hattori, M., Northemann, W., Abraham, L. J., Baumann, M., Braciak, T. A., Fletcher, R. G., Gauldie, J., Lee, F., and Reymond, M. F. (1989). Regulation of rat liver acute phase genes by interleukin-6 and production of hepatocyte stimulating factors by rat hepatoma cells. *Ann. N.Y. Acad. Sci.* **557**, 317–331.

Fowlkes, D. M., Mullis, N. T., Comeau, C. M., and Crabtree, G. R. (1984). Potential basis for regulation of the coordinately expressed fibrinogen genes: homology in the 5' flanking regions. *Proc. Natl. Acad. Sci. USA* **81**, 2313–2316.

Frankel, F. R., Steeger, J. R., Damiano, V. V., Sohn, M., Oppenheim, D., and Weinbaum, G. (1991). Induction of unilateral pulmonary fibrosis in the rat by cadmium chloride. *Am. J. Respir. Cell. Mol. Biol.* **5**, 385–394.

Fuller, G., and Grenett, H. (1989). The structure and function of the mouse hepatocyte stimulating factor. *Ann. N.Y. Acad. Sci.* **557**, 31–45.

Gauldie, J. (1991). Acute phase response. *In* "The Encyclopedia of Human Biology" (R. Dulbecco, ed.), pp. 1–11. Academic Press, San Diego.

Gauldie, J., Lamontagne, L., and Stadnyk, A. (1985). Acute phase response in infectious disease. *Surv. Synth. Pathol. Res.* **4**, 126–151.

Gauldie, J., Richards, C., Harnish, D., Lansdorp, P., and Baumann, H. (1987a). Interferon-beta2/B-cell stimulatory factor type 2 shares identity with monocyte hepatocyte-stimulating factor and regulates the major acute phase protein response in liver cells. *Proc. Natl. Acad. Sci. USA* **84**, 7251–7255.

Gauldie, J., Sauder, D. N., McAdam, K. P. W. J., and Dinarello, C. A. (1987b). Purified interleukin-1 (IL-1) from human monocytes stimulates acute-phase protein synthesis by rodent hepatocytes *in vitro*. *Immunol.* **60**, 203–207.

Gauldie, J., Northemann, W., and Fey, G. H. (1990). IL-6 functions as an exocrine hormone in inflammation. *J. Immunol.* **144**, 3804–3808.

Gauldie, J., Geisterfer, M., Richards, C., and Baumann, H. (1992). IL-6 regulation of the hepatic acute phase response. *In "Proceedings of the International Symposium on IL-6: Physiopathology and Clinical Potentials,"* pp. 151–162. Raven Press, New York.

Gearing, D. P., and Bruce, A. G. (1991). Oncostatin M binds the high-affinity leukemia inhibitory factor receptor. *New Biologist* **4**, 61–65.

Geiger, T., Andus, T., Klapproth, J., Northoff, H., and Heinrich, P. C. (1988a). Induction of alpha 1-acid glycoprotein by recombinant human interleukin-1 rat hepatoma cells. *J. Biol. Chem.* **263**, 7141–7176.

Geiger, T., Andus, T., Klapproth, J., Hirano, T., Kishimoto, T., and Heinrich, P. C. (1988b). Induction of rat acute-phase proteins by interleukin 6 in vivo. *Eur. J. Immunol.* **18**, 717–721.

Geisterfer, M., Richards, C. D., Baumann, M., Fey, G., Gwynne, D., and Gauldie, J. (1993). Regulation of IL-6 and the hepatic IL-6 receptor in acute inflammation in vivo. *Cytokine* **5**, 1–7.

Goldman, N. D., and Liu, T. Y. (1987). Biosynthesis of human C-reactive protein in cultured hepatoma cells is induced by a monocyte factor(s) other than interleukin-1. *J. Biol. Chem.* **262**, 2363–2368.

Goldstein, H., Koerholz, D., Chesky, L., Fan, X.-D., and Ambrus, J. L., Jr. (1990). Divergent activities of protein kinases in IL-6-induced differentiation of a human B cell line. *J. Immunol.* **145**, 952–961.

Gosset, P., Lassalle, P., Vanhee, D., Wallaert, B., Aerts, C., Voisin, C., and Tonnel, A.-B. (1991). Production of tumor necrosis factor-alpha and interleukin-6 by human alveolar macrophages exposed in vitro to coal mine dust. *Am. J. Resp. Cell. Mol. Biol.* **5**, 431–436.

Gross, V., Andus, T., and Tran-Thi, T. A. (1984). Induction of acute phase proteins by dexamethasone in primary rat hepatocyte cultures. *Exp. Cell. Res.* **151**, 46–54.

Hattori, M., Abraham, L. J., Northemann, W., and Fey, G. H. (1990). Acute-phase reaction induces a specific complex between hepatic nuclear proteins and the interleukin 6 response element of the rat alpha2-macroglobulin gene. *Proc. Natl. Acad. Sci. USA* **87**, 2364–2368.

Hibi, M., Murakami, M., Saito, M., Hirano, T., Taga, T., and Kishimoto, T. (1990). Molecular cloning and expression of an IL-6 signal transducer, gp130. *Cell* **63**, 1149–1157.

Hirano, T., Yasaukawa, K., Harada, H., Taga, T., Watanabe, Y., Matsuda, T., Kashiwamura, S.-i., Nakajima, K., Koyama, K., Iwamatsu, A., Tsunasawa, S., Sakiyama, F., Matsui, H., Takahara, Y., Taniguchi, T., and Kishimoto, T. (1986). Complementary DNA for a novel human interleukin (BSF-2) that induces B lymphocytes to produce immunoglobulin. *Nature (London)* **324**, 73–76.

Hirano, T., Taga, T., Yamasaki, F., Matsuda, T., Yasukawa, K., Kirata, Y., Yawata, H., Tanable, O., Akira, S., and Kishimoto, T. (1989). Molecular cloning of the cDNAs for IL-6 and its receptor. *Ann. N.Y. Acad. Sci.* **557**, 167–180.

Hoffman, M., Feldman, S. R., and Pizzo, S. V. (1983). Alpha$_2$-macroglobulin "fast" forms inhibit superoxide production by activated macrophages. *Biochim. Biophys. Acta* **760**, 421–426.

Homburger, F. (1945). A plasma fibrinogen-increasing factor obtained from sterile abscesses in dogs. *J. Clin. Invest.* **24**, 43–45.

Hooper, D. C., Steer, C. J., Dinarello, C. A., and Peacock, A. C. (1981). Inhibition of human natural cytotoxicity by macromolecular antiproteases. *J. Immunol.* **126**, 1569–1574.

Hudig, D., Haverty, T., Fulcher, C., Redelman, D., and Mendelsohn, J. (1981). Inhibition of human natural cytotoxicity by macromolecular antiproteases. *J. Immunol.* **126**, 1569.

Isshiki, H., Akira, S., Tanabe, O., Nakajima, T., Shimamoto, T., Hirano, T., and Kishimoto,

T. (1990). Constitutive and interleukin-1 (IL-1)-inducible factors interact with the IL-1-responsive element in the IL-6 gene. *Mol. Cell. Biol.* **10**, 2757–2764.

Jablons, D. M., Mule, J. J., McIntosh, J. K., Sehgal, P. B., May, L. T., Huang, C. M., Rosenberg, S. A., and Lotze, M. T. (1989). IL-6/IFN-beta2 as a circulating hormone. Induction by cytokine administration in humans *J Immunol.* **142**, 1542 1547.

Jordana, M., Richards, C. D., and Gauldie, J. (1988). Spontaneous release of alveolar macrophage cytokines after the intratracheal instillation of bleomycin in rats. *Am. Rev. Resp. Dis.* **137**, 1135–1140.

Kampschmidt, R. F., and Mesecher, M. (1985). Interleukin-1 from P388D: Effects upon neutrophils plasma iron, and fibrinogen in rats, mice, and rabbits. *Proc. Soc. Exp. Biol. Med.* **179**, 197–200.

Kampschmidt, R., and Upchurch, H. F. (1974). Effect of leukocytic endogenous mediator on plasma fibrinogen and haptoglobin. *Proc. Soc. Exp. Biol. Med.* **146**, 904–907.

Kampschmidt, R. F., Upchurch, H. P., and Pulliam, L. A. (1982). Characterisation of a leukocyte-derived endogenous mediator responsible for increased plasma fibrinogen. *Ann. N.Y. Acad. Sci.* **389**, 338–353.

Kaur, P., and Saklatvala, J. (1988). Interleukin 1 and tumour necrosis factor increase phosphorylation of fibroblast proteins. *FEBS Lett.* **241**, 6–10.

Kaur, P., Welch, W. J., and Saklatvala, J. (1989). Interleukin 1 and tumour necrosis factor increase phosphorylation of the small heat shock protein. *FEBS Lett.* **258**, 269–273.

Kishimoto, T. (1989). The biology of interleukin-6. *Blood* **74**, 1–10.

Koj, A. (1974). Acute phase reactants—Their synthesis, turnover and biological significance. *In* "Structure and Function of Plasma Proteins" (A. C. Allison, ed.), pp. 73–125. Plenum Press, London.

Koj, A., and Gordon, A. H. (1985). The acute-phase response to injury and infection (Introduction). *In* "Research Monographs in Cell and Tissue Pathology" (J. T. Dingle and J. L. Gordon, eds.), Vol. 10, pp. xxi–xxix. Elsevier, Amsterdam.

Koj, A., Gauldie, J., Regoeczi, E., Sauder, D. N., and Sweeney, G. D. (1984). The acute-phase response of cultured rat hepatocytes. System characterisation and the effect of human cytokines. *Biochem. J.* **224**, 505–514.

Koj, A., Kurdowska, A., Magielska-Zero, D., Rokita, H., Sipe, J. D., Dayer, J.-M., Demczuk, S., and Gauldie, J. (1987). Limited effects of recombinant human and murine interleukin-1 and tumour necrosis factor on production of acute phase proteins by cultured rat hepatocytes. *Biochem. Int.* **14**, 553–560.

Kushner, I. (1982). The phenomenon of the acute phase response. *Ann. N.Y. Acad. Sci.* **389**, 39–48.

Kushner, I., and Mackiewicz, A. (1987). Acute phase proteins as disease markers. *Disease Markers* **5**, 1–11.

Le, J., and Vilcek, J. (1987). Biology of disease. Tumor necrosis factor and interleukin I: Cytokines with multiple overlapping biological activities. *Lab. Invest.* **56**, 234–248.

Le, P. T., and Mortensen, R. F. (1984). In vitro induction of hepatocyte synthesis of the acute phase reaction mouse serum amyloid P-component by macrophages and IL-1. *J. Leuk. Biol.* **35**, 587–603.

Liberman, T. A., and Baltimore, D. (1990). Activation of interleukin-6 gene expression through NF-kappa B transcription factor. *Mol. Cell. Biol.* **10**, 2327–2334.

Linsley, P. S., Bolton-Hanson, M., Horn, D., Malik, N., Kallestad, J. C., Ochs, V., Zarling, J. M., and Shoyab, M. (1989). Identification and characterization of cellular receptors for the growth regulator, oncostatin M. *J. Biol. Chem.* **264**, 4282–4289.

Mackiewicz, A., and Kushner, I. (1989). Role of IL-6 in acute phase protein glycosylation. *Ann. N.Y. Acad. Sci.* **557**, 515–517.

Mackiewicz, A., Ganapathi, M. K., and Schultz, D. (1987). Monokines regulate glycosylation of acute phase proteins. *J. Exp. Med.* **166**, 253–258.

Magielska-Zero, D., Bereta, J., Czuba-Pelech, P. V., Gauldie, J., and Koh, A. (1988). Inhibitory effect of recombinant human interferon gamma on synthesis of some acute phase proteins in human hepatoma Hep G2 cells. *Biochem. Int.* **17,** 17–23.

Malik, N., Kallestad, J. C., Gunderson, N. L., Austin, S. D., Neubauer, M. G., Ochs, V., Marquardt, H., Zarling, J. M., Shoyab, M., Wei, C.-M., Linsley, P. S., and Rose, T. M. (1989). Molecular cloning, sequence analysis, and functional expression of a novel growth regulator, oncostatin M. *Mol. Cell. Biol.* **9,** 2847–2853.

May, L., Ghrayeb, J., Santhanam, U., Tatter, S., Sthoeger, Z., Helfgott, D., Chiorazzi, N., Greninger, G., and Sehgal, P. (1988). Synthesis and secretion of multiple forms of beta2-interferon/B-cell differentiation factor-2/hepatocyte stimulating factor by human fibroblasts and monocytes. *J. Biol. Chem.* **263,** 7760–7766.

May, L. T., Santhanam, U., Tatter, S. B., Ghrayeb, J., and Sehgal, P. B. (1989). Multiple forms of human interleukin-6: Phosphoglycoproteins secreted by many different tissues. *Ann. N.Y. Acad. Sci.* **557,** 114–121.

Morrone, G., Ciliberto, G., Oliviero, S., Arcones, R., Dente, L., Content, J., and Cortese, R. (1988). Recombinant interleukin-6 regulates the transcriptional activation of a set of human acute phase genes. *J. Biol. Chem.* **263,** 12554–12558.

Musso, T., Espinoza-Delgado, I., Pulkki, K., Gusella, G. L., Longo, D. L., and Varesio, L. (1990). Transforming growth factor beta downregulates interleukin-1 (IL-1)-induced IL-6 production by human monocytes. *Blood* **76,** 2466–2469.

Naitoh, Y., Fukata, J., Tominaga, T., Nakai, Y., Tamai, S., Mori, K., and Imura, H. (1988). Interleukin-6 stimulates the secretion of adrenocorticotropic hormone in conscious, freely-moving rats. *Biochem. Biophys. Res. Commun.* **155,** 1459.

Nakajima, K., and Wall, R. (1991). Interleukin-6 signals activating junB and TIS11 gene transcription in a B-cell hybridoma. *Mol. Cell. Biol.* **11,** 1409–1418.

Nijsten, M., deGroot, E., TenDuuis, H., Klensen, H., Hack, C., and Aarden, L. (1987). Serum levels of interleukin-6 and acute phase responses. *Lancet* **2,** 921.

Northemann, W., Braciak, T. A., Hattori, M., Lee, F., and Fey, G. H. (1990a). Structure of th rat interleukin 6 gene and its expression in macrophage-derived cells. *J. Biol. Chem.* **264,** 16072–16082.

Northemann, W., Hattori, M., Baffet, G., Braciak, T. A., Fletcher, R. G., Abraham, L. J., Gauldie, J., Baumann, M., and Fey, G. H. (1990b). Production of interleukin 6 by hepatoma cells. *Mol. Biol. Med.* **7,** 273–285.

Overall, C. M., Wrana, J. L., and Sodek, J. (1989). Independent regulation of collagenase, 72-kDa progelatinase, and metalloendoproteinase inhibitor expression in human fibroblasts by transforming growth factor-beta. *J. Biol. Chem.* **264,** 1860–1869.

Paul, S. R., Bennett, F., Calvetti, J. A., Kelleher, K., Wood, C. R., O'Hara, Jr., R. M., Leary, A. C., Sibley, B., Clark, S. C., Williams, D. A., and Yang, Y.-C. (1990). Molecular cloning of a cDNA encoding interleukin 11, a stromal cell-derived lymphopoietic and hematopoietic cytokine. *Proc. Natl. Acad. Sci. USA* **87,** 7512–7516.

Pepys, M. B., and Baltz, M. L. (1983). Acute phase proteins with special reference to C-reactive protein and related proteins (Pentaxins) and serum amyloid A protein. *Adv. Immunol.* **34,** 141–211.

Perlmutter, D. H., Dinarello, C. A., Punsal, P. I., and Coltent, H. R. (1986). Cachectin/tumor necrosis factor regulates hepatic acute phase gene expression. *J. Clin. Invest.* **78,** 1349.

Poli, V., Mancini, F. P., and Cortese, R. (1990). IL-6DBP, a nuclear protein involved in interleukin-6 signal transduction, defines a new family of leucine zipper proteins related to C/EBP. *Cell* **63,** 643–653.

Poupart, P., Vandenabeele, P., Cayphas, S., Van Snick, J., Haegeman, G., Kruys, V., Fiers, W., and Content, J. (1987). B cell growth modulating and differentiating activity of recombinant human 26-kd protein (BSF-2, HuIFN-beta2, HPGF). *EMBO J.* **6,** 1219–1224.

Prowse, K. R., and Baumann, H. (1988). Hepatocyte-stimulating factor, beta-2 interferon, and interleukin-1 enhance expression of the rat alpha-1-acid glycoprotein gene via a distal upstream regulatory region. *Mol. Cell. Biol.* **8,** 42–51.

Prowse, K. R., and Baumann, H. (1990). Molecular characterization and acute phase expression of the multiple *Mus caroli* alpha$_1$-acid glycoprotein (AGP) genes. *J. Biol. Chem.* **265,** 10201–10209.

Ramadori, G., Sipe, J. D., Dinarello, C. S., Mizel, S. B., and Colten, H. R. (1985). Pretranslational modulation of acute phase hepatic protein synthesis by murine recombinant interleukin-1 (IL-1) and purified human IL-1. *J. Exp. Med.* **162,** 930–942.

Ray, A., LaForge, K. S., and Sehgal, P. B. (1990). On the mechanism for efficient repression of the interleukin-6 promoter by glucocorticoids: Enhancer, TATA box, and RNA start site (Inr motif) occlusion. *Mol. Cell. Biol.* **10,** 5736–5746.

Richards, C. D., and Saklatvala, J. (1991). Molecular cloning and sequence of porcine interleukin-6 cDNA and expression of mRNA in synovial fibroblasts in vitro. *Cytokine* **3,** 269–276.

Richards, C. D., Brown, T. J., Shoyab, M., Baumann, H., and Gauldie, J. (1992). Recombinant oncostatin-M stimulates the production of acute phase proteins in hepatocytes in vitro. *J. Immunol.* **148,** 1731–1736.

Ritchie, D. G., and Fuller, G. M. (1983). Hepatocyte-stimulating factor: A monocyte-derived acute-phase regulatory protein. *Ann. N.Y. Acad. Sci.* **408,** 490–502.

Rokita, H., Bereta, J., Koj, A., Gordon, A. H., and Gauldie, J. (1990). Epidermal growth factor and transforming growth factor-beta differently modulate the acute phase response elicited by interleukin-6 in cultured liver cells from man, rat and mouse. *Comp. Biochem. Physiol.* **95A,** 41–45.

Rose, T. M., and Bruce, A. G. (1991). Oncostatin M is a member of the cytokine family which includes LIF, GM-CSF and IL-6. *Proc. Natl. Acad. Sci. USA* **88,** 864–8645.

Rose-John, S., Schooltink, H., Lenz, D., Hipp, E., Dufhues, G., Schmitz, H., Schiel, X., Hirano, T., Kishimoto, K., and Heinrich, P. C. (1990). Studies on the structure and regulation of the human hepatic interleukin-6 receptor. *Eur. J. Biochem.* **190,** 79–83.

Saito, M., Yoshida, K., Hibi, M., Taga, T., and Kishimoto, T. (1992). Molecular cloning of a murine IL-6 receptor-associated signal transducer, gp130, and its regulated expression in vivo. *J. Immunol.* **148,** 4066–4071.

Scales, W. E., Chensue, S. W., Otterness, I., and Kunkel, S. L. (1989). Regulation of monokine gene expression: Prostaglandin E2 suppresses tumor necrosis factor but not interleukin-1alpha or beta-mRNA and cell-associated bioactivity. *J. Leuk. Biol.* **45,** 416–421.

Schooltink, H., Schmitz-Van de Leur, H., Heinrich, P. C., and Rose-John, S. (1992). Upregulation of the interleukin-6 signal transducing protein (gp130) by interleukin 6 and dexamethasone in HepG2 cells. *FEBS Lett.* **297,** 263–265.

Schreiber, G. (1987). Synthesis, processing and secretion of plasma proteins by the liver (and other organs) and their regulation. *In* "The Plasma Proteins" (F. W. Putnam, ed.), pp. 294–363. Academic Press, New York.

Schreiber, G., Tsykin, A., Aldred, A. R., Thomas, T., Fung, W.-P., Dickson, P. W., Cole, T., Birch, H., De Jong, F. A., and Milland, J. (1989). The acute phase response in the rodent. *Ann. N.Y. Acad. Sci.* **557,** 61–86.

Schroeder, J. J., and Cousins, R. J. (1990). Interleukin 6 regulates metallothionein gene expression and zinc metabolism in hepatocyte monolayer cultures. *Proc. Natl. Acad. Sci. USA* **87,** 3137–3141.

Scuderi, P. (1990). Differential effects of copper and zinc on human peripheral blood monocyte cytokine secretion. *Cell. Immunol.* **126,** 391–405.

Sehgal, P. B., Grieninger, G., and Tosato, G. (1989). Regulation of the acute phase and immune responses: Interleukin-6. Introduction: A merging of disciplines. *Ann. N.Y. Acad. Sci.* **557,** xv–xvi.

Sims, J. E., March, C. J., Cosman, D., Widmer, M. B., MacDonald, H. R., McMahan, C. J., Grubin, C. E., Wignall, J. M., Jackson, J. L., Call, S. M., Friend, D., Alpert, A. R., Gillis,

S., Urdal, D. L., and Dower, S. K. (1988). cDNA expression cloning of the IL-1 receptor, a member of the immunoglobulin superfamily. *Science* **241**, 585–588.

Sironi, M., Breviario, F., Prosperpio, P., Biondi, A., Vecchi, A., Van Damme, J., Dejana, E., and Mantovani, A. (1989). IL-1 stimulates IL-6 production in endothelial cells. *J. Immunol.* **142**, 549–553.

Sporn, M. B., Roberts, A. B., Wakefield, L. M., and Assoian, R. K. (1986). Transforming growth factor-B: Biological function and chemical structure. *Science* **233**, 532–534.

Stadnyk, A. W., Baumann, H., and Gauldie, J. (1990). The acute-phase protein response in parasite infection. *Nippostrongylus brasiliensis* and *Trichinella spiralis* in the rat. *Immunol.* **69**, 588–595.

Stepien, H., Agro, A., Crossley, J., Padol, I., Richards, C., and Stanisz, A. (1993). Immunomodulatory properties of diazepam-binding inhibitor: Effect on human Interleukin-6 secretion, lymphocyte proliferation and natural killer cell activity in vitro. *Neuropeptides* **25**, 207–211.

Sternberg, E. M., Hill, J. M., Chrousos, G. P., Kamilaris, T., Listwak, S. J., Gold, P. W., and Wilder, R. L. (1989a). Inflammatory mediator-induced hypothalamic-pituitary-adrenal axis activation is defective in streptococcal cell wall arthritis-susceptible Lewis rats. *Proc. Natl. Acad. Sci. USA* **86**, 2374–2378.

Sternberg, E. M., Young, W. S., III, Bernardini, R., Calogero, A. E., Chrousos, G. P., Gold, P. W., and Wilder, R. L. (1989b). A central nervous system defect in biosynthesis of corticotropin-releasing hormone is associated with susceptibility to streptococcal cell wall-induced arthritis in Lewis rats. *Proc. Natl. Acad. Sci. USA* **86**, 4771–4775.

Taga, T., Hibi, M., Hirata, Y., Yamasaki, K., Yasukawa, K., Matsuda, T., Hirano, T., and Kishimoto, T. (1989). Interleukin-6 triggers the association of its receptor with a possible signal transducer, gp130. *Cell* **58**, 573–581.

Taga, T., and Kishimoto, T. (1992). Cytokine receptors and signal transduction. *FASEB J.* **6**, 3387–3396.

Tanabe, O., Akira, S., Kamiya, T., Wong, G., Hirano, T., and Kishimoto, T. (1989). Genomic structure of the murine IL-6 gene. *J. Immunol.* **141**, 3875–3880.

Taupin, V., Herbelin, A., Descamps-Latscha, B., and Zavala, F. (1991). Endogenous anxiogenic peptide, ODN-diazepam-binding inhibitor, and benzodiazepines enhance the production of interleukin-1 and tumor necrosis factor by human monocytes. *Lymphokine Cytokine Res.* **10**, 7–13.

Travis, J., and Salvesen, G. S. (1983). Human plasma proteinase inhibitors. *Ann. Rev. Biochem.* **52**, 665–709.

Tsuchiya, Y., Hattori, M., Hayashida, K., Ishibashi, H., Okubo, H., and Sakaki, Y. (1987). Sequence analysis of the putative regulatory region of rat alpha$_2$-macroglobulin gene. *Gene* **57**, 73–80.

Van Snick, J., Cayphas, S., Szikora, J.-P., Renauld, J.-C., Roost, E., and Simpson, R. (1988). cDNA cloning of murine interleukin-HP1: Homology with human interleukin 6. *Eur. J. Immunol.* **18**, 193–197.

Van Vugt, H., van Gool, J., and de Ridder, L. (1986). Alpha$_2$-macroglobulin of the rat, an acute phase protein mitigates the early course of endotoxin shock. *Br. J. Exp. Pathol.* **67**, 313–319.

Wilson, D. R., Juan, T. S.-C., Wilde, M. D., Fey, G. H., and Darlington, G. J. (1990). A 58-base-pair region of the human C3 gene confers synergistic inducibility by interleukin-1 and interleukin-6. *Mol. Cell Biol.* **10**, 6181–6191.

Woloski, B. M. R. N. J., and Fuller, G. M. (1985b). Identification and partial characterisation of hepatocyte-stimulating factor from leukemia cell lines: comparison with interleukin-1. *Proc. Natl. Acad. Sci. USA* **82**, 1443–1447.

Woloski, B. M. R. N. J., Smith, E. M., Meyer, W. J., III, Fuller, G. M., and Blalock, J. E. (1985). Corticotropin-releasing activity of monokines. *Science* **230**, 1035–1037.

Won, K.-A., and Baumann, H. (1990). The cytokine response element of the rat alpha 1-acid glycoprotein gene is a complex of several interacting regulatory sequences. *Mol. Cell Biol.* **10**, 3965–3978.

Yamasaki, K., Taga, T., Hirata, Y., Yawata, H., Kawanishi, Y., Seed, B., Taniguchi, T., Hirano, T., and Kishimoto, T. (1988). Cloning and expression of the human interleukin-6 (BSF-2/IFNbeta 2) receptor. *Science* **241**, 825–828.

Zarling, J. M., Shoyab, M., Marquardt, H., Hanson, M. B., Lioubin, M. N., and Todaro, G. J. (1986). Oncostatin M: A growth regulator produced by differentiated histiocyte lymphoma cells. *Proc. Natl. Acad. Sci. USA* **83**, 9739–9743.

Zhang, Y., Lin, J.-X., and Vilcek, J. (1988). Synthesis of interleukin 6 (interferon-beta2/B cell stimulatory factor 2) in human fibroblasts is triggered by an increase in intracellular cyclic AMP. *J. Biol. Chem.* **263**, 6177–6182.

5

Role of Tumor Necrosis Factor α in Acute and Chronic Inflammatory Responses: Novel Therapeutic Approaches

Carl K. Edwards, III, Shawn M. Borcherding, Jun Zhang, and David R. Borcherding

I. Introduction

In the last decade, the understanding of immunopathological reactions has evolved greatly as a result of the characterization of cytokines and interleukins that regulate the interactions not only between cells of the immune system but also between the immune system and other tissues and cells, such as endothelial cells, fibroblasts, and adipocytes. One cytokine that is increasingly recognized as a central mediator in a wide spectrum of physiological and immune functions is macrophage-derived tumor necrosis factor (TNF) or cachectin. Although much remains to be elucidated about this molecule, TNF has been found to mediate effects as diverse as tumoricidal activity (Carswell et al., 1975; Dressler et al., 1992), wasting associated with chronic disease (Tracey et al., 1988), and the recruitment of both immune and nonimmune cells to participate more effectively in the host response to an invasive agent (Old, 1990). In addition, an increasingly large body of evidence indicates that TNF serves as a proximal mediator in the evolution of septic shock (Beutler and Cerami, 1989). Although a lymphocyte-derived molecule called lymphotoxin or TNFβ possesses overlapping biological activities and 30% homology at the amino acid level, this chapter focuses on macrophage-derived TNF, or TNFα. Historical background, physical properties, interactions with various cell types, in vivo effects, and finally pharmacological regulation of the expression of this cytokine are discussed.

Xenobiotics and Inflammation
Copyright 1994 © by Academic Press, Inc. All rights of reproduction in any form reserved.

II. General Properties of Tumor Necrosis Factor α

Interferon γ (IFNγ) is the most completely characterized macrophage-activating factor (MAF) for *in vitro* and *in vivo* systems (Schultz and Kleinschmidt, 1983; Svedersky *et al.*, 1984; Nathan, 1986; Murray, 1988). Other MAFs are also thought to exist (Sharp *et al.*, 1985; Wing *et al.*, 1985; Crawford *et al.*, 1987; Hoffman and Weinberg, 1987; Reed *et al.*, 1987). Properties of activated macrophages include enhanced respiratory burst activity (Johnson and Baglioni, 1988), increased killing of microbial pathogens (Nathan, 1986; Johnston, 1988), increased expression of major histocompatibility complex (MHC) class II antigens (Unanue and Allen, 1987), enhanced abilities to kill tumor cells (Unanue and Allen, 1987), and production of cytokines such as interleukin 1 (IL-1; Dinarello, 1985, 1987) and TNFα (Carswell *et al.*, 1975; Beutler and Cerami, 1989).

As stated in the introduction, TNFα is also referred to as cachectin (Beutler *et al.*, 1985a). This cytokine has a wide range of biological effects (Beutler and Cerami, 1987, 1988), including antitumor activity (Balkwell *et al.*, 1986; Price *et al.*, 1987; Schiller *et al.*, 1987; Talmadge *et al.*, 1987), reduction of malarial parasite infection in mice (Clark *et al.*, 1987; Grau *et al.*, 1987), mediation of endotoxic shock and cachexia in infectious disease (Beutler *et al.*, 1985a; Torti *et al.*, 1985; Tracey *et al.*, 1987, 1988), augmentation of superoxide anion (O_2^-) and hydrogen peroxide (H_2O_2) release by neutrophils and macrophages (Berkow *et al.*, 1987; Ding and Nathan, 1987; Figari *et al.*, 1987; Hoffman and Weinberg, 1987; Berkow and Dodson, 1988), inhibition of viral replication (Wong and Goeddel, 1986), and potentiation of nonviral pathogen destruction by macrophages *in vitro* (De Titto *et al.*, 1986; Esparza *et al.*, 1989; Bermudez and Young, 1988) and *in vivo* (Scuderi *et al.*, 1986; Havell, 1987; Waage *et al.*, 1987; Jacob and McDevitt, 1988; Nakane *et al.*, 1988). Although IFNγ alone is incapable of stimulating TNFα release from macrophages, it is able to augment TNFα biosynthesis in response to lipopolysaccharide (LPS) at the transcriptional and posttranscriptional levels (Nedwin *et al.*, 1985a; Gifford and Lohman-Matthes, 1987; Koerner *et al.*, 1987; Scuderi *et al.*, 1987). Investigations have demonstrated that many of the physiological effects of TNFα may be elevated through its intrinsic ion-channel-forming activity (Kagan *et al.*, 1992).

III. Regulation of TNFα Gene Expression

TNFα and TNFβ (or lymphotoxin) have single-copy genes, closely linked within the cluster of MHC genes located at the boundary of the class I and class II MHC region on the short arm of human chromosome 6 (Spies *et al.*, 1986, 1989) and murine chromosome 17 (Muller *et al.*, 1987; Figure 1).

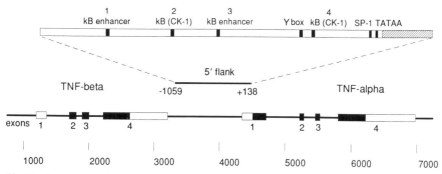

Fig. 1 Structure of the murine TNF locus. Reproduced from Shakov et al. (1990), by copyright permission of the Rockefeller University Press.

In all animal species examined (human, murine, rat, and rabbit), certain characteristics of the TNFα and TNFβ genes have been consistently observed: TNFβ genes are 5' to TNFα genes, TNFα and TNFβ genes are each approximately 3 kb in length, and each gene consists of four exons and three introns (reviewed by Vilcek and Lee, 1991). These similarities strongly suggest that, through genetic duplication, TNFα and TNFβ genes were derived from a common ancestral gene. Although the organization and coding regions of TNFα and TNFβ genes display a high degree of homology (particularly the fourth exons, which encode 80–90% of the mature proteins), little similarity is observed in the 5' flanking regions for the TNFα and TNFβ genes. These flanking regions are thought to contain most of the elements responsible for transcriptional regulation (Nedwin et al., 1985b; Shakov et al., 1990).

A. Transcriptional Regulation

LPS is the most potent stimulus for biosynthesis of TNFα in monocytes and macrophages, and can enhance TNF gene transcription as much as 3-fold (Beutler et al., 1986). Studies employing inhibitors of protein kinase C suggest that LPS-induced transcription of the TNFα gene is moderated by protein kinase C (Kovacs et al., 1988), although this viewpoint has been challenged (Celada and Maki, 1991).

IL-1 is an LPS-inducible cytokine that possesses multiple overlapping biological activities with TNFα (Beutler and Cerami, 1986; Dinarello, 1987, 1991; Le and Vilcek, 1987). Interestingly, inhibition of calmodulin-dependent kinase has no measurable effect on inhibition of LPS-induced expression of TNFα, although inhibition of IL-1 expression is observed (Kovacs et al., 1988). LPS induces binding of various DNA-binding proteins to enhancer elements in the regulatory region of the TNFα gene (Shakov et al., 1990). These enhancer elements include promoters with sequence homology to κB (Collart *et al.*, 1990; Molitar *et al.*, 1990; Pessara and Koch, 1990); Y-box, a DNA sequence usually located in the promoters of MHC class II genes (Drouet *et al.*, 1991); and an IL-1 responsive element in the interleukin 6 (IL-6) gene (Akira *et al.*, 1990). Other studies have indicated that regulation of the TNF promoter can be mediated by TNF itself (Leitman *et al.*, 1991).

Drouet and colleagues (1991) analyzed the protein-binding characteristics and enhancer activity of four κB-like enhancers and an MHC class II-like Y-box found in the mouse TNFα promoter. In addition to members of the NF-κB/*rel* transcription factor family, at least two of the κB sites also contained a nuclear protein identified as NF-GMa, a factor that binds to promoter sequences in response to action of TNFα and many other cytokines. When inserted upstream of an enhancerless promoter, two κB sites were active as LPS-inducible enhancers in primary macrophages and the other two κB sites were not active. Variations in nucleotides known to contain nuclear factors severely reduced the affinity of κB sites for NF-κB. Introduction of the same modulators into a construct containing 1059 bp TNFα promoter coupled to a chloramphenicol acetyltransferase (CAT) reporter gene resulted in a stepwise reduction in LPS induction of gene expression; mutation of all 4 sites (11 bp of 1059 bp) reduced LPS inducibility of gene expression by 90%. These results suggest that transcription factors belonging to the NF-κB/*rel* family are important in TNFα promoter activities. Other studies have examined mechanisms of TNF mRNA expression using mRNA half-life, DNase sensitivity, and DNA-binding factor assays (Hensel *et al.*, 1989; Sung *et al.*, 1991). These results indicate that phorbol esters increase TNF mRNA half-life and increase NF-κB binding activities. Increases in mRNA expression of c-*fos*, *jun*B, and *jun*D (the subunits of AP-1), but not that of c-*jun*, preceded or paralleled increases in TNFα genetic transcription. Phorbol 12-myristate 13-acetate (PMA) increased binding activities of nuclear extracts to TNF κB, AP-1, and AP-2 motifs. In addition, a DNase hypersensitivity site present only in TNF-producing cell lines was mapped to the TNF gene promoter region.

Additional studies have demonstrated effects of viral infections and TNFα production (Mestan *et al.*, 1986; Wong and Goeddel, 1986; Wong and Goeddel, 1988; Gong *et al.*, 1991). In an investigation of viral triggering of TNFα production, Nain and co-workers (1990) observed that different types of mononuclear phagocytes were susceptible to infection by influenza type A virus. Each cell type permitted viral replication and responded to the infection with a high level of TNFα mRNA accumulation which, however, was accompanied by surprisingly low levels of TNFα secreted protein (<1 ng/ml). When small amounts of LPS were added, a strong TNFα release from virus-infected macrophages occurred. Note that a viral infection appeared to precondition, or "prime," the macrophages to release large amounts of TNFα in response to secondary triggering signals such as bacterial products. One group of investigators (Gong *et al.*, 1991) demonstrated that high levels of TNFα mRNA accumulation in influenza type A virus-primed macrophages is primarily the result of enhanced gene transcription and prolonged TNFα mRNA stability.

B. Posttranscriptional Regulation

In addition to transcriptional activation, compelling evidence exists for regulation of the TNFα gene at the translational level. The presence of TNFα mRNA in cells does not necessarily lead to protein synthesis (Beutler *et al.*, 1986; Collart *et al.*, 1986). For example, IFNγ can induce TNFα transcription, but other stimuli are needed for protein biosynthesis (Collart *et al.*, 1986; Sariben *et al.*, 1988; Zuckerman *et al.*, 1989, 1991; Han *et al.*, 1990a). LPS induces approximately 3-fold increases in transcriptional activity of the TNFα gene, a 100-fold increase in cellular TNFα mRNA content, and a 10,000-fold increase in the quantity of protein secreted from activated mononuclear cells. Thus, TNFα biosynthesis appears to be highly regulated at a posttranscriptional level (Jäättelä, 1991).

Transcriptional regulation of TNFα is likely to involve a distinct structural element in the 3' untranslated region of TNFα mRNA (Caput *et al.*, 1986; Han *et al.*, 1990a). This region contains various repeated and overlapping copies of the consensus octamer sequence UUAUUUAU. This AU-rich sequence is also present in the mRNA sequences of several other potent inflammatory mediators including TNFβ, the interferons, IL-1, and granulocyte–macrophage colony stimulating factor (GM-CSF), as well as in the mRNA sequences for c-*myc* and c-*fos* oncoproteins (Gessani *et al.*, 1991; Leitman *et al.*, 1991; Zuckerman *et al.*, 1991). These AU-rich sequences, in conjunction with surrounding sequences, are very responsive to LPS (Han *et al.*, 1990a) and control the half-life and translation of mRNAs (Shaw and Kamen, 1986). Therefore, a ribonuclease present in macrophages and other mammalian cells selectively degrades mRNAs at a rate that depends on the number of AU sequence copies. This phenomenon may play an important role in the control of TNFα biosynthesis (Beutler *et al.*, 1988).

Constructs in which the CAT coding sequence was followed by varying segments of the TNF 3' untranslated region have been used to study the function of these sequences (Han *et al.*, 1990a; Beutler and Brown, 1991). Investigators demonstrated that downstream sequences present in TNF mRNA are sufficient to mediate a >200-fold induction of CAT synthesis in response to activation by endotoxin. Induction of CAT activity was not attributable to changes in cytoplasmic mRNA concentration, but to a marked enhancement of translational efficiency. The response to endotoxin represents "derepression" and is conferred chiefly by the translational expressive TTATTTAT element, acting in concert with essential flanking sequences (Han *et al.*, 1990a).

Finally, another mechanism by which TNFα is regulated involves tolerance to LPS by macrophages (Takusaka *et al.*, 1991). Macrophages pretreated with low doses of LPS *in vitro* failed to produce TNFα when they were restimulated with LPS. These results suggest that macrophage exposure to low doses of LPS suppresses TNFα production, but not IL-1 production, by inhibition of mRNA expression. This inhibition occurs through a monocyclooxygenase-dependent mechanism. Other reports, including one by Haas and colleagues (1990), have suggested that, in LPS-desensitized macrophage cell lines, two distinct pathways of signal transduction—generation of prostaglandin E_2 (PGE_2) and activation of protein kinase C—are required. Collectively, these studies indicate that pathways known to be involved in triggering TNF production may at the same time be involved in its down-regulation.

IV. Role of TNFα in Acute and Chronic Inflammatory Processes

Enhanced synthesis and release of cytokines has been observed during many acute and chronic inflammatory processes. Investigators increasingly realize that, in many cases, overproduction of TNFα is a major contributor to inflammation, cellular injury, and cell death (Figure 2). Note that the mere presence of cytokines such as TNFα in physiological compartments (such as plasma) does not necessarily imply that an inflammatory process is occurring in that compartment or elsewhere in the body. Careful investigation into the complex functions and contributions of individual cytokines in particular disease states is necessary to design and apply novel immunotherapeutic interventions effectively. Combination therapy including immunomodulation and supportive treatment may be the best approach. Animal and human investigations into pathophysiological contributions of cytokines to acute and chronic inflammatory processes are not standardized in design or study populations. Therefore, comparisons across studies should be carefully evaluated. However, the following section provides evidence to support the claim that TNFα immunomodulation may fill a therapeutic niche when conventional interventions have failed. Table I provides additional disease states and syndromes in which TNFα is implicated and inhibition of TNFα overproduction may be useful.

A. Septicemia

A need exists to standardize definitions of bacteremia, sepsis, septic shock, and refractory septic shock and to employ standard criteria when designing and conducting investigations. Readers should refer to these terms as defined according to the criteria of Bone *et al.* (1991a). Remember that the severity and duration of septic shock may vary in different clinical

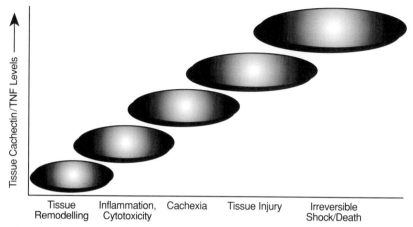

Fig. 2 Net biological effects of cachectin/TNF according to tissue levels. Reproduced from Tracey (1989) by permission of Lancet Ltd.

investigations and can contribute to variations in outcome across investigations.

The incidence of sepsis, the leading cause of morbidity and mortality in hospitalized patients, increased 2-fold in the United States from 1979 to 1987, making septicemia the thirteenth leading cause of death in the United States (Centers for Disease Control, 1990). Although septic shock is usually recognized to be a consequence of gram-negative bacteremia, the condition may also be caused by gram-positive organisms, fungi, viruses, and parasites (Glauser *et al.*, 1991). The highest lethality occurs in patients with gram-negative infections who develop septic shock, with mortality rates as high as 50–80% (Bone *et al.*, 1987; Calandra *et al.*, 1988). Patients at increased risk for developing gram-negative sepsis and septic shock include immunocompromised patients, the elderly, and patients subject to invasive device usage such as intravenous and urinary catheters or respirators (Bone *et al.*, 1989; Parker and Parrillo, 1983; Mizock, 1984).

Endotoxin is an LPS component of the gram-negative bacterial outer membrane that is released into the circulation and initiates adverse systemic events associated with sepsis and bacteremia (Figure 3). Bacterial LPS is a lipid bilayer composed of three regions: oligosaccharide side chains, core polysaccharide, and lipid A. LPS aggregation *in vivo* depends on its microenvironment; the degree of this aggregation may influence the degree of complement activation (Wilson and Morrison, 1982). Endotoxin is not directly toxic to human tissues and does not appear to induce metabolic derangements or norepinephrine release directly (Beutler and Cerami, 1987; Lunn *et al.*, 1990; Michalek *et al.*, 1980). Instead, endotoxin, and lipid A in particular, appears to activate macrophages for the biosynthesis and release

Table I   Additional Diseases and Syndromes in Which TNFα Is Implicated

Disease or syndrome	References
Vascular injury/atherosclerosis	Hansson *et al.* (1989); Warner and Libby (1989); Barath *et al.* (1990); Ip *et al.* (1990)
Diabetes mellitus type I	Bendtzen (1990); Campbell and Harrison (1990); Campbell (1991); Mandrup-Poulsen *et al.* (1990); Rabinovitch (1991)
Kawasaki disease	Furukawa *et al.* (1988)
Starvation	Vaisman *et al.* (1989)
Leprosy	Kaplan and Cohn (1991)
Multiple sclerosis	Brosnan *et al.* (1988); Sharief and Hentges (1991)
Anemia of chronic disease	Schilling (1991)
Ultraviolet radiation	Köck *et al.* (1990)
Dermatological disease	Cooper (1990); Mckay and Leigh (1991); Piguet *et al.* (1991)
Helicobacter pylori gastritis/ulcer disease	Crabtree *et al.* (1991); Wyle (1991); Blaser (1992)
Paracoccidioidomycosis	Silva and Figueiredo (1991)
Septic melioidosis	Suputtamongkol *et al.* (1992)
Respiratory disease	Kelley (1990); Nohynek *et al.* (1990); Corrigan and Kay (1991); Holtzman (1991); Schleimer *et al.* (1991)
Heart failure	Levine *et al.* (1990)
Familial Mediterranean fever	Schattner *et al.* (1991)
Toxic shock syndrome	Ikejima *et al.* (1988); Jupin *et al.* (1988); Parsonnet and Gillis (1988); Miethke *et al.* (1992)
Chronic fatigue syndrome	Chao *et al.* (1991)
Gastrointestinal disease	Nelson *et al.* (1989a); Bird *et al.* (1990); Schmiegel *et al.* (1991); Treon *et al.* (1991); Whiting *et al.* (1991); Zeni *et al.* (1991)
Allograft rejection/graft-versus-host disease	Halloran *et al.* (1989); Deeg and Henslee-Downey (1990); Krams *et al.* (1992); Nestel *et al.* (1992); Tsuchida *et al.* (1992)
Schistosomiasis	Amiri *et al.* (1992)

of endogenous cytokines (refer to Section III). Leukocyte receptors for endotoxin have been identified that up-regulate and degrade LPS (Hampton *et al.*, 1991; Wright, 1991). One receptor type, CD14, appears to bind a complex of LPS and LPS-binding protein, thereby initiating release of TNFα. The intracellular mechanisms of CD14-mediated TNFα release from macrophages remain to be elucidated. In addition, endotoxin and TNFα release *in vivo* may be augmented by administration of antibiotics to patients with gram-negative infections (Shenep and Mogan, 1984; Shenep *et al.*, 1985; Hurley *et al.*, 1991; Simon *et al.*, 1991).

Evidence that TNFα is a primary mediator of septic shock has accumulated from animal and human studies demonstrating that TNFα administra-

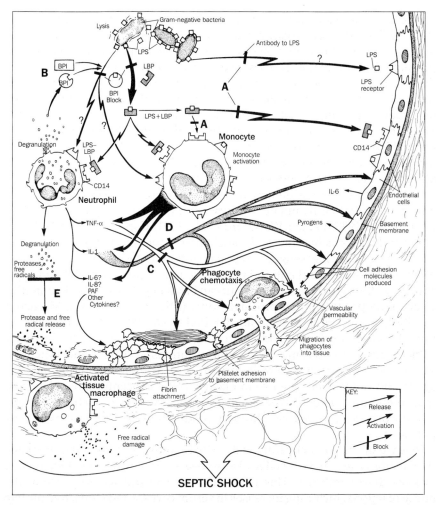

Fig. 3 Cellular and molecular events leading to septic shock. Reproduced from Johnson (1991), ©1991 *The Journal of NIH Research*, Washington, D.C. Reprinted with permission.

tion provoked the signs and symptoms of endotoxin-induced septic shock. Cytokines, including TNFα, trigger inflammatory and metabolic responses attributed to sepsis and septic shock, including the adult respiratory distress syndrome (ARDS), fever, and disseminated intravascular coagulation (Beutler and Cerami, 1987; Michie *et al.*, 1988a; Stephens *et al.*, 1988; Suffredini *et al.*, 1989a; van der Poll *et al.*, 1990).

When recombinant human TNFα was administered to rats in dosages similar to those produced endogenously in response to endotoxin administration, metabolic acidosis, hyperkalemia, and hyperglycemia were observed after infusion, with death occurring minutes to hours later (Tracey *et al.*, 1987a). Multiple organ damage was observed, including diffuse pulmonary and intestinal inflammation as well as acute tubular necrosis. Pathophysiological and histological changes noted after TNFα infusion mimicked those observed after lethal doses of endotoxin (Tracey *et al.*, 1987a). In contrast, animals passively immunized against TNFα were afforded protection against potentially lethal doses of TNFα or LPS (Beutler *et al.*, 1985; Tracey *et al.*, 1987a,b; Mathison *et al.*, 1988). Humans administered recombinant TNFα have also experienced hemodynamic and metabolic derangements resembling responses noted with endotoxinemia (Warren *et al.*, 1987; Sherman *et al.*, 1988; Spriggs *et al.*, 1988).

Several studies have demonstrated that cytokines, particularly TNFα, may contribute to inflammatory injury through eicosanoid activation (Kettelhut *et al.*, 1987; Leeper-Woodford *et al.*, 1991; Carey *et al.*, 1991). These TNFα-induced arachidonic acid metabolites appear to function intracellularly as secondary messengers to escalate inflammatory processes. Pretreatment with nonsteroidal anti-inflammatory agents prior to endotoxin exposure may alter cytokine responses but can block negative feedback inhibition of cytokine production by prostaglandins (Michie *et al.*, 1988a; Martich *et al.*, 1991; Spinas *et al.*, 1991; van der Poll *et al.*, 1991). In one study, an intravenous bolus dose of endotoxin (4 ng/kg body weight) to healthy male subjects increased plasma TNFα concentrations at least 7-fold (Michie *et al.*, 1988b). Pretreatment with ibuprofen, a nonsteroidal antiinflammatory agent, did not prevent the rise in plasma TNFα concentrations. However, ibuprofen attenuated TNFα-mediated responses of fever, tachycardia, and adrenocorticotropin release through modulation of the cyclooxygenase pathway.

Release of platelet activating factor (PAF) appears to be TNFα mediated (Bonavada *et al.*, 1989). TNFα also appears to activate hepatocytes and increase IL-6 synthesis. This effect has been postulated to cause acute-phase reactions, including increases in serum cortisol and C-reactive protein (Andus *et al.*, 1988; Geiger *et al.*, 1988; Michie *et al.*, 1988b; Ramadori *et al.*, 1988; Shalaby *et al.*, 1989; Calandra *et al.*, 1991).

The inflammatory glycopeptide IL-1 also mediates signs and symptoms of septic shock. TNFα can induce IL-1 release from monocytes and endothelial cells, and IL-1 appears to synergize with TNFα (Dinarello *et al.*, 1986; Nawroth *et al.*, 1986a; Waage and Espevik, 1988; Dinarello and Thompson, 1991; McIntyre *et al.*, 1991; Wakabayashi *et al.*, 1991a). Endogenously produced polypeptides inhibitory to IL-1 have been detected in human serum after injection of endotoxin (Dinarello *et al.*, 1981). Endogenous IL-1 antibody was investigated in healthy humans after intravenous boluses of 3–4 ng/kg U.S. standard reference endotoxin (Granowitz *et al.*, 1991). A 100-fold greater increase in IL-1 antibody production was noted relative to IL-1 production; the peak concentration of IL-1 antibody occurred 1–2 hr after the peak concentration of IL-1. Investigators postulated that synthesis of IL-1 antibody was not a consequence of induction by IL-1 alone. Treatment of animals with an exogenous IL-1 receptor antagonist (IL-1ra) has prevented death from endotoxin-induced septic shock (Ohlsson *et al.*, 1990; Alexander *et al.*, 1991). Rabbits pretreated with IL-1ra prior to intravenous injection of *Escherichia coli* experienced mild transient hypotension, compared with sustained profound hypotension observed for untreated controls, and was lethal 50% of the time (Wakabayashi *et al.*, 1991b).

Myocardial depression often accompanies severe septic shock (Parker *et al.*, 1984; Suffredini *et al.*, 1989b). TNFα may be a major contributor to cardiovascular demise (Natanson *et al.*, 1989). In a small uncontrolled study, murine anti-TNFα antibody (2 mg/kg) was administered to 10 patients with septic shock who were unresponsive to conventional treatment (Vincent *et al.*, 1992). Of these patients, 5 were also diagnosed with ARDS. Left ventricular stroke work index was monitored for 8 hr postinfusion, and was statistically increased at 1 and 2 hr postinfusion (from a mean ± SD of 26.5 ± 5.6 g·m^2 at baseline to 31.5 ± 10.5 g·m^2 at 2 hr). However, 8 of 10 patients did not survive more than 17 days after diagnosis of septic shock, including all 5 patients with ARDS. Although more study is needed, treatment of septic shock with anti-TNFα regimens may attenuate and/or reverse some of the adverse cardiovascular events observed in patients. How these improvements may translate into improved survival are unclear.

Although a detailed review of these agents is beyond the scope of this chapter, various agents useful or potentially useful in the treatment of sepsis have been developed that are directed against endotoxin, IL-1, and TNFα (Bone, 1991b). These agents include monoclonal antibodies against TNFα and TNFα receptors (Calandra and Glauser, 1990; Cohen, 1990; Espevik *et al.*, 1990; Exley *et al.*, 1990; Shalaby *et al.*, 1990), TNFα receptor immunoadhesion molecule (Ashkenazi *et al.*, 1991), limulus antilipopolysaccharide factor (Alpert *et al.*, 1992), and soluble receptors for TNFα, which could sequester TNFα *in vivo* (Veterans Administration Systemic Sepsis Cooperative Study Group, 1987). Some evidence exists that these soluble receptors may augment, rather than inhibit, TNFα activity in a concentration-dependent manner (Aderka *et al.*, 1992). Additional studies are needed to clarify the potential clinical usefulness of soluble TNFα receptors. Glucocorticoids inhibit TNFα biosynthesis by inhibiting mRNA transcription and preventing its translation (Beutler *et al.*, 1986). However, TNFα production appears to be inhibited only if corticosteroids are administered prior to LPS-induced macrophage activation. Human trials to date using high dose corticosteroids have not uniformly prevented mortality in patients with sepsis and septic shock (Bone and the Methylprednisolone Severe Sepsis Study Group, 1987; Engelmann *et al.*, 1989).

Considerable controversy and conjecture exists over when best to administer therapeutic interventions against TNFα. Aggressive intervention before documentation of bacteremia or shock has been proposed as the optimal therapeutic window (Bone, 1991c). Although TNFα has a short half-life of approximately 14–18 min, patients with septic shock may have chronically elevated plasma TNFα concentrations (Calandra *et al.*, 1990; Vincent *et al.*, 1992). TNFα also plays a part in arming the immune system as a host defense mechanism (Czuprynski *et al.*, 1992), but variable concentrations of TNFα interact with individual factors of host response to bacteremia, sepsis, and septic shock caused by a variety of organisms. Therefore, identifying a uniformly predictable niche for optimal therapeutic intervention with varying antisepsis agents, including those directed against TNFα, is inherently difficult.

B. Adult Respiratory Distress Syndrome

ARDS manifests itself after certain pulmonary and systemic disorders such as smoke inhalation, pancreatitis, the sepsis syndrome, and long-bone fractures. This syndrome is characterized by increased pulmonary capillary permeability resulting in noncardiogenic pulmonary edema, decreased lung compliance, and decreased lung volume. In addition, multiple organ dysfunction can occur that can deteriorate into multiple organ failure (Bone *et al.*, 1992). Approximately 150,000 cases of ARDS occur in the United States annually, with a mortality rate of about 50% (Murray *et al.*, 1988).

ARDS is frequently associated with sepsis, occurring in 5–40% of septic patients (Bone *et al.*, 1992). Evidence suggests that endogenous cytokines enhance and sustain the pulmonary inflammatory responses observed in patients with sepsis and ARDS (Tabor *et al.*, 1988; Jacobs *et al.*, 1989; refer also to Section IV,A). In particular, TNFα appears to be an important mediator of sepsis-induced ARDS. A TNFα receptor has been identified in human lung tissue (Shepherd and Abdolrasulnia, 1989). Alveolar macrophages are believed to account for production of TNFα and other inflammatory mediators observed in sepsis-induced ARDS. These macrophages secrete chemotactic peptides that sequester neutrophils into pulmonary interstitium and air spaces. Some of the peptides identified are monocyte-derived chemotactic factor, monocyte-derived neutrophil-activating peptide, neutrophil activating peptide 1, macrophage inflammatory proteins 1 and 2, and interleukin 8 (Rinaldo and Christman, 1990; Nahum *et al.*, 1991). TNFα contributes to acute lung injury through mechanisms such as induction of IL-1 production (Nawroth *et al.*, 1986b; Tracey *et al.*, 1988), activation of polymorphonuclear leukocytes (PMNs) (Shalaby *et al.*, 1985), and endothelial cell monolayer rearrangement (Stolpen *et al.*, 1986). Proinflammatory mediators, including TNFα, have been observed to initiate and amplify the production of factors responsible for the pathophysiological processes of ARDS. These factors include procoagulants, neutrophil oxygen radicals, endothelial activation antigens, and eicosanoids (Stolpen *et al.*,

1986; Kettelhut *et al.*, 1987; Leeper-Woodford *et al.*, 1991; Carey *et al.*, 1991). PGE$_2$, in turn, has been demonstrated to inhibit TNFα production transcriptionally through increases in intracellular cyclic AMP (cAMP; Kunkel *et al.*, 1988; Lehmmann *et al.*, 1988; Renz *et al.*, 1988). The synthesis and release of PAF from macrophages, PMNs, and vascular endothelial cells appears to be induced by TNFα (Camussi *et al.*, 1987; Bussolini *et al.*, 1988; Thivierge and Rola-Pleszczynski, 1991). TNFα also synthesizes endothelial cell-surface adhesive glycoproteins (ELAM-1) that bind leukocytes capable of injuring vascular endothelial cells (Bevilacqua *et al.*, 1987).

Several animal and human studies have documented adverse effects of PAF on pulmonary function, the net effect of which is acutely decreased lung compliance and increased total pulmonary resistance, as well as increased airway hyperresponsiveness (McManus and Deavers, 1989). Sheep prepared with chronic lung lymph fistulas were challenged with TNFα to assess the effects of a PAF receptor antagonist on TNFα-induced vasoconstriction and plasma–lymph protein transport (Horvath *et al.*, 1991). Results showed that initial increases in pulmonary arterial pressure and pulmonary vascular resistance were prevented after TNFα challenge. The possibility that pulmonary vasoconstriction was due to cyclooxygenase metabolites was not ruled out. TNFα-induced increases in pulmonary lymph flow and transvascular protein clearance were not affected by PAF antagonism.

When recombinant human TNFα (rHuTNFα) was infused into mice in quantities similar to those produced endogenously in response to endotoxin, extensive end-organ damage occurred. Gross and histopathological damage to the lungs included diffuse inflammation, arterial occlusion, and punctate hemorrhages (Tracey *et al.*, 1986). Guinea pigs injected with rHuTNFα developed increased pulmonary permeability, peripheral neutropenia, systemic hypotension, and pulmonary edema similar to that observed in *E. coli*-induced septic guinea pigs (Stephens *et al.*, 1988). In an investigation of LPS induction of TNFα activity and the pulmonary inflammatory response, rats were challenged intravenously or intratracheally with *E. coli* LPS (Nelson *et al.*, 1989b). TNFα detected in serum and bronchoalveolar fluid was confined to the respective LPS-challenged compartments. A pulmonary inflammatory response with migration of PMNs into alveoli occurred with intratracheally but not intravenously administered LPS. TNFα was detected in the bronchopulmonary secretions of 5 patients diagnosed with septic and nonseptic ARDS (a mean TNFα level of 13.1 ng/ml compared with undetectable TNFα in 24 control patients; Millar *et al.*, 1989). In another small study, elevated TNFα levels were found in bronchoalveolar lavage fluid (range, 62–94 pg/ml) and not plasma from 3 of 4 patients with ARDS (Roberts *et al.*, 1989).

Another study demonstrated an association between plasma TNFα concentrations and development of ARDS (Marks *et al.*, 1990). In this study, early steroid treatment of patients in septic shock was not found to decrease plasma TNFα concentrations. Another study determined TNFα levels in bronchoalveolar lavage fluid or serum of 22 patients with ARDS and 20 patients determined to be at high risk for ARDS (Hyers *et al.*, 1991). Of these 22 ARDS patients, 14 were described as having sepsis or serious infection, and 10 of 20 high risk patients were described as having sepsis or serious infection. Mean bronchoalveolar fluid TNFα levels for ARDS patients were significantly higher than those in normal subjects. Mean bronchoalveolar levels of TNFα for high-risk ARDS patients were not statistically different from those of normal subjects, possibly because of greater variability in the data. TNFα levels in patients with ARDS or at high risk for ARDS were not statistically different from those in normal subjects. Levels of TNFα in serum and bronchoalveolar lavage fluid of survivors and nonsurvivors were not statistically different. Caution must be used in interpreting the relationship between cytokine concentrations in body fluids and outcome, because biological effects of cytokines may not be directly correlated with their concentration. A porcine model demonstrated that plasma TNFα and TNFβ were elevated in septic animals (Leeper-Woodford *et al.*, 1991). The increase in plasma TNFα and TNFβ activity, which peaked at 90–120 min postinfusion, correlated with development of increased lung water, pulmonary artery hypertension, decreased lung compliance, and deteriorating gas exchange.

In summary, TNFα plays a significant role in enhancing the inflammatory processes of ARDS and contributes to vascular leakiness as a consequence of endothelial tissue reorganization. Agents that inhibit TNFα activity are anticipated to be useful for effective prevention and treatment of ARDS.

C. Acquired Immunodeficiency Syndrome

Patients infected with the human immunodeficiency virus (HIV) enter a long period of clinical latency prior to developing clinically apparent disease. Estimates of the average time from infection to progression into the acquired immunodeficiency syndrome (AIDS) have varied, but the average time appears to be between 8 and 11 yr (Lifson *et al.*, 1988). After infection with HIV, patients become clinically asymptomatic. A portion of the viral population enters biological latency or chronic, low-level viral expression because of decreased or absent posttranscriptional protein production. The complex mechanisms by which clinically stable, asymptomatic HIV infection deteriorates to rapidly progressing disease with an increased cellular HIV deoxyribonucleic acid burden are under investigation. Progression of AIDS is a result of continued functional impairment of the immune system, especially in the CD4$^+$ T cell helper/inducer subset, by HIV. HIV integrates itself into the immunoregulatory network, altering hemeostatic mechanisms of resistance through manipulation of cytokine secretion. HIV infects

T cells as well as monocytes and macrophages. Activation of latent or marginally active HIV-infected cells may be promoted in part by cytokines, including TNFα (Ito *et al.*, 1989; Matsuyama *et al.*, 1989; Vayakarnam *et al.*, 1990).

Cultured monocytes infected with HIV and treated with macrophage colony stimulating factor (M-CSF) demonstrated a transcriptional block in interferon α gene expression, indicating that HIV replication may also be enhanced by viral inhibition of interferon α (Gendelman *et al.*, 1990). This impairment is proposed to cause increased immune complex formation and inflammatory tissue damage as a result of HIV infection and activation of monocytes. An increase in TNFα secretion and lymphotoxins appears to result (Morrow *et al.*, 1991). Resting T cells do not contain actively replicating HIV, but the virus becomes transcriptionally active as a result of exposure of the T cell to various stimuli, including cytokines (such as IL-1 and TNFα), mitogens, and the gene products of certain viruses such as herpesvirus, adenovirus, cytomegalovirus, human T cell leukemia virus type I, Epstein–Barr virus, and hepatitis B virus (Lifson *et al.*, 1988; Meltzer *et al.*, 1990; Rosenberg and Fauci, 1990).

Determining activation of HIV expression in latent or chronically infected host cells has been facilitated by investigating cytokine-triggered induction of HIV expression in T cell and monocyte cell lines. A promonocyte cell line (U937) and a T lymphocyte cell line (A3.01) were infected with HIV, then cloned to form chronically HIV-infected U1 and ACH-2 cell lines, respectively. These cell lines constitutively express low-to-undetectable levels of HIV, as determined by reverse transcriptase (RT) and antigen capture assays. Expression of HIV by these cell lines can be induced by exposure to cytokine-rich crude supernatant from mononuclear cells activated with phytohemagglutinin (PHA) or from LPS-activated monocytes, or by exposure to PMA (Rosenberg and Fauci, 1990; Fauci, 1991). Reports have also indicated that TNFα and TNFβ have antiviral activity, but the overall benefits of this characteristic in HIV infection are unknown. *In vitro*, this activity has been postulated to vary according to the particular cultured cell line used in experimentation (Matsuyama *et al.*, 1988).

TNFα, as opposed to IL-6 or GM-CSF, induces HIV expression in chronically infected U1 and ACH-2 cell lines. IL-6 and GM-CSF have induced HIV expression in the U1 cell line only. In an investigation of the regulatory effects of recombinant TNFα and TNFβ, ACH-2 cells were exposed to selected cytokines and RT activity was measured. TNFα and TNFβ induced HIV expression by roughly 400%, whereas interleukins 1–4, platelet-derived growth factor (PDGF), and IFNγ had no effect on HIV expression (Folks *et al.*, 1989).

Up-regulation of HIV expression by TNFα also appears to be synergistic with other cytokines, including IL-6, in an autocrine and paracrine manner similar to the cytokine regulation of the normal immune response (Poli *et* al., 1990a). An investigation of the autocrine mechanisms of TNFα-mediated HIV induction revealed that stimulation of U1 and ACH-2 cells with PMA induced production of TNFα mRNA as well as TNFα secretion. Expression of HIV was suppressed by anti-TNFα antibodies in PMA-stimulated U1 and ACH-2 cells, and in the chronically infected promonocytic clone U33.3 with or without PMA stimulation (Poli et al., 1990b). Primary human macrophages infected with HIV in vitro have yielded similar results (Mellors et al., 1991).

Mechanisms of TNFα-induced HIV expression appear to include transcriptional activation of HIV mRNA. Initiation of HIV mRNA synthesis has been activated by TNFα in the chronically infected ACH-2 cell line. This effect was attributed to transcriptional activation of HIV long terminal repeat sequences (Osborn et al., 1989). Genomic HIV long terminal repeat contains regulatory sequences that are recognized by host transcription factors for expression of HIV genes. Nuclear factor κB binds in the core enhancer region of the HIV proviral long terminal repeat (Duh et al., 1989; Osborn et al., 1989); TNFα enhances HIV up-regulation by inducing production of host-derived NF-κB-binding proteins to initiate transcription of HIV mRNA (Osborn et al., 1989). Up-regulation of lymphocyte-tropic (human T lymphotropic virus type III_B) and macrophage-tropic (human T lymphotropic virus type III_{BaL}) HIV production in primary blood monocyte-derived macrophages has been observed by incubation of these cells with recombinant TNFα starting before or after viral infection. Concentrations of TNFα used were similar to serum levels produced endogenously in response to various human diseases, including AIDS and AIDS-related complex (ARC). Conflicting findings were observed by Kornbluth et al. (1989) for a similar model of $HTLV-III_{BaL}$ replication; these differences were postulated to result from methodological differences and a difference in duration of monocyte treatment with TNFα.

Some evidence suggests that adrenocorticotropic hormone (ACTH) and melanocyte-stimulating hormone (MSH) production are produced intracellularly by HIV-infected H9 T lymphoma cells, resulting in inactivation of human granulocytes (Smith et al., 1992). These immunomodulatory actions of ACTH and MSH may enhance HIV replication, possibly through their influence on enhancing cytokine production, including release of TNFα (Smith et al., 1992).

Various studies have been conducted to detect the presence of TNFα in HIV-infected patients. TNFα has been detected in the serum of patients with AIDS and generalized lymphadenopathy (Lähdevirta et al., 1988; Reddy et al., 1988). This cytokine has been implicated in the pathogenesis of fever and cachexia (wasting syndrome) in AIDS patients (Lähdevirta et al., 1988). A study of the association of serum TNFα concentrations with AIDS clinically classified patients into four groups according to Centers for Disease Control criteria: asymptomatic patients, or patients with lymphadenopathy syndrome, ARC, or AIDS. Serum levels of TNFα were measured in patients using a double-antibody radioimmunoassay. Of 8 asymptomatic patients and 13 lymphadenopathy subjects, 8 and 11, respectively, had serum TNFα levels within control values. In contrast, TNF serum levels were increased relative to controls for 5 of 9 ARC patients and 9 of 9 AIDS patients. Follow-up of the AIDS and ARC patients revealed persistently increased but fluctuating TNF serum concentrations. Mean serum TNF concentrations were higher for AIDS patients than for ARC patients, although the TNF levels were not qualitatively related to degrees of weight loss. Because AIDS patients are usually co-infected with several different opportunistic organisms, the increased TNF concentrations probably were related to the presence of these secondarily acquired microbes as well and not to HIV infection alone. TNFα has also been detected in rectal mucosal tissue of HIV-infected patients, most likely from intestinal macrophage secretion (Reka and Kotler, 1991). In addition, TNFα has been detected in peripheral blood monocytes (PBMCs) isolated from AIDS patients (Wright et al., 1988; Roux-Lombard et al., 1989). In another investigation, isolated PBMCs, infected with HIV in vivo and in vitro spontaneously secreted more TNFα than PBMCs from uninfected controls (Merrell et al., 1989; Roux-Lombard et al., 1989). IL-1β levels secreted from PBMCs of symptomatic HIV-infected patients and from monocytes infected in vitro were also elevated relative to uninfected controls. Monocytes infected with HIV in vivo with IFNγ and E. coli LPS increased TNFα production; the highest production was noted for symptomatic HIV-infected patients (Roux-Lombard et al., 1989). Other studies showed that macrophages infected with HIV in vitro failed to produce detectable IL-1β, IL-6, or TNFα prior to stimulation with LPS (Molina et al., 1989, 1990; Munis et al., 1990; Peters et al., 1991).

The number of Mycobacterium tuberculosis cases reported annually in the United States has dramatically increased since 1984. This unprecedented resurgence is largely related to the HIV epidemic, and has been referred to as one of the greatest public health disasters since the bubonic plague (Chaisson and Slutkin, 1989; Barnes et al., 1991). In patients with tuberculosis, perturbations in the immunoregulatory pathway are observed that appear to include IFNγ and calcitriol activation of macrophages, thus inducing the synthesis and release of TNFα from these cells (Rook and Attiyah, 1991). Inhibition of lipoprotein lipase by TNFα has been associated with hypertriglyceridemia in patients with pulmonary tuberculosis, resulting in a hypercatabolic state and cachexia (Silva et al., 1988). Efforts are being made to develop improved skin test reagents and to identify vaccines against M. tuberculosis, but AIDS patients with tuberculosis represent a particularly difficult challenge in diagnosis. Reduction of TNFα attributed to concomitant HIV and tuberculosis infection has been identified as a major target of therapeutic intervention worldwide. Anti-TNFα regimens in combination with chemotherapy or immunotherapy may be effective for the prophylaxis and containment of tuberculosis by reducing progression and spread of the disease.

D. Inflammatory Bowel Disease

Ulcerative colitis and Crohn's disease represent two common forms of inflammatory bowel disease, and share many pathophysiological properties. The cause of inflammatory bowel disease is unknown. Ulcerative colitis inflammation is confined to the mucosa and superficial submucosa of the large bowel. Nonspecific histopathological features include microabscesses within crypts, depletion of mucin from goblet cells, and dense infiltration of the lamina propria with neutrophils, lymphocytes, and other inflammatory constituents (Podolski, 1991a). Crohn's disease is also characterized by an inflammatory infiltrate, and collagen deposition is common. This disease typically includes areas of patchy inflammation with transmural involvement of the terminal ileum, colon, or both (Podolski, 1991a). Extraintestinal complications of inflammatory bowel disease include axial arthritis, oligoarticular arthritis, and inflammation of the eyes and skin (Podolski, 1991b).

Alterations in the intestinal immunoregulatory network have been implicated in inflammatory bowel disease. Whether these alterations in immune function are partly or wholly responsible for the initiation of inflammatory bowel disease, or whether they are the reactive manifestations of other causative factors, remains unknown. The altered immune response observed in inflammatory bowel disease may be attributable to overactivity of this response in addition to a lack of normally occurring down-regulation processes. The number and constitution of intestinal immunoactive cells is altered in ulcerative colitis and Crohn's disease and includes increases in tissue macrophages, lymphocytes, and PAF (Eliakim *et al.*, 1988; Arato *et al.*, 1989; Mahida, 1990). A decreased number of suppressor/inducer T cells has also been reported (Moore *et al.*, 1988; Mayer and Eisenhart, 1990).

Cytokines, including TNFα, play an important role in the pathogenic processes of inflammatory bowel disease. Cytokine-mediated chronic alterations in the morphology and renewal of epithelial cells associated with inflammatory bowel disease may contribute to the increased risk of cancer, particularly colorectal cancer, in these patients (Jarry *et al.*, 1991; Mansour *et al.*, 1991; Podolski, 1991b; Schürer-Maly *et al.*, 1991). Increases in cytokine-mediated induction of tissue and peripheral blood cytolytic T lymphocytes and lymphokine-induced activated killer cells have also been implicated as pathophysiological mechanisms of inflammatory bowel disease; however, current supporting evidence is controversial (Mayer, 1990; Ogata *et al.*, 1991; Podolski, 1991a).

Several investigations have detected TNFα and IL-1β in mucosal tissue and serum of patients with inflammatory bowel disease (Deusch *et al.*, 1991; Duclos *et al.*, 1991; Mansour *et al.*, 1991; Noguchi *et al.*, 1991; Podolski, 1991a; Pullman *et al.*, 1991; Reimund *et al.*, 1991). Interleukin 2 (IL-2) and soluble IL-2 receptors isolated from the lamina propria have been found to be decreased in patients with Crohn's disease and ulcerative colitis (Fiocchi *et al.*, 1984). Identification of the factors that may be responsible for this phenomenon have revealed that inflammatory bowel disease may produce a deficiency in the number of IL-2-secreting mucosal helper T cells or may generate the production of inhibitory factors (Kusagami *et al.*, 1991). In contrast, serum samples from patients with active Crohn's disease have been found to have increased IL-2 and soluble IL-2 receptor concentrations (Brynskov and Tvede, 1990). Mucosal biopsy specimens from patients with ulcerative colitis and Crohn's disease have been found to contain increased local concentrations of IL-1β, IL-2, and soluble Il-2 receptors (Brynskov *et al.*, 1992). Another investigation has identified increased mucosal concentrations of IL-8, a neutrophil-attracting chemotactic molecule, during active ulcerative colitis (Mahida *et al.*, 1991). Expression of the cytokine-activated endothelial cell surface glycoprotein ELAM and intercellular adhesion molecule 1 (ICAM-1) on mononuclear phagocytes has also been identified (Malizia *et al.*, 1991; Podolski, 1991a).

An *in vitro* experiment investigated the morphological effects of TNFα and IFNγ on a fully differentiated goblet cell line (CL.16E; Jarry *et al.*, 1991). Treatment of the cells with IFNγ and TNFα produced a synergistic dose-related necrosis, with formation of a mucoid cap over viable epithelial cells. Neither cytokine induced these changes when employed alone.

Increased stool TNFα concentrations have been identified in children with moderate to severe active Crohn's disease or active ulcerative colitis (Braegger *et al.*, 1992). Concentrations of TNFα in the stools of patients with inactive inflammatory bowel disease as a consequence of right hemicolectomy or steroid treatment did not differ from TNFα levels detected in control patients. Whether stool TNFα concentrations fluctuate predictably with the degree of inflammatory bowel disease severity is currently unknown.

E. Bacterial Meningitis

Endotoxin is associated with gram-negative bacterial meningitis. Some antibiotics may liberate endotoxin and cell wall products that induce an inflammatory response (Berman *et al.*, 1976; Shenep and Mogan, 1984; Shenep *et al.*, 1985; Tuomanen *et al.*, 1985a,b; Täuber *et al.*, 1987; Hurley *et al.*, 1991; Simon *et al.*, 1991). Diffuse cerebral swelling and edema may be a prominent feature of bacterial meningitis in some patients, although the pathogenesis is unclear (Swartz, 1984). One possible mechanism is cytotoxic edema, in which diffusible inflammatory products originate in the meningeal exudate and exert cytotoxic effects on the cerebellum (Täuber *et al.*, 1987).

TNFα and other cytokines have been detected locally in cerebrospinal fluid in patients with bacterial meningitis (Leist *et al.*, 1988; Mustafa *et al.*, 1989b; Waage *et al.*, 1989b). TNF was detected in serum from 79 patients with meningococcal meningitis, sepsis (not defined), or both (Waage *et al.*,

1987). Of these patients, TNF was detected in 10 of 11 nonsurvivors and in 8 of 68 survivors. None of the patients with serum TNF concentrations >440 units/ml (>0.1 ng/ml recombinant TNF) survived.

Complex patterns of interacting cytokines and products of arachidonic acid metabolism produced locally in the central nervous system have been implicated in contributing to adverse sequelae of bacterial meningitis (Kadurugamuwa et al., 1987; Tureen et al., 1987; Saukkonen et al., 1990). Waage and colleagues (1989b) detected elevated levels of TNFα, IL-1, and IL-6 in serum of 79 patients with meningococcal septic shock. These patients were considered to have septic shock if their systolic blood pressure was ≤70 mm Hg (patients ≤12 years old) or ≤100 mm Hg (patients >12 years old). Researchers concluded that high levels of these cytokines interacted and potentiated their individual contributions to fatal outcome (Waage et al., 1989a). In addition, analysis of the relative time course of cytokine release indicated that TNFα was released prior to IL-6.

Inhibition of inflammatory pathways appears to be beneficial in treatment of bacterial meningitis. The nonsteroidal anti-inflammatory agent indomethacin decreased serum protein influx into the cerebrospinal fluid and prevented brain edema in rabbits, presumably by inhibition of the cyclooxygenase pathway (Tureen et al., 1987). Corticosteroids may be useful as adjunct therapy for bacterial meningitis because of their anti-inflammatory effects. These beneficial effects may ultimately be through modulation of the activated cytokine network, including TNFα (Lebel et al., 1988). Studies of systemic corticosteroids have not always had favorable outcomes, possibly because of difficulties in methodology and interpretation (Lebel et al., 1988).

Cerebrospinal fluid samples were obtained on hospital admission from 106 infants and children with bacterial meningitis (Mustafa et al., 1989a). On admission, the samples contained increased levels of IL-1β for 95% of the patients and increased levels of TNFα for 75% of the patients. The mean IL-1β concentration in cerebrospinal fluid was 944 ± 1293 pg/ml and the mean TNFα concentration was 787 ± 3358 pg/ml. In cerebrospinal fluid samples obtained 18–30 hr after admission, IL-1β and TNFα were still detectable for roughly half the patients. Dexamethasone therapy was started at the time of diagnosis for 47 of 106 patients (0.6 mg/kg/day in 4 divided doses over 4 days). Statistically significantly lower mean IL-1β concentrations in cerebrospinal fluid were found for the dexamethasone-treated group compared with the placebo group; no difference between these two groups for TNFα concentrations was detectable. In addition, a statistically signficant inverse correlation existed between cerebrospinal fluid IL-1β concentrations and improvement in meningeal inflammation indices and outcome from disease. Investigators postulated that dexamethasone was beneficial because of inhibition of IL-1β production, although dexamethasone was administered after macrophage activation by LPS.

Cerebrospinal fluid concentrations of PGE_2, PGI_2, IL-1β, and TNF were measured on diagnosis and approximately 24 hr later in 80 infants and children with bacterial meningitis (Mustafa *et al.*, 1989c). Dexamethasone was administered as adjunct therapy to 40 patients (0.6 mg/kg/day in 4 divided doses for 4 consecutive days). All patients with detectable IL-1β activity in their first cerebrospinal fluid sample continued to have this activity 18–30 hr later. PGE_2, TNF, and PGI_2 were still detected to a lesser extent compared to the first cerebrospinal fluid sample. Patients with no detectable PGE_2, PGI_2, or IL-1β activity 18–30 hr after their first cerebrospinal fluid sample had statistically shorter fever duration, a lower incidence of neurological sequelae, lower cerebrospinal fluid protein concentrations, and higher cerebrospinal fluid glucose concentrations. The 18 to 30-hr cerebrospinal fluid samples obtained from dexamethasone-treated patients contained statistically higher glucose and lower lactate concentrations; these patients had shorter fever duration and a lower incidence of neurological sequelae than placebo-treated patients. In summary, further studies are needed to evaluate different cytokine modulators and anti-inflammatory agents for treatment of bacterial meningitis.

F. Rheumatoid Arthritis

Rheumatoid arthritis is a heterogeneous systemic disease of unknown etiology. Persons with rheumatoid arthritis typically develop inflammation of joint synovium (synovitis; see Section VI). Clinical symptoms become apparent with progression of synovitis because of production and release of cytokines from activated macrophages as well as activation of T lymphocytes, angiogenesis, and attraction of neutrophils to the joint cavities (Harris, 1990). Cytokines induce synovial cell proliferation, resulting in invasion and destruction of articular cartilage (Figure 4). Synovial fibroblasts are thought to become activated by pro-inflammatory mediators such as TNFα to secrete a large variety of cytokines and growth factors (Bucala *et al.*, 1991). TNFα activity in rheumatoid arthritis includes recruitment and activation of PMNs, cellular proliferation, increased prostaglandin and matrix-degrading protease activity, fever, and bone and cartilage resorption (Beutler and Cerami, 1987). Rheumatoid synovial fluid appears to include predominantly macrophage-derived products such as IL-1α, IL-1β, IL-6, TNFα, and IL-8, although disagreement has arisen over the exact cytokine composition (Westacott *et al.*, 1990; Feldmann *et al.*, 1992). The relative composition of cytokine presence in synovial fluid may be influenced *in vivo* by variables such as disease severity and stage of progression. Pro-inflammatory mediators such as TNFα and TNFα-induced IL-1 induce synthesis of collagenase and stromelysin by synoviocytes (Case *et al.*, 1989; McCachren *et al.*, 1990), contributing to loss of normal joint integrity and function. Cellular expression of MHC class II molecules within the joint microenvironment is a

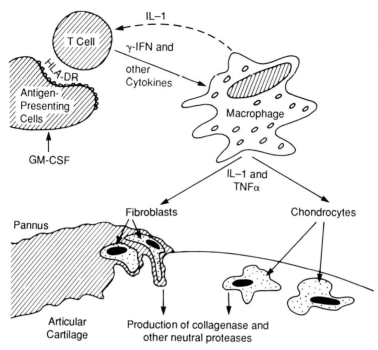

Fig. 4 Cytokine interactions in rheumatoid arthritis. Reproduced with permission from Arend and Dayer (1990).

predominant feature of rheumatoid arthritis. This expression induces production of a complex network of cytokines. IL-8 may be responsible for accumulation of neutrophils in the joint cavity, and its production may be stimulated by IL-1 and TNFα (Brennan *et al.*, 1990).

Significant differences may exist between effects of cytokines on the systemic immune response and their local influences in the joint. These differences remain to be determined. A study of lung involvement as an extraarticular manifestation of rheumatoid arthritis examined TNFα release from alveolar macrophages in 31 patients with and without interstitial lung disease (Gosset *et al.*, 1991). Similar amounts of biologically active alveolar macrophage-derived TNFα were detected in 14 patients with and 17 patients without interstitial lung disease, compared with healthy controls. LPS-stimulated alveolar macrophages from both patient groups also released statistically higher TNFα levels relative to healthy controls. IL-1 production and release was not statistically different in either group of rheumatoid arthritis patients from that in healthy controls. Although the data were not published, Gosset and colleagues (1991) also reported that LPS did not increase IL-1 release from stimulated alveolar macrophages in either patient group relative to healthy controls.

G. Malaria

Throughout the tropics and subtropics, between 200 and 400 million people are infected with malaria (Cox, 1991). Malarial parasites are protozoa belonging to the genus *Plasmodium*. Four species infect humans: *P. falciparum*, *P. vivax*, *P. malariae*, and *P. ovale*. The most severe complication of *P. falciparum* malaria is cerebral malaria, which is responsible for over 1 million deaths annually in sub-Saharan African children (Grau *et al.*, 1987). In The Gambia, West Africa, *P. falciparum* malaria is responsible for approximately 25% of all deaths in children aged 1–4 yr (Brewster *et al.*, 1990). Resistance by the mosquito vector to insecticides, and increasing parasite resistance to conventional antimalarial drugs, makes development of effective new therapeutic strategies an urgent goal.

TNFα has been identified as a major cytokine responsible for the pathobiology of malaria and cerebral malaria. TNFα, possibly in combination with other cytokines and mediators yet to be identified, has also been demonstrated to be toxic to malarial parasites, but this concentration- and time-dependent effect has not been demonstrated to be an antimalarial treatment (Haidaris *et al.*, 1983; Clark *et al.*, 1989; Mendis *et al.*, 1990; Cook, 1991; Naotunne *et al.*, 1991). Kwaitkowski and co-workers (1989) proposed that TNFα mediates malarial fever in humans, and also concluded that ruptured schizonts paroxysmally release TNFα from monocytes and activated macrophages in patients with malaria.

The pathobiological mechanisms of cerebral malaria are unknown, but researchers have theorized that neurological deficits due to cerebral malaria are caused by metabolic derangements associated with parasitized erythrocyte adherence to cerebral capillaries and subsequent oxygen depletion (Grau *et al.*, 1987; Warrell, 1987; Cook, 1991). In addition, TNFα-induced thrombospondin secretion has also been proposed to increase sequestration of erythrocytes indirectly (Clark *et al.*, 1989). However, the erythrocyte adherence theory by itself may not adequately explain the mechanism(s) involved. As an alternative mechanism, cerebral accumulation and activation of macrophages, with subsequent TNFα production and release, have been proposed as major factors in the observed predominance of lesions within the central nervous system. However, currently no definitive evidence for this proposal exists (Haidaris *et al.*, 1983; Brewster *et al.*, 1990). TNFα has been implicated in altering endothelial permeability and promoting endothelial adherence of parasitized erythrocytes, which could promote cerebral edema and vascular stasis in brain tissue (Wyler, 1988). Cytokines such as TNFα, present locally in high concentrations, have also been proposed to influence neurological sequelae through induction of nitric oxide from endothelial cells and vascular smooth muscle (Clark *et al.*, 1991). Nitric oxide, through diffusion into nearby neurons, has been theorized to interfere with neurotransmission and to contribute to cerebral vasodilation observed in cerebral malaria (Clark *et al.*, 1991).

The mechanisms by which TNFα potentially contributes to morbidity and mortality of malaria are under investigation. Investigators have demonstrated that, in mice, TNFα is secreted from macrophages in response to malarial infection (Bate et al., 1988). Exogenous TNFα administered to P. berghei-infected mice accelerates development of the cerebral syndrome (Curfs et al., 1990). Treatment with anti-TNFα antibodies protects mice from cerebral complications of this organism (Grau et al., 1987). Serum TNFα has been detected in patients with parasitic infections, including malaria (Scuderi et al., 1986). In another study, elevated serum levels of TNFα were detected in 65 children with P. falciparum malaria. These increased TNFα levels were correlated with increased severity of illness and increased mortality (Grau et al., 1989). Likewise, Shaffer and co-workers (1991) detected higher TNFα concentrations in 61 children with detectable P. falciparum parasitemia compared with 26 aparasitemic ill children (TNFα geometric means of 71 pg/ml and 10 pg/ml, respectively). In addition, TNFα levels increased directly with increasing P. falciparum parasite densities. Plasma TNFα concentrations were equally elevated in 9 children with cerebral malaria and in 31 children with severe malaria.

In a study conducted by Kern and co-workers (1989), the roles of IL-6, TNFα, and IFNγ were investigated in 40 adults with malaria caused by P. falciparum or P. vivax. In this investigation, elevated levels of all three cytokines were detected in over half the patients infected with P. falciparum. In addition, increased serum levels of TNFα and IL-6 were correlated with increasing organ involvement, including infection of brain tissue, in 12 of 18 patients. Although its role is uncertain, host IL-6 production in response to infection with malarial parasites may be induced in part by TNFα (Grau et al., 1990). In another investigation, elevated levels of serum TNFα, increased plasma thrombin–antithrombin III levels, and decreased levels of plasma anticoagulant protein C were described in patients with P. falciparum malaria. High serum TNFα levels correlated with higher degrees of parasitemia, lower protein C activity, and increased prothrombin time, partial thromboplastin time, and plasma fibrinogen levels (Hemmer et al., 1991). Parasitized erythrocytes and malarial proteins have been demonstrated to interact with macrophages in vivo and in vitro to induce TNFα production. Attempts to develop effective treatments for cerebral malaria include a vaccine directed against TNFα, which has been reported to have equivocal results in humans (Cox, 1991; Naotunne et al., 1991).

V. Design of TNFα Inhibitors

Although TNFα appears to play a direct role in a number of diseases and syndromes, TNFα has been most extensively investigated as a causative agent in the pathogenesis of septic shock. The most advanced therapies undergoing preclinical and clinical evaluations for sepsis are with anti-

TNF monoclonal antibodies, TNFα binding proteins, and soluble TNFα receptors. In addition, Xoma and Centacor are two companies that have sought Food and Drug Administration (FDA) approval for clinical testing using anti-LPS monoclonal antibodies for the treatment of gram-negative sepsis. The use of biotechnology products in long-term treatment regimens or in chronic diseases might be limited because of their potentially prohibitive expense to hospitals and patients (Schulman *et al.*, 1991), as well as the potential immunogenicity of large molecular weight proteins. Therefore, the synthesis of small molecular weight inhibitors of TNFα biosynthesis, processing, and release is predicted to become a major focus for rational drug design. Ideally, these drugs should exert inhibitory effects as a consequence of their interaction with the target without affecting the viability or normal function of resident macrophages.

A. Potential Targets for the Design of TNFα Inhibitors

Several inhibitors of TNFα biosynthesis have been published over the last several years. However, their molecular mechanisms of action are not well known or understood. A list of molecular targets for which some TNFα inhibitors have been demonstrated to exert an effect, or potential targets for future drug design, is given in Table II. Table III lists compounds currently under development for the treatment of TNFα-related diseases which interfere with several of these targets.

B. Signal Transduction, Transcription, and Translation of the TNFα Gene

Pentoxifylline (PNF; Figure 5) has been shown to prevent LPS-induced lethality in mice and rabbits (Schönharting and Schade, 1989; Noel *et al.*, 1990). This reduction in lethality has been attributed to the ability of PNF to inhibit TNFα production selectively without affecting IL-1 (Berman *et al.*, 1990). PNF does not appear to be working at adenosine receptors. PNF is an inhibitor of phosphodiesterase, which causes an increase in cyclic adenosine monophosphate (cAMP) levels. The increased levels of cAMP have been shown to block accumulation of TNFα mRNA (Noel *et al.*, 1990). Cyclic AMP analogs such as dibutryl cAMP have also been shown to inhibit TNFα production (Han *et al.*, 1990b). Increased levels of cAMP have been

Table II Potential Targets for the Design of TNFα Inhibitors

Signal transduction
Transcription and translation of TNFα
TNFα processing
TNF receptor down-regulation and inhibition
Inhibition of TNFα cytotoxicity

Table III Agents That Attenuate TNF and Are under Development for Septic Shock Treatment

Developer	Compound	Phase of development (WW/US)[a]	Comments
Monoclonal antibodies (MAb) against TNF			
Chiron/Cetus/Bayer	Bay-x-1351	P3/P3	Murine IgG MAb to TNF
Centocor	CenTNF	P2/P2	Humanized chimeric MAb
Celltech	CDP-571	PC(U.K.)/UC	Humanized IgG MAb; IND to be filed in 1992; patient WO9101755 (2-21-91)
Celltech	CB0006	DC/DC	Murine MAb
TNF binding protein			
Synergen	TNF-BP	PC/PC	Lead compound for clinicals has been chosen
Interpharma (Serono)	rTBP-1	PC(Switz)/UC	
Weitzmann Institute/Yeda R&D	TNF-BP1 and TNF-BP2	PC(Israel)/UC	Has cloned the genes for TNF-BP1 and TNF-BP2; patents; EP412486A (2-13-91), EP398327A (11-22-90), EP308378A (3-22-89)
Monoclonal antibody against TNF receptor			
Genentech/Roche	TNFr MAb	PC/PC	
Soluble TNF receptors as TNF antagonists			
Immunex (Receptech)	Soluble TNF receptor	PC/PC	Patents: WO9105553A (3-21-91), EP418014 (3-20-91)
Synergen	Soluble TNF receptor	PC/PC	Patent: EP422339A (4-17-91)
Affymax	Soluble TNF receptor	PC/PC	

Company	Agent	Phase	Comments
Other			
Sandoz	SDZ-MRL-953	PC/PC	Lipid A-derived monosaccharide which decreases release of IL-1, IL-6, and TNF from macrophages
SmithKline Beecham	SKF-86002	PC/PC	Dual cyclo-oxygenase/5-lipoxygenase inhibitor claimed to decrease TNF also
Genentech	anti-rMu-TNF	PC/PC	Antibody against recombinant murine TNF for graft vs host disease
Zambon (Italy)	N-acetyl-cytsteine (NAC)	PC/PC	Claimed to antagonize TNF production; intended for HIV infection
Hoechst	Pentoxifylline	P1/P1	Launched as Trental® for peripheral vascular disease; has been shown to decrease TNF levels (mechanism unknown); targeted for HIV infection
Xenova	TNF antagonist	PC(UK)/UC	Targeted for rheumatoid arthritis
Roche (Switzerland)	Recombinant TNF receptor	PC(Switz)/UC	Targeted for cancer
Schering Plough	Mometasone furoate	UC/UC	Steroid that inhibits *in vitro* production of TNF, IL-1 and IL-6

[a] The phases of development listed are for the disease state indicated in the comments section. Abbreviations: R, Registered; PR, preregistered; P3, phase 3; P2, phase 2; P1, phase 1; PC, preclinical; UC, unconfirmed; DC, discontinued; WW, worldwide; US, United States.

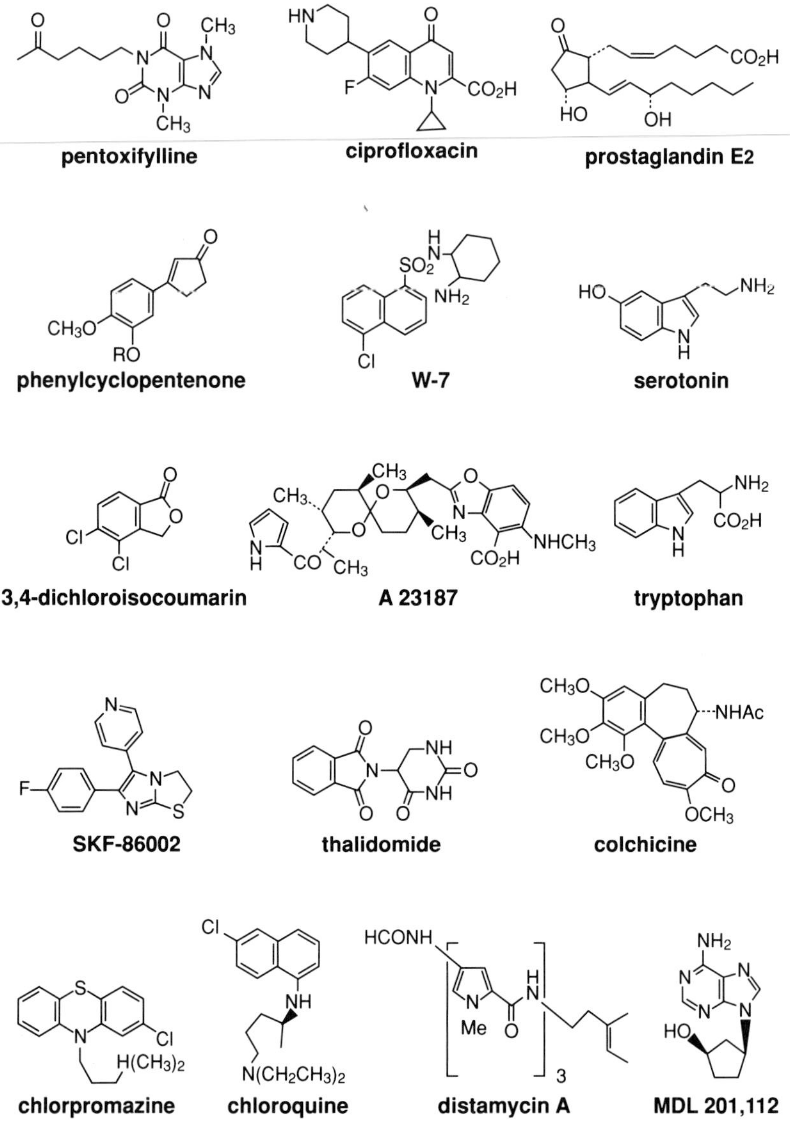

Fig. 5 TNFα inhibitors.

demonstrated to decrease the rate of transcription of available transcripts and do not appear to have any effects at the posttranscriptional level (Doherty *et al.*, 1991). PNF inhibits LPS-induced transcription of the TNFα gene, rather than enhancing mRNA breakdown. In addition, PNF does not exert control over TNF production at the translational level, as assessed using translational reporter constructs (Han *et al.*, 1990a).

Several other compounds that inhibit phosphodiesterase or increase cAMP also inhibit TNFα production, including: PGE$_2$ (Kunkel et al., 1988), misoprostol (Mahatama et al., 1991), quinilone antibiotics such as ciprofloxacin (Bailly et al., 1990), and a new series of phenylcyclopentenone derivatives (Maschler and Christenson, 1991; see Figure 5). Investigators have suggested that TNFα signal transduction may also be mediated by a calmodulin-dependent protein kinase (Crowly et al., 1990). TNFα induces transmembrane calcium influx and stimulates protein phosphorylation. The calmodulin inhibitor W-7 (Figure 5) has been shown to inhibit calmodulin-dependent phosphorylation and protein kinase C. W-7 subsequently inhibits TNFα-induced chemiluminescence and inhibits TNFα-induced cell death at 25 μM. Serotonin seems to play an important immunomodulatory role in directing macrophage function. TNFα inhibitory actions of serotonin have been speculated to work through 5-hydroxytryptamine-2 and/or 5-hydroxytryptamine-1c receptors (Arzt et al., 1991). This result suggests that serotonin receptors may mediate part of the TNFα signal transduction pathway. Additionally, steroids such as dexamethasone inhibit TNFα mRNA accumulation, presumably by inhibiting early transduction proteins.

Another possible target for inhibition of TNFα production is through direct effects on transcription and translation of the TNFα gene. Using antisense oligonucleotide techniques, Braham and colleagues (1991) have synthesized several antisense mRNA oligonucleotides containing a constant region—TCA TGG TGT CCT TTG CAG X—as well as a variable region containing 1–17 nucleotides. When X is CC TCA TGC TTT CAG TAG, a 63.5% decrease in production of TNFα at 6 μM is detected. Thus, the use of oligonucleotides will probably become an important part of controlling TNFα gene expression.

Vannier and co-workers (1991) have investigated mechanisms of TNFα inhibition by histamine, which appears to occur at the translational level. When mononuclear cells were isolated from healthy subjects and stimulated with LPS, histamine markedly suppressed TNFα synthesis by 83% in unfractionated PBMCs. This effect was not reversed by H$_1$ antagonists, but was reversed by the H$_2$ antagonists cimetidine and ranitidine. Decreased TNFα production by histamine appeared to be a result of PGE$_2$ synthesis, since the cyclooxygenase inhibitor indomethacin and the H$_1$ antagonist diphenhydramine did not reverse this effect.

C. TNFα Processing

TNFα is biosynthesized as a 26-kDa prohormone that is converted to a 17-kDa mature protein. Specifically, an enzyme referred to as TNF convertase removes a 76-amino-acid signal sequence from the 26-kDa molecule to produce the mature TNFα molecule (Kriegler, 1991). The major cleavage site of the enzyme appears to be between alanine and valine residues. The

17-kDa fragment has been shown to contain a valine residue as the terminal amino acid. Kriegler (1991) demonstrated that TNF convertase is inhibited by 3,4-isocoumarin (Figure 5), elastinal, and 6R-cis-1-{3-[(acetyloxy)-7-methoxy-8-oxy-5-thio-1-azabicyclo(4.2.0)oct-2-en-2-yl]carbonyl}morpholino, S,S-dioxide. Kriegler (1991) also demonstrated that the 26-kDa prohormone is biologically inactive; thus, novel inhibitors of this enzyme may have important clinical applications.

D. Down-regulation of TNFα Receptors

Human cells express two distinct TNF receptor types that differ in molecular weight, ligand binding affinity, glycosylation, immunoreactivity, and proteolytic fragmentation patterns (Hohmann et al., 1989). These receptors have been purified and are referred to as TNFRα, a 75-kDa protein, and TNFRβ, a 55-kDa protein. Both receptor types bind TNFα and TNFβ (Loetscher et al., 1990a; Schoenfeld et al., 1990). Several groups have cloned the TNFα and TNFβ receptors from cDNA (Dembic et al., 1990; Loetscher et al., 1990b, 1991). Phospholipase C and cAMP major signal transduction pathways have been implicated in cellular effects observed as a consequence of TNF binding to its receptor (Loetscher et al., 1991).

TNFα receptors are found on many cell types. When cells are exposed to TNFα, the cytokine elicits a large variety of biological responses including (1) secretion of collagenase and PGE_2 by synovial cells (Dayer et al., 1985); (2) activation of neutrophils and mononuclear cells (Dinarello et al., 1986; Klebanoff et al., 1986); and (3) induction of MHC class I antigens on endothelial cells (Collins et al., 1986).

Researchers have well established that protein kinase C is a Ca^{2+}- and phospholipid-dependent enzyme involved in transmembrane signal transduction (Nishizuka, 1986). Johnson and Baglioni (1988) reported that, in vitro, affinity of TNFα for its receptors was decreased when target cells were treated with protein kinase C activators. When HeLa cell cultures were treated with PMA, the calcium ionophore A23187, and diacylglycerol (all known protein kinase C activators), a dose-dependent decrease in TNFα binding to its receptor was observed. In addition, effects of the protein kinase C activators were reversed with addition of the protein kinase C inhibitors H-7 and staurosporine. Protection afforded from the activators was most effective when the inhibitors were added to the cell cultures prior to TNFα treatment. As a result, investigators concluded that the TNFα receptor is phosphorylated, resulting in a decrease of ligand affinity. However, this TNFα receptor down-regulation by protein kinase C activators apparently must occur early in the process of TNFα signal transduction.

E. Inhibition of TNFα Cytotoxicity

Although inhibition of TNFα cytotoxicity does not alter TNFα production, this approach should be considered a potential target area for treating TNF-related diseases. Cells killed by TNFα possess enhanced ADP ribosylation (Agarwal et al., 1988). DNA fragmentation takes place as part of the killing process and, as a result of excessive ADP ribosylation, NAD and ATP stores are reduced to very low levels (Berger, 1985; Yuhas et al., 1990). ADP ribosylation is thought to be involved in the repair of DNA strand breaks. Tryptophan may affect cell killing by enhancing metabolic pathways in which it serves as a precursor to NAD synthesis. Two inhibitors of ADP ribosylation, 3-aminobenzamide and nicotinamide, have inhibited TNFα cytotoxicity (Agarwal et al., 1988). Tryptophan (Figure 5) indole, indole acetic acid, and monomethylated indoles have also been speculated to prevent cell death by inhibition of chymotrypsin-like proteases (Ruggiero et al., 1987), as well as by reducing oxygen-derived radicals that have been found to protect against cell killing by TNFα.

In endotoxic shock, oxygen-derived radicals are generated from PMNs primed by TNFα (Weiss, 1989). Radical scavengers such as UF4006 and U78517F provide moderate protection against septic shock, but only if administered as a pretreatment prior to cecal ligation and puncture in experimental animal models (Powell et al., 1991). TEMP01, a spin trap reagent, mimics superoxide dismutase detoxification of superoxide, and has been shown to protect L929 and WEHI cells from TNFα-induced cytotoxicity in vitro (Pogrebniak et al., 1991). Note that, experimentally, these radical scavengers appear to be effective in preventing mortality caused by septic shock only when administered 30 min prior to LPS pretreatment. Therefore, their clinical utility is questionable at this time. This requirement for pretreatment may be shared by other potential therapeutic agents such as TNFα receptor immunoadhesions (Ashkenazi et al., 1991).

Inhibition of TNFα-mediated effects has also been accomplished through the development of biotechnological products such as anti-TNFα antibodies (Tracey et al., 1988), TNFα binding proteins (Peetre et al., 1988; Seckinger et al., 1989; Porteau and Nathan, 1990), and soluble TNF receptors (Aderka et al., 1992).

F. TNFα Inhibitors with Unknown Mechanisms of Action

Many pharmaceutical products with unknown mechanisms of action demonstrate TNFα inhibition. Examples include colchicine, chloroquine, and thalidomide. Colchicine significantly reduced TNFα release and increased IL-1 release when LPS was administered to 6 normal subjects (Allen et al., 1990). Picot and co-workers (1991) demonstrated that chloroquine (at a dose of approximately 0.75 μg/ml) blocks, in a dose-dependent fashion, TNFα release from human monocytes *in vitro*. TNFα appears to play a role in the pathogenesis of malaria; thus, Chloroquine may produce beneficial effects through inhibition of TNFα production (Picot *et al.*, 1991). *In vitro*, the nonteratogenic R enantiomer of thalidomide has also inhibited human monocyte TNFα release by 40% relative to controls at clinically attainable plasma concentrations of 1.0 μg/ml (Sampaio *et al.*, 1991). In this study, thalidomide did not affect IL-1, IL-6, or GM-CSF concentrations.

Other TNFα inhibitors include cyclosporin A (Bokulic *et al.*, 1989), picotamide (Altavilla *et al.*, 1991), lipid X (Cornwall *et al.*, 1989), polymyxin B (Bysani *et al.*, 1989), nisoldipine (Currin *et al.*, 1991), distamycin A and its analogs (Mongelli *et al.*, 1991), and chlorpromazine (Schleuning *et al.*, 1989).

Lipoxygenase and cyclooxygenase inhibitors of TNFα production include SK&F 86002, SK&F 201-610, SK&F 208-199, ibuprofen, and indomethacin. Endogenous macrophage lipoxygenase catalyzes the formation of 13-hydroxyoctadecadienoic acid (13-HODD). Once formed, 13-HODD remains inside macrophages, where it is covalently bound. Further, LPS activation substantially increases macrophage 13-HODD synthesis. Invesigators have suggested that inhibition of lipoxygenase may result in decreased formation of 13-HODD and TNFα (Schade *et al.*, 1989). Compounds such as SK&F 86002 dually inhibit lipoxygenase and cyclooxygenase through an unknown mechanism, resulting in multiple biological actions (Smith *et al.*, 1991). The cyclooxygenase inhibitors ibuprofen and indomethacin appear to inhibit TNFα production through prostaglandin inhibition (Schade *et al.*, 1989; Griffin *et al.*, 1991).

Adenosine and its analog MDL 201,112 have inhibited TNFα production by selective inhibition of TNFα mRNA synthesis through an unknown mechanism (Parmely *et al.*, 1993; Edwards *et al.*, 1993). This agent has also been shown to inhibit IFNγ priming of rat macrophages and PMNs for an enhanced respiratory burst (Borcherding *et al.*, 1994). Table IV shows data that indicate inhibitory effects of adenosine and MDL 201,112 on TNFα production in LPS-stimulated murine macrophages *in vitro*. This investigation demonstrated that inhibition of TNFα production by MDL 201,112 and adenosine probably occurs by fundamentally different mechanisms. Although MDL 201,112 reduced steady-state peak TNFα mRNA levels in LPS-stimulated RAW.264 and J774 cells, adenosine did not affect peak steady-state TNFα mRNA levels in these cells. When adenosine and MDL 201,112 were tested against LPS-induced lethality in D-galactosamine treated mice (Table V), only MDL 201,112 provided protection at 100 mg/kg. Protection afforded against lethality with anti-TNFα antibodies confirmed that lethality was the result of TNFα overproduction and that the inability of adenosine to protect mice from LPS-induced lethality was probably caused by its rapid metabolism *in vivo*. Conversely, the more metaboli-

Table IV TNFα Bioactivity[a] Inhibition (%)

Drug concentration (μM)	ADO ($\bar{x} \pm$ SEM)	MDL201,112 ($\bar{x} \pm$ SEM)
1000	12 ± 1 (99%)	7 ± 2 (99%)
100	9 ± 1 (99%)	114 ± 2 (87%)
10	161 ± 5 (82%)	770 ± 134 (12%)
1	547 ± 23 (38%)	1517 ± 140 (0%)
0	876 ± 159 (100%)	

[a] Mouse peritoneal macrophages were stimulated with *E. coli* LPS (10 ng/ml) and IFNγ (10 U/ml) for 6 hr. Culture supernatants were assayed for TNFα by cytotoxicity of actinomycin D-treated L929 cells. Results are the average of triplicate determinations ± SEM (Parmely *et al.*, 1992).

cally stable analog (MDL 201,112) demonstrated protection against LPS-induced lethality over a 48-hr period following a single 100 mg/kg intraperitoneal dose.

VI. Evidence of a Pro-inflammatory Role for TNFα in Superantigen-Induced Arthritis

Autoimmune diseases are thought to result from a loss of tolerance of self-reactive lymphocytes, leading to either autoantibody production or

Table V Effect of ADO, MDL201112, or Anti-TNFα Antibody on Endotoxin Lethality in D-GalNH₂-Treated Mice

Experimental	Pretreatment[a]	Challenge[b]	Lethality (deaths/total)
1	Vehicle control	LPS + D-galNH₂	8/10
	MDL201,112	LPS + D-galNH₂	1/10*
2	Vehicle control	LPS + D-galNH₂	5/6
	MDL201,112	LPS + D-galNH₂	0/6*
3	Vehicle control	LPS + D-galNH₂	8/8
	MDL201,112	LPS + D-galNH₂	1/8*
	ADO	LPS + D-galNH₂	8/8
4	Rat IgG1	LPS + D-galNH₂	5/5
	Anti-TNFα	LPS + D-galNH₂	0/5*

[a] All nucleosides were injected ip 1 hr prior to challenge at a dose of 100 mg/kg. The drug vehicle was carboxymethyl cellulose. Anti-TNFα MAb was given iv at a dose of 500 μg/mouse.
[b] Mice were challenged with 15–50 ng *S. enteriditis* LPS + 20 mg D-galNH₂ ip and lethality was recorded over the following 48 hr. LPS, Lipopolysaccharide.
* $p < 0.01$ (Chi Square) compared with controls (Parmely *et al.*, 1992).

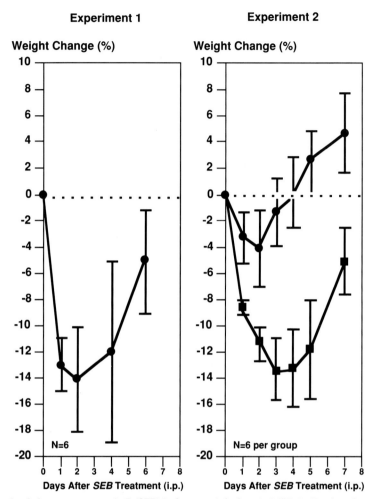

Fig. 6 *Staphylococcus enterotoxin B* (SEB) induces weight loss in MRL *lpr/lpr* female mice. In Experiment 1, ● indicates mean weight loss percent. In Experiment 2, ● indicates mean percent heat-denatured SEB and ■ indicates mean percent SEB. Data from Zhang *et al.* (1991).

cytokine release from T cells, macrophages, and additional inflammatory responses (Cohen and Eisenberg, 1991). However, demonstrating an increase in autoreactive T cells, or an oligoclonal expansion of T cells with limited specificity, in autoimmune disease has been difficult. Several reports have shown that rheumatoid arthritis patients exhibit a clonal expansion of selected T cell receptor (TCR) Vβ-expressing T cells in the synovial fluid relative to the peripheral blood, suggesting that bacterial enterotoxins or superantigens may be involved in initial phases of chronic arthritis (Paliard *et al.*, 1991).

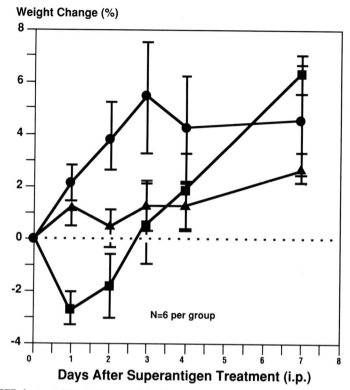

Fig. 7 SEB, but not SEA, induces weight loss in MRL *lpr/lpr* female mice. ●, Mean percent heat-denatured SEB; ▲, mean percent SEA; ■, mean percent SEB. Data from Zhang *et al.* (1991).

Superantigens are important in the development of toxic shock syndrome, enteritis, and heat shock protein-associated diseases (Miethke *et al.*, 1992). These diseases have been proposed to be caused by activation of large numbers of T cells through an interaction with the TCR Vβ region, because early expansion followed by late deletion of T cells expressing superantigen-reactive TCR Vβ regions has been observed in these diseases. However, why some individuals are more predisposed to the development of superantigen-related diseases is currently unknown, although the predisposition appears to be the result of a T cell functional defect rather than the absence of T cells bearing superantigen-reactive Vβ regions (Kim *et al.*, 1991). Since not all rheumatoid arthritis patients exhibit preferential expression of Vβ14 in synovial fluids (Howell *et al.*, 1991; Paliard *et al.*, 1991), induction of rheumatoid arthritis appears to be of multifactorial origin. Thus, development of rheumatoid arthritis can probably be attributed to genetic and environmental factors as well.

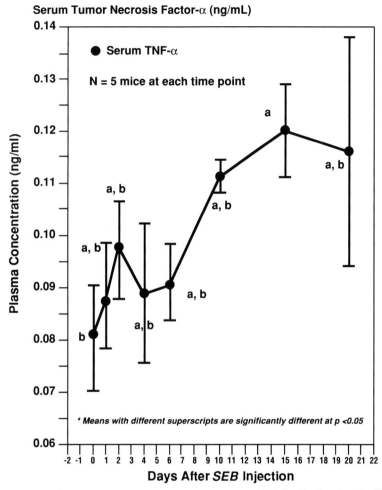

Fig. 8 SEB induces tumor necrosis factor α production in MRL *lpr/lpr* female mice (kinetic time course of study for days 0–20). Data from Zhang *et al.* (1991).

MRL-*lpr/lpr* mice develop autoimmune diseases and lymphadenopathy (Koopman and Gay, 1988; Cohen and Eisenberg, 1991). The *lpr* gene results in intrinsic defects in T cell tolerance and B cell hyperactivity (Mountz *et al.*, 1991). An *lpr* locus encoding Fas antigen (a cell-surface protein mediating apoptosis) has been identified (Watanabe-Fukunaga *et al.*, 1992). Because superantigens have been proposed to play a role in initiating autoimmune diseases, MRL-*lpr/lpr* mice and a Vβ8.2 TCR MRL-*lpr/lpr* transgenic mouse model have been used to study acute and chronic responses after mice were injected intraarticularly into the knee joints with Vβ8-reactive Staphylococcal enterotoxin B (SEB), as well as with Vβ8-nonreactive Staphylococcal

PCR Amplification/Southern Hybridization

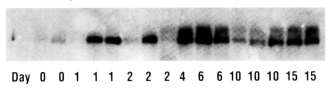

Day 0   0   1   1   1   2   2   2   4   6   6 10 10 10 15 15

Image Analysis Densitometry

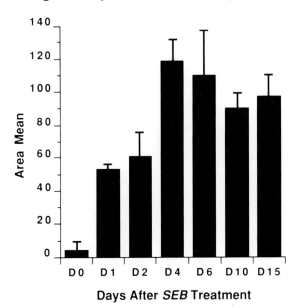

Fig. 9 SEB-induced TNFα expression in MRL *lpr/lpr* spleen: time course kinetics. Data from Zhang *et al.* (1992).

enterotoxin A (SEA). The acute response in SEB-injected MRL-*lpr/lpr* mice was manifested by a 5–15% weight loss, PMN infiltration, and fibrin formation in the injected joint (Figure 6; Zhang *et al.*, 1991, 1993). Chronic arthritis was observed by 30 days postsuperantigen injection, and was characterized by synovial cell hyperplasia, proliferation of cartilage, and bone destruction (Mountz *et al.*, 1994). Interestingly, different bacterial superantigens appear to have dissimilar effects in these models because SEA did not cause acute weight loss after intraperitoneal injection (Figure 7; Zhang *et al.*, 1992).

Because TNFα has been implicated as a pro-inflammatory cytokine important in the pathogenesis of rheumatoid arthritis (Boswell *et al.*, 1988; Jacob and McDevitt, 1988, 1990; Brennan *et al.*, 1989; Yochum *et al.*, 1989;

Northern Blot Hybridization
Using RNA-RNA Riboprobes

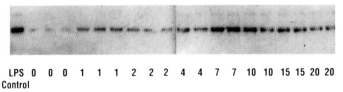

LPS 0   0   0   1   1   1   2   2   2   4   4   7   7   10 10 15 15 20 20
Control

Image Analysis Densitometry

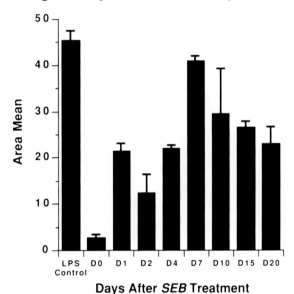

Days After *SEB* Treatment

Fig. 10 SEB-induced TNFα expression in MRL *lpr/lpr* spleen: time course kinetics. Data from Zhang *et al.* (1992).

Houssiau and Nagant De Deaxcharsone, 1990; Macnaul *et al.*, 1990; Bucala *et al.*, 1991; Jacob and McDevitt, 1991; Mourad *et al.*, 1992), serum levels of TNFα in mouse MRI *lpr/lpr* transgenic models were measured after a single SEB injection (Figure 8; Zhang *et al.*, 1991). Serum TNFα levels appeared to correlate qualitatively with acute and chronic cycling phases of SEB-induced autoimmune disease. These data are further reinforced by experiments documenting that splenic TNFα gene expression in SEB-injected *lpr/lpr* mice increased over time (Figures 9, 10; Zhang *et al.*, 1992). Other investigations have addressed the *in vitro* ability of SEB to activate peritoneal macrophages obtained from autoimmune diseased mice (Figure 11) (Zhang *et al.*, 1992, 1994). The data indicate that SEB induces TNFα in

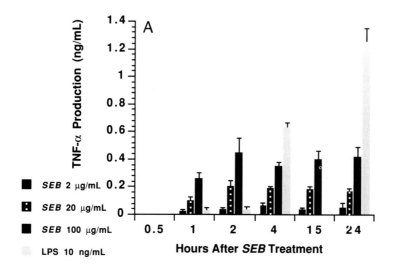

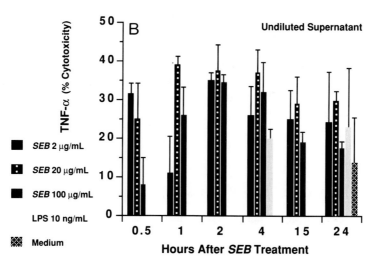

Fig. 11 (A) *In vitro* production of TNFα by MRL *lpr/lpr* peritoneal macrophages stimulated with SEB. (B) Cytotoxicity of supernatant of peritoneal macrophage treated with SEB *in vitro* from MRL *lpr/lpr* mice. Data from Zhang *et al.* (1992).

both kinetic and dose-related fashions. Collectively, these data suggest that bacterial superantigens are potent macrophage-activating substances *in vivo* and *in vitro*. The ability of superantigens to produce a pro-inflammatory response characterized by the production and secretion of TNFα and other cytokines may provide one explanation for unknown triggering antigens that stimulate the pathogenesis of autoimmune diseases such as rheumatoid arthritis.

VII. Conclusion

The biological function of TNFα extends well beyond its initial discovery as a mediator of tumor necrosis. Increasingly, researchers realize that the interacting milieu of host cytokines existing locally and systemically is an extremely important network that dictates the pathogenesis of many immune and inflammatory events. In particular, TNFα appears to play a critically important role in this regard because of its ability to activate a wide range of cell types to promote production of several key cytokines (such as IL-1) and bioactive eicosanoids. In particular, many studies described in this chapter have implicated TNFα as a pivotal mediator for events culminating in progression of sepsis to septic shock. Currently, medical treatment for septic shock remains primarily supportive. Morbidity and mortality attributed to septic shock have not decreased appreciably over the past decade, emphasizing the need for a greater understanding of (1) mechanisms regulating TNFα gene expression (including production and inhibition of TNFα, (2) the cascade of events set in motion by the burst of TNFα production elicited by live microorganisms or LPS, and (3) development and appropriate use of pharmacological interventions that are effective in blocking TNFα production or ameliorating the untoward sequelae of septic shock or other inflammatory diseases subsequent to elaboration of TNFα.

References

Aderka, D., Engelmann, H., Maor, Y., Brakebusch, C., and Wallach, D. (1992). *J. Exp. Med.* **175**, 323–329.

Agarwal, S., Drysdale, B.-E., and Shin, H. S. (1988). *J. Immunol.* **140**, 4187–4192.

Akira, S., Isshiki, H., Sugita, T., *et al.* (1990). *EMBO J* **9**, 1897–1906.

Alexander, H. R., Doherty, G. M., Buresh, C. M., Venzon, D. J., and Norton, J. A. (1991). *J. Exp. Med.* **173**, 1029–1032.

Allen, J. N., Herzyk, D. I., and Wewers, M. D. (1990). *Am. Rev. Resp. Dis.* **141**, A677. (Abstract)

Alpert, G., Baldwin, G., Thompson, C., *et al.* (1992). *J. Infect. Dis.* **165**, 494–500.

Altavilla, D., Costa, G. B., Zumma, S., Ianello, D., and Mastroeni, P. (1991). *Am. Soc. Microbiol.* **91**, 62 (Abstract).

Amiri, P., Locksley, R. M., Parslow, T. G., Sadick, M., Rector, E., Ritter, D., and McKerrow, J. H. (1992). *Nature (London)* **356**, 604–607.

Andus, T., Geiger, T., Hirano, T., Kishimoto, T., and Heinrich, P. C. (1988). *Eur. J. Immunol.* **18**, 739–746.

Arato, A., Savilahti, E., Tainio, V. M., and Klemola, T. (1989). *J. Pediatr. Gastroenterol. Nutr.* **8**, 172–180.

Arend, W. P., and Dayer, J-M. (1990). *Arthritis Rheum.* **33,** 305–315.
Arzt, E., Costas, M., Finkielman, S., and Nahmod, V. (1991). *Life Sci.* **48,** 2557–2562.
Ashkenazi, A., Marsters, S. A., Capon, D. J., *et al.* (1991). *Proc. Natl. Acad. Sci. USA* **88,** 10535–10539.
Bailly S., Roche, F. Y., and Gougerot-Pocidalo, M. A. (1990). *Int. J. Immunopharmacol.* **12,** 31–36.
Balkwell, F. R., Lee, A., Aldam, G., *et al.* (1986). *Cancer Res.* **46,** 3990–3993.
Barath, P., Fishbein, M. C., Cao, J., Berenson, J., Helfant, J. H., and Forrester, J. S. (1990). *Am. J. Cardiol.* **65,** 297–302.
Barnes, P. F., Bloch, A. B., Davidson, P. T., and Snider, D. E. (1991). *N. Engl. J. Med.* **324,** 1644–1650.
Bate, C. A. W., Laverne, J., and Playfair, J. H. L. (1988). *Immunology* **64,** 227–231.
Bendtzen, K. (1990). *Scand. J. Clin. Lab. Invest.* **50** (Suppl. 202), 163–167.
Berger, N. (1985). *Radiation Res.* **101,** 4–15.
Berkow, R. L., and Dodson, M. R. (1988). *J. Leuk. Biol.* **44,** 345–352.
Berkow, R. L., Wang, D., Larrick, J. W., Dodson, R. W., and Howard, T. H. (1987). *J. Immunol.* **139,** 3783–3791.
Berman, N. S., Siegel, S. E., Nachum, R., Lipsey, A., and Leedom, J. (1976). *J. Pediatr.* **88,** 553–556.
Berman, B., Wietzerbin, J., Sanceau, J., Merlin, G., and Duncan, M. R. (1990). *J. Interferon Res.* **10** (Suppl. 1), S143 (Abstract).
Bermudez, L. E. M., and Young, L. S. (1988). *J. Immunol.* **140,** 3006–3013.
Beutler, B., and Brown, T. (1991). *J. Clin. Invest.* **87,** 1336–1344.
Beutler, B., and Cerami, A. (1986). *Nature (London)* **320,** 584–588.
Beutler, B., and Cerami, A. (1987). *N. Engl. J. Med.* **316,** 379–385.
Beutler, B., and Cerami, A. (1988). *Endocrin. Rev.* **9,** 57–66.
Beutler, B., and Cerami, A. (1989). *Ann. Rev. Immunol.* **7,** 625–655.
Beutler, B., Greenwald, D., Holmes, J. D., *et al.* (1985a). *Nature (London)* **316,** 552–554.
Beutler, B., Milsark, I. W., and Cerami, A. (1985b). *Science* **229,** 869–871.
Beutler, B., Krochin, N., Milsark, I. W., Luedke, C., and Cerami, A. (1986). *Science* **232,** 977–980.
Beutler, B., Thompson, P., Keyer, J., Hagerty, K., and Crawford, D. (1988). *Biochem. Biophys. Res. Commun.* **152,** 973–980.
Bevilacqua, M. P., Pober, J. S., Mendrick, D. L., Cotran, R. S., and Gimbrone, M. A., Jr. (1987). *Proc. Natl. Acad. Sci. USA* **84,** 9238–9242.
Bird, G. L. A., Sheron, N., Goka, J., Alexander, G. J., and Williams, R. S. (1990). *Ann. Int. Med.* **112,** 917–920.
Blaser, M. (1992). *Gastroenterology* **102,** 720–727.
Bokulic, R., Nelson, S., Bagby, G., Noel, P., and Summer, W. (1989). *Am. Rev. Resp. Dis.* **139,** A355.
Bonavida, B., Paubert-Braquet, M., Hosford, D., *et al.* (1989). *Prog. Clin. Biol. Res.* **308,** 485–489.
Bone, R. C. (1991a). *Ann. Intern. Med.* **114,** 332–333.
Bone, R. C. (1991b). *J. Am. Med. Assoc.* **266,** 1686–1691.
Bone, R. C. (1991c). *Chest* **100,** 802–808.
Bone, R. C., and the Methylprednisolone Severe Sepsis Study Group (1987). *N. Engl. J. Med.* **317,** 653–658.
Bone, R. C., Fisher, C. J., Jr., Clemmer, T. P., *et al.* (1989). *Crit. Care. Med.* **17,** 389–393.
Bone, R. C., Balk, R., Slotman, G., *et al.*, and the Prostaglandin E$_1$ Study Group (1992). *Chest* **101,** 320–326.
Borcherding, D. B., Butler, T. T., Linnik, M. D., Mehdi, S., and Edwards III, C. K. (1994). *J. Med. Chem.* (In press).
Boswell, J. M., Yui, M. A., Burt, D. W., and Kelley, V. E. (1988). *J. Immunol.* **141,** 3050–3054.

Braegger, C. P., Nicholls, S., Murch, S. H., Stephens, S., and MacDonald, T. T. (1992). *Lancet* **339**, 89–91.

Braham, A. K., Smets, D., and Zalisz, R. (1991). Patent #EPO 414607A2. European Patent Office.

Brennan, D. C., Yui, M. A., Wuthrich, R. P., and Kelley, V. E. (1989). *J. Immunol.* **143**, 3470–3475.

Brennan, F. M., Zachariae, C. O. C., Chantry, D., *et al.* (1990). *Eur. J. Immunol.* **20**, 2141–2144.

Brewster, D. R., Kwiatkowski, D., and White, N. J. (1990). *Lancet* **336**, 1039–1043.

Brosnan, C. F., Selmaj, K., and Raine, C. S. (1988). *J. Neuroimmunol.* **18**, 87–94.

Brynskov, J., and Tvede, N. (1990). *Gut* **31**, 795–799.

Brynskov, J., Tvede, N., Anderson, C. B., and Vilien, M. (1992). *Gut* **33**, 55–58.

Bucala, R., Ritchlin, C., Winchester, R., and Cerami, A. (1991). *J. Exp. Med.* **173**, 569–574.

Bussolini, F., Camussi, G., and Baglioni, C. (1988). *J. Biol. Chem.* **263**, 11856–11861.

Bysani, G. K., Stokes, D. C., Shenep, J. L., Fishman, M., Hildner, W. K., and Rufus, K. L. (1989). *Am. Rev. Resp. Dis.* **139**, A158.

Calandra, T., and Glauser, M. P. (1990). *Circ. Shock* **31**, 244. (Abstract)

Calandra, T., and the Swiss-Dutch J5 Study Group (1988). *J. Infect. Dis.* **158**, 312–319.

Calandra, T., Baumgartner, J. D., Grau, G. E., *et al.* (1990). *J. Infect. Dis.* **161**, 982–987.

Calandra, T., Gerain, J., Heumann, D., Baumgartner, J-D., Glauser, M. P., and the Swiss-Dutch J5 Immunoglobulin Study Group (1991). *Am. J. Med.* **91**, 23–29.

Campbell, I. L. (1991). Cytokines and the molecular pathology of IDDM. *In* "Diabetes 1991" (H. Rifkin, J. A. Colwell, and S. I. Taylor, eds.), pp. 578–581. Exerpta Medica, Amsterdam, The Netherlands.

Campbell, I. L., and Harrison, L. C. (1990). *Mol. Biol. Med.* **7**, 299–309.

Camussi, G., Bussolino, F., Salvidio, G., and Baglioni, C. (1987). *J. Exp. Med.* **166**, 1390–1404.

Caput, D., Beutler, B., Hartog, R., Thayer, S., Brown-Shirmer, S., and Cerami, A. (1986). *Proc. Natl. Acad. Sci. USA* **83**, 1670–1674.

Carey, P. D., Leeper-Woodford, S. K., Walsh, C. J., Byrne, K., Fowler, A. A., and Sugerman, H. J. (1991). *J. Trauma* **31**, 733–741.

Carswell, E. A., Old, E. J., Kassel, R. L., Green, S., Fiore, N., and Williamson, B. (1975). *Proc. Natl. Acad. Sci. USA* **72**, 3666–3670.

Case, J. P., Lafyatis, R., Remmers, E. F., Kumkumian, G. K., and Wilder, R. L. (1989). *Am. J. Pathol.* **135**, 1055–1064.

Celada, A., and Maki, R. A. (1991). *J. Immunol.* **146**, 114–120.

Centers for Disease Control (1990). *Morbid. Mortal. Wkly. Rep.* **39**, 31–34.

Chaisson, R. E., and Slutkin, G. (1989). *J. Infect. Dis.* **159**, 96–100.

Chao, C. C., Janoff, E. N., Hu, S., *et al.* (1991). *Cytokine* **3**, 292–298.

Clark, I. A., Hunt, N. H., Butcher, G. A., and Cowden, W. B. (1987). *J. Immunol.* **139**, 3493–3496.

Clark, I. A., Chaudri, G., and Cowden, W. B. (1989). *Trans. R. Soc. Trop. Med. Hyg.* **83**, 436–440.

Clark, I. A., Rockett, K. A., and Cowden, W. B. (1991). *Parasitol. Today* **7**, 205–207.

Cohen, J. (1990). *Circ. Shock* **31**, 245. (Abstract)

Cohen, P. L., and Eisenberg, R. A. (1991). *Ann. Rev. Immunol.* **9**, 243–269.

Collart, M. A., Belin, D., Vassalli, J-D., de Kossodo, S., and Vassalli, P. (1986). *J. Exp. Med.* **164**, 2113–2118.

Collart, M. A., Baeuerle, P., and Vassalli, P. (1990). *Mol. Cell. Biol.* **10**, 1498–1506.

Collins, T., Lapierre, L. A., Fiers, W., Strominger, J. L., and Pober, J. S. (1986). *Proc. Natl. Acad. Sci. USA* **83**, 446–450.

Cook, G. C. (1991). *Postgrad. Med. J.* **67**, 798–822.

Cooper, K. D. (1990). *Dermatol. Clin.* **8**, 737–745.

Cornwall, R. D., Golenbock, D. T., and Proctor, R. A. (1989). *Am. Rev. Resp. Dis.* **139**, A356.

Corrigan, C. J., and Kay, A. B. (1991). *Am. Rev. Resp. Dis.* **143,** 1165–1168.

Cox, F. E. G. (1991). *Trends Biotechnol.* **9,** 389–394.

Crabtree, J. E., Shallcross, T. M., Heatley, R. V., and Wyatt, J. I. (1991). *Gut* **32,** 1473–1477.

Crawford, R. M., Finbloom, D. S., Ohara, J., Paul, W. E., and Meltzer, M. S. (1987). *J. Immunol.* **139,** 135–141.

Crowley, J., Zheng, H., Yonemaru, M., and Raffin, T. A. (1990). *Am. Rev. Resp. Dis.* **141,** A919. (Abstract)

Curfs, J. H. A., van der Meer, J. W. M., Sauerwein, R. W., and Eling, W. M. C. (1990). *J. Exp. Med.* **11,** 1287–1291.

Currin, R. T., Lichtman, S. N., Thurman, R. G., and Lemasters, J. J. (1991). *Hepatology* **14,** 165A. (Abstract)

Czuprynski, C. J., Haak-Frenscho, M., Maroushek, N., and Brown, J. F. (1992). *Antimicrob. Agents Chemother.* **36,** 68–70.

Dayer, J. M., Beutler, B., and Cerami, A. (1985). *J. Exp. Med.* **162,** 2163–2168.

Deeg, H. J., and Henslee-Downey, P. J. (1990). *Bone Marrow Transplant.* **6,** 1–8.

Dembic, Z., Loetscher, H., Gubler, U., *et al.* (1990). *Cytokines* **2,** 231–239.

De Titto, E. H., Catterall, J. R., and Remington, J. S. (1986). *J. Immunol.* **137,** 1342–1345.

Deusch, K., Köhne, I., Dähne, I., Daum, S., and Classen, M. (1991). *Gastroenterology* **100,** A573. (Abstract)

Dinarello, C. A. (1985). *J. Clin. Immunol.* **5,** 287–297.

Dinarello, C. A. (1987). *Immunol. Lett.* **16,** 227–232.

Dinarello, C. A. (1991). *J. Infect. Dis.* **163,** 1177–1184.

Dinarello, C. A., and Thompson, R. C. (1991). *Immunol. Today* **12,** 404–410.

Dinarello, C. A., Rosenwasser, L. J., and Wolff, S. M. (1981). *J. Immunol.* **127,** 2517–2519.

Dinarello, C. A., Cannon, J. G., Wolff, S. M., *et al.* (1986). *J. Exp. Med.* **163,** 1433–1450.

Ding, A. H., and Nathan, C. F. (1987). *J. Immunol.* **139,** 1971–1977.

Doherty, G. M., Jensen, J. C., Alexander, H. R., Buresh, C. M., and Norton, J. A. (1991). *Surgery* **110,** 192–198.

Dressler, K. A., Mathias, S., and Kolesnick, R. N. (1992). *Science* **255,** 1715–1718.

Drouet, C., Shakov, A. N., and Jongeneel, C. V. (1991). *J. Immunol.* **147,** 1694–1700.

Duclos, B., Reimund, J. M., Lehr, L., *et al.* (1991). *Gastroenterology* **100,** A576 (Abstract)

Duh, E. J., Maury, W. J., Folks, T. M., Fauci, A. S., and Rabson, A. B. (1989). *Proc. Natl. Acad. Sci. USA* **86,** 5974–5978.

Edwards, C. K., III, Zhou, T., Zhang, J., Long, R. E., Borcherding, D. R., and Mountz, J. D. (1992). *J. Cell. Biochem.* **160,** 46. (Abstract 0315)

Edwards, III, C. K., Hoeper, B. J., Borcherding, D. R., Bowlin, T. R., and Parmely, M. J. (1993). *J. Cell. Biochem.* **178,** 104 (abstract).

Edwards, III, C. K., Watts, L. M., Parmely, M. J., Linnik, M. D., Long, R. E., and Borcherding, D. R. (1994). *J. Leuk. Biol.* (*In press*).

Eliakim, R., Karmell, F., Razin, E., and Rachmilewitz, D. (1988). *Gastroenterology* **95,** 1176–1182.

Engelmann, H., Aderka, D., Rubinstein, M., Rotman, D., and Wallach, D. (1989). *J. Biol. Chem.* **264,** 11974–11980.

Ertal, W., Morrison, M. H., Ayala, A., and Chawdry, I. H. (1991). *J. Trauma* **31,** 609–616.

Esparza, I., Mannel, D., Ruppel, A., Falk, W., and Krammer, P. H. (1989). *J. Exp. Med.* **166,** 589–594.

Espevik, T., Brockhaus, M., Loetscher, H., Nonstad, U., and Shalaby, R. (1990). *J. Exp. Med.* **171,** 415–426.

Exley, A. R., Cohen, J., Buurman, W., *et al.* (1990). *Lancet* **335,** 1275–1277.

Fauci, A. S. (1991). *Ann. Intern. Med.* **114,** 678–693.

Feldmann, M., Brennan, F. M., Field, M., and Maini, R. N. (1992). *In* "Recent Advances in Rheumatoid Arthritis" (J. Smolen, J. R. Kalden, and R. N. Maini, eds.). Springer-Verlag, Berlin.

Figari, J. S., Mori, N. A., and Palladino, M. A., Jr. (1987). *Blood* **70**, 979–984.

Fiocchi, C., Hilfiker, M. L., Youngman, K. R., Doerder, N. C., and Finke, J. H. (1984). *Gastroenterology* **86**, 734–742.

Folks, T. M., Clouse, K. A., Justement, J., *et al.* (1989). *Proc. Natl. Acad. Sci. USA* **86**, 2365–2368.

Furukawa, S., Matsubara, T., Jujoh, K., *et al.* (1988). *Clin. Immunol. Immunopathol.* **48**, 247–251.

Geiger, T., Andus, T., Klapproth, J., Hirano, T., Kishimoto, T., and Heinrich, P. C. (1988). *Eur. J. Immunol.* **18**, 717–721.

Gendelman, H. E., Friedman, R. M., Joe, S., *et al.* (1990). *J. Exp. Med.* **172**, 1433–1442.

Gessani, S., DiMarzio, P., Rizza, P., Belurdelli, F., and Baglioni, C. (1991). *J. Virol.* **65**, 989–991.

Gifford, G. E., and Lohmann-Matthes, M-L. (1987). *J. Natl. Cancer Inst.* **78**, 121–124.

Glauser, M. P., Zanetti, G., Baumgartner, J-D., and Cohen, J. (1991). *Lancet* **338**, 732–736.

Gong, J-H., Sprenger, H., Hinder, F., *et al.* (1991). *J. Immunol.* **147**, 3507–3513.

Gosset, P., Perez, T., Lassalle, P., Duquesnoy, B., *et al.* (1991). *Am. Rev. Resp. Dis.* **143**, 593–597.

Granowitz, E. V., Santos, A. A., Poutsiaka, D. D., *et al.* (1991). *Lancet* **338**, 1423–1424.

Grau, G. E., Fajardo, L. F., Piguet, P. F., Allet, B., Lambert, P. H., and Vassali, P. (1987). *Science* **237**, 1210–1212.

Grau, G. E., Taylor, T. E., Molyneux, M. E., *et al.* (1989). *N. Engl. J. Med.* **320**, 1586–1591.

Grau, G. E., Frei, K., Piguet, P-F., *et al.* (1990). *J. Exp. Med.* **172**, 1505–1508.

Griffin, M. P., Gore, D. C., Lobe, T. E., Flynn, J. F., Traber, D. L., and Herndon, D. N. (1991). *Resuscitation* **22**, 75–83.

Haas, J. G., Baeuerle, P. A., Riethmüller, G., and Zeigler-Heitbrock, H. W. L. (1990). *Proc. Natl. Acad. Sci. USA* **87**, 9563–9567.

Haidaris, C. G., Haynes, J. D., Meltzer, M. S., and Allison, A. C. (1983). *Infect. Immun.* **42**, 385–393.

Hampton, R. Y., Golenbock, D. T., Penman, M., Krieger, M., and Raetz, C. R. H. (1991). *Nature (London)* **352**, 342–344.

Han, J., Brown, T., and Beutler, B. (1990a). *J. Exp. Med.* **171**, 465–475.

Han, J., Thompson, P., and Beutler, B. (1990b). *J. Exp. Med.* **172**, 391–394.

Hansson, G. K., Jonasson, L., and Stemme, S. (1989). *Arteriosclerosis* **9**, 567–578.

Harris, E. D. (1990). Rheumatoid arthritis. *N. Engl. J. Med.* **322**, 1277–1289.

Havell, E. A. (1987). *J. Immunol.* **139**, 4225–4231.

Helloran, P. F., Cockfield, S. M., and Madrenas, J. (1989). *Transplant Proc.* **21**, 26–30.

Hemmer, C. J., Kern, P., Holst, F. G. E., *et al.* (1991). *Am. J. Med.* **91**, 37–44.

Hensel, G., Meichle, A., Pfizenmaier, K., and Krönke, M. (1989). *Lymph. Res.* **8**, 347–351.

Hoffman, M., and Weinberg, J. B. (1987). *J. Leuk. Biol.* **42**, 704–707.

Hohmann, H. P., Remy, R., Brockhaus, M., and van Loon, A. P. G. M. (1989). *J. Biol. Chem.* **264**, 14927–14934.

Holtzmann, M. J. (1991). *Am. Rev. Resp. Dis.* **143**, 188–203.

Horvath, C. J., Kaplan, J. E., and Malik, A. B. (1991). *Am. Rev. Resp. Dis.* **144**, 1337–1441.

Houssiau, F. A., and Nagant De Deaxcharsone, C. (1990). *Clin. Exp. Rheum.* **8**, 531–533.

Howell, M. D., Dively, J. P., Lundeen, K. A. *et al.* (1991). *Proc. Natl. Acad. Sci. USA* **88**, 10921–10925.

Hurley, J. C., Lois, W. J., Tosolini, F. A., and Carlin, J. B. (1991). *Antimicrob. Agents Chemother.* **35**, 2388–2394.

Hyers, T. M., Tricomi, S. M., Dettenmeier, P. A., and Fowler, A. A. (1991). *Am. Rev. Resp. Dis.* **144**, 268–271.

Ikejuma, T., Okusawa, S., van der Meer, J. W. M., and Dinarello, C. A. (1988). *J. Infect. Dis.* **158**, 1017–1125.

Ip, J. M., Fuster, V., Badimon, L., Badimon, J., Taubman, M. B., and Chesebro, J. H. (1990). *J. Am. Coll. Cardiol.* **15**, 67–87.

Ito, M., Baba, M., and Sato, A. (1989). *Biochem. Biophys. Res. Commun.* **158**, 307–312.

Jäätelä, M. (1991). *Lab. Invest.* **64**, 724–742.

Jacob, C. O., and McDevitt, H. O. (1991). Interferon gamma and tumor necrosis factor in autoimmune disease models: Implications for immunoregulation and genetic susceptibility. *In* "Molecular Autoimmunity" (N. Talal, ed.), pp. 107–126. Academic Press, New York.

Jacob, C. O., and McDevitt, H. O. (1988). *Nature (London)* **331,** 356–358.

Jacob, C. O., Aiso, S., Michie, S. A., McDevitt, H. O., and Arha-Orbea, H. (1990). *Proc. Natl. Acad. Sci. USA* **87,** 968–972.

Jacobs, K. H., Fletcher, J., and Barnett, A. H. (1991). *Diabetologia* **34,** 576–578.

Jacobs, R. F., Tabor, D. R., Burks, A. W., and Campbell, G. D. (1989). *Am. Rev. Resp. Dis.* **40,** 1686–1692.

Jarry, A., Mezeau, F., and Laboisse, C. L. (1991). *Gastroenterology* **100,** A691. (Abstract)

Johnson, J. (1991). *J. NIH Res.* **3,** 61–65.

Johnson, S. E., and Baglioni, G. (1988). *J. Biol. Chem.* **263,** 5686–5692.

Johnston, R. B., Jr. (1988). Monocytes and macrophages. *N. Engl. J. Med.,* **318,** 747–752.

Jupin, C., Anderson, S., Damais, C., Alouf, J. E., and Parant, M. (1988). *J. Exp. Med.* **167,** 752–761.

Kadurugamuwa, J. L., Hengstler, B., and Zak, O. (1987). *Pediatr. Infect. Dis. J.* **6,** 1152–1154.

Kagan, B. L., Baldwin, R. L., Munoz, D., and Wisnieski, B. J. (1992). *Science* **255,** 1427–1430.

Kaplan, G., and Cohn, Z. A. (1991). *Curr. Opin. Immunol.* **3,** 91–96.

Kelley, J. (1990). *Am. Rev. Resp. Dis.* **141,** 765–788.

Kern, P., Hemmer, C. J., van Damme, J., Gruss, H-J., and Dietrich, M. (1989). *Am. J. Med.* **87,** 139–143.

Kettelhut, I. C., Fiers, W., and Goldberg, A. L. (1987). *Proc. Natl. Acad. Sci. USA* **84,** 4273–4277.

Kim, C., Siminovitch, K. A., and Ochi, A. (1991). *J. Exp. Med.* **174,** 1431–1434.

Klebanoff, S. J., Vudas, M. A., Harlan, J. M., Sparks, L. H., Gamble, J. R., Agosti, J. M., and Wultersdorph, A. M. (1986). *J. Immunol.* **136,** 4220–4225.

Köck, A., Schwarz, T., Kirnbauer, R., *et al.* (1990). *J. Exp. Med.* **172,** 1609–1614.

Koerner, T. J., Adams, D. O., Hamilton, T. A. (1987). *Cell. Immunol.* **109,** 437–443.

Koopman, W. J., and Gay, S. (1988). *Scand. J. Rheumatol.* **75,** 284–289.

Kornbluth, R. S., Oh, P. S., Munis, J. R., Cleveland, P. H., and Richman, D. D. (1989). *J. Exp. Med.* **169,** 1137–1151.

Kovaks, E., Radzioch, D., Young, H. A., and Varesio, L. (1988). *J. Immunol.* **141,** 3101–3105.

Krams, S. M., Falco, D. A., and Villanueva, J. C. (1992). *Transplantation* **53,** 151–156.

Kriegler, M. P. (1991). Patent #W091/02540. U.S. Patent Office, Washington, D.C.

Kunkel, S. L., Spengler, M., May, M. A., Spengler, R., Remick, J., and Remicle, D. (1988). *J. Biol. Chem.* **263,** 5380–5384.

Kusagami, K., Matsuura, T., West, G., Youngman, K. R., Rachmilewitz, D., and Fiocchi, C. (1991). *Gastroenterology* **101,** 1594–1605.

Kwaitkowski, D., Cannon, J. G., Manogue, K. R., Cerami, A., Dinarello, C. A., and Greenwood, B. M. (1989). *J. Exp. Immunol.* **77,** 361–366.

Lähdevirta, J., Maury, C. P. J., Teppo, A-M., and Repo, H. (1988). *Am. J. Med.* **85,** 289–291.

Le, J., and Vilcek, J. (1987). *Lab. Invest.* **56,** 234–248.

Lebel, M. H., Freij, B. J., Syrogiannopoulos, G. A., *et al.* (1988). *N. Engl. J. Med.* **319,** 964–971.

Leeper-Woodford, S., Carey, P. D., Fisher, B. J., *et al.* (1990). *Am. Rev. Resp. Dis.* **144,** A919. (Abstract)

Leeper-Woodford, S. K., Carey, P. S., Byrne, K., *et al.* (1991). *Am. Rev. Resp. Dis.* **143,** 1076–1082.

Lehmmann, V., Finninghoff, B., and Droege, W. (1988). *J. Immunol.* **141,** 587–591.

Leist, T. P., Frei, K., Kam-Hansen, S., Zinkernagel, R. M., and Fontano, A. (1988). *J. Exp. Med.* **167,** 1743–1748.

Leitman, D. C., Ribeiro, R. C. J., Mackow, E. R., Baxter, J. D., West, B. L. (1991). *J. Biol. Chem.* **266,** 9343–9346.

Levine, B., Kalman, J., Mayer, L., Fillit, H. M., and Packer, M. (1990). *N. Engl. J. Med.* **323,** 236–241.

Lifson, A. R., Rutherford, G. W., and Jaffe, H. W. (1988). *J. Infect. Dis.* **158**, 1360–1367.

Loetscher, H., Schlaeger, E. J., Lahm, H-W., Pan, Y.-C. E., Lesslauer, W., and Brockhaus, M. (1990a). *J. Biol. Chem.* **265**, 20131–20138.

Loetscher, H., Pan, Y.-C. E., Lahn, H. W., *et al.* (1990b). *Cell* **61**, 351–357.

Loetscher, H., Steinmetz, M., and Lesslauer, W. (1991). *Cancer Cells* **3**, 221–226.

Lunn, J. J., Murray, M. J., and Rorie, D. K. (1990). *Crit. Care Med.* **18**, 1408–1412.

Macnaul, K. L., Hutchinson, N. I., Parsons, J. N., Bayne, E. K., and Tocci, M. J. (1990). *J. Immunol.* **145**, 4154–4166.

Mahatama, M., Agrawal, N., Dajani, E. Z., Nelson, S., Nakamuna, C., and Sitter, J. (1991). *Digest. Dis. Sci.* **36**, 1562–1568.

Mahida, Y. R. (1990). *Eur. J. Gastroenterol. Hepatol.* **2**, 251–255.

Mahida, Y. R., Ceska, M., Lindley, I., and Hawkey, C. J. (1991). *Gastroenterology* **100**, A595. (Abstract)

Malizia, G., Calabrese, A., Cottone, M., *et al.* (1991). *Gastroenterology* **100**, 150–159.

Mandrup-Poulsen, T., Helqvist, S., Wogensen, L. D., *et al.* (1990). *Curr. Top. Microbiol. Immunol.* **164**, 169–193.

Mansour, A. M., Gurbindo, C., Mehran, E., and Seidman, E. (1991). *Gastroenterology* **100**, A833. (Abstract)

Marks, J. D., Marks, C. B., Luce, J. M., *et al.* (1990). *Am. Rev. Resp. Dis.* **141**, 94–97.

Martich, G. D., Danner, R. L., Ceska, M., and Suffredini, A. F. (1991). *J. Exp. Med.* **173**, 1021–1024.

Maschler, H., and Christenson, S. B. (1991). Patent #WO91/15451. U.S. Patent Office, Washington, D.C.

Mathison, J. C., Wolfson, E., and Ulevitch, R. J. (1988). *J. Clin. Invest.* **81**, 1925–1937.

Matsuyama, T., Hamamoto, Y., Okamoto, T., Shimotohno, K., Kobayashi, N., and Yamamoto, N. (1988). *Lancet* **ii**, 364.

Matsuyama, T., Yoshiyama, H., Hamamoto, Y., *et al.* (1989). *AIDS Res. Hum. Retroviruses* **5**, 139–146.

Mayer, L. (1990). *Curr. Opin. Gastroenterol.* **614**, 556–560.

Mayer, L., and Eisenhart, D. (1990). *J. Clin. Invest.* **86**, 1255–1260.

McCachren, S. S., Haynes, B. F., and Neidel, J. F. (1990). *J. Clin. Immunol.* **10**, 19–27.

McIntyre, K. W., Stepan, G. J., Kolinsky, K. D., *et al.* (1991). *J. Exp. Med.* **173**, 931–939.

McKay, I. A., and Leigh, I. M. (1991). *J. Dermatol.* **124**, 513–518.

McManus, L. M., and Deavers, S. I. (1989). *Clin. Chest Med.* **10**, 107–118.

Mellors, J. W., Griffith, B. P., Ortiz, M. A., Landry, M. L., and Ryan, J. L. (1991). *J. Infect. Dis.* **163**, 78–82.

Meltzer, M. S., Skillman, D. R., Hoover, D. L., *et al.* (1990). *Immunol. Today* **11**, 217–223.

Mendis, K. N., Naotunne, T. deS., Karunaweena, N. D., Giudice, G. D., Grau, G. E., and Carter, R. (1990). *Immunol. Lett.* **25**, 217–220.

Merrell, J. E., Koyanagi, Y., and Chen, I. (1989). *J. Virol.* **63**, 4404–4408.

Mestan, J., Digel, W., Mittnacht, S., *et al.* (1986). *Nature (London)* **323**, 816–819.

Michalek, S. M., Moore, R. N., McGhee, J. R., Rosenstriech, D. L., and Mergenhagen, S. E. (1980). *J. Infect. Dis.* **141**, 55–63.

Michie, H. R., Manogue, K. R., Spriggs, D. R., *et al.* (1988a). *N. Engl. J. Med.* **318**, 1481–1486.

Michie, H. R., Spriggs, D. R., Manogue, K. R., *et al.* (1988b). *Surgery (St. Louis)* **104**, 280–286.

Miethke, T., Wahl, C., Heeg, K., Echtenacher, B., Krammer, P. H., and Wagner, H. (1992). *J. Exp. Med.* **175**, 91–98.

Millar, A. B., Singer, M., Meager, A., Foley, N. M., Johnson, N. M., and Rook, G. A. W. (1989). *Lancet* **ii**, 712–714.

Mizock, B. (1984). *Arch. Intern. Med.* **144**, 579–585.

Molina, J-M., Scadden, D. T., Byrn, R., Dinarello, C. A., and Groopman, J. E. (1989). *J. Clin. Invest.* **84**, 733–737.

Molina, J-M., Scadden, D. T., Amirault, C., *et al.* (1990). *J. Virol.* **64**, 2901–2906.

Molitor, J. A., Walker, W. H., Doerre, S., Ballard, D. W., and Greene, W. C. (1990). *Proc. Natl. Acad. Sci. USA* **87**, 10028–10032.

Mongelli, N., Biasolli, G., Grandi, M., and Ciomei, M. (1991). Patent #W091/10699. U.S. Patent Office, Washington, D.C.

Moore, K., Walters, M. T., Jones, D. B., *et al.* (1988). *Immunology* **65**, 457–463.

Morrow, W. J. W., Isenberg, D. A., Sobol, R. E., Stricker, R. B., and Kieber-Emmons, T. (1991). *Clin. Immunol. Immunopathol.* **58**, 163–180.

Mountz, J. D., Gause, W. C., and Jonsson, R. (1991). *Curr. Opin. Rheum.* **3**, 738–756.

Mountz, J. D., Zhou, T., Long, R. E., Blüthmann, H., Koopman, W. J., and Edwards, C. K., III (1994). *Arthritis Rheum.* **37**, 113–124.

Mourad, W., Mehindata, K., Schall, T. J., and McCall, S. R. (1992). *J. Exp. Med.* **175**, 613–616.

Muller, U., Jongeneel, C. V., Nedospasor, S. A., Lindahl, K. F., and Steinmetz, M. (1987). *Nature (London)* **325**, 265–267.

Munis, J. R., Richman, D. D., and Kornbluth, R. S. (1990). *J. Clin. Invest.* **85**, 591–596.

Murray, H. W. (1988). *Ann. Intern. Med.* **108**, 595–608.

Murray, J. F., Matthay, M. A., Luce, J. M., *et al.* (1988). *Am. Rev. Resp. Dis.* **138**, 720–723 [Erratum, (1989), *Am. Rev. Resp. Dis.* **139**, 1065].

Mustafa, M. M., Lebel, M. H., Ramilo, O., *et al.* (1989a). *J. Pediatr.* **115**, 208–213.

Mustafa, M. M., Ramilo, O., Olsen, K. D., *et al.* (1989b). *J. Clin. Invest.* **84**, 1253–1259.

Mustafa, M. M., Ramilo, O., Saez-Llorens, X., Mertsola, J., Magness, R. R., and McCracken, G. H. (1989c). *Pediatr. Infect. Dis. J.* **8**, 921–922.

Nahum, A., Chamberlin, W., and Sznajder, J. I. (1991). *Am. Rev. Resp. Dis.* **143**, 1083–1087.

Nain, M., Hinder, F., Garg, J. H., *et al.* (1990). *J. Immunol.* **145**, 1921–1928.

Nakane, A., Minagawa, T., and Kato, K. (1988). *Infect. Immun.* **56**, 2563–2569.

Naotunne, T. deS., Karunaweera, N. D., del Giudice, G., *et al.* (1991). *J. Exp. Med.* **173**, 523–529.

Natanson, C., Eichenholtz, P. W., Danner, R. L., *et al.* (1989). *J. Exp. Med.* **169**, 823–832.

Nathan, C. F. (1986). Interferon-gamma and macrophage activation in cell-mediated immunity. *In* "Mechanisms of Host Resistance to Infectious Agents, Tumors, and Allografts" (R. M. Steinman and R. J. North, eds.), 165–184. Rockefeller University Press, New York.

Nawroth, P. P., Bank, I., Handley, D., Cassimeris, J., Chess, L., and Stern, D. (1986a). *J. Exp. Med.* **163**, 1363–1375.

Nawroth, P. P., Bank, I., Handley, D., Cassimeris, J., Chess, L., and Stern, D. (1986b). *J. Exp. Med.* **163**, 1363–1375.

Nedwin, G. E., Naylor, S. L., Sakaguchi, A. Y., *et al.* (1985a). *Nucl. Acids Res.* **13**, 6361–6373.

Nedwin, G. E., Sverdersky, L. D., Bringman, T. S., Palladino, M. A., and Goeddel, D. V. (1985b). *J. Immunol.* **135**, 2492–2497.

Nelson, S., Bagby, G. J., Bainton, B. G., and Summer, W. R. (1989a). *J. Infect. Dis.* **160**, 422–429.

Nelson, S., Bagby, G. J., Bainton, B. G., Wilson, L. A., Thompson, J. J., and Summer, W. R. (1989b). *J. Infect. Dis.* **159**, 189–194.

Nestel, F. P., Price, K. S., Seemayer, T. A., and Lapp, W. S. (1992). *J. Exp. Med.* **175**, 405–413.

Nishizuka, Y. (1986). *Science* **233**, 305–312.

Noel, P., Nelson, S., Bukulic, R., *et al.* (1990). *Life Sci.* **47**, 1023–1029.

Noguchi, M., Sasaki, T., Hiwatashi, N., and Toyota, T. (1991). *Gastroenterology* **100**, A604. (Abstract)

Nohynek, H., Teppo, A-M., Laine, E., Leinonen, M., and Eskola, J. (1990). *J. Infect. Dis.* **163**, 1029–1032.

Ogata, H., Hibi, T., Ohara, M., *et al.* (1991). *Gastroenterology* **100**, A604. (Abstract)

Ohlsson, K., Bjork, P., Bergenfeldt, M., Hageman, R., and Thompson, R. C. (1990). *Nature (London)* **348**, 550–552.

Old, L. J. (1990). Tumor necrosis factor. *In* "Tumor Necrosis Factor: Structure, Mechanism of Action, Role in Disease and Therapy" (B. Bonavida and G. Granger, eds.), pp. 1–30. Karger, Basel.

Osborn, L., Kunkel, S., and Nabel, G. J. (1989). *Proc. Natl. Acad. Sci. USA* **86,** 2336–2340.

Paliard, X., West, S. G., Lafferty, J. A., *et al.* (1991). *Science* **253,** 325–329.

Parker, M. M., and Parrillo, J. E. (1983). *J. Am. Med. Assoc.* **250,** 3324–3327.

Parker, M. M., Schelhamer, J. H., Bacharach, S. L., *et al.* (1984). *Ann. Intern. Med.* **100,** 483–490.

Parmely, M. J., Zho, W. W., Edwards, C. K., III, Borcherding, D., Silverstein, R., and Morrison, D. C. (1993). *J. Immunol.* **151,** 389–396.

Parsonnet, J., and Gillis, Z. A. (1988). *J. Infect. Dis.* **158,** 1026–1033.

Peetre, C., Thysell, H., Grubb, A., and Olsson, I. (1988). *Eur. J. Hematol.* **41,** 414–419.

Pessara, U., and Koch, N. (1990). *Mol. Cell. Biol.* **10,** 4146–4154.

Peters, A. M. J., Jager, F.-S., Warneke, A., *et al.* (1991). *Clin. Immunol. Immunopathol.* **61,** 343–352.

Picot, S., Peyron, F., Vuillez, J. P., Polack, B., and Ambroise-Thomas, P. (1991). *J. Infect. Dis.* **164,** 830.

Piguet, P. F., Graw, G. E., Hauser, C., and Vassalli, P. (1991). *J. Exp. Med.* **173,** 673–679.

Podolsky, D. K. (1991a). *N. Engl. J. Med.* **325,** 928–937.

Podolsky, D. K. (1991b). *N. Engl. J. Med.* **325,** 1008–1016.

Pogrebniak, H., Matthews, W., Mitchell, J., Russo, A., Samuni, A., and Pass, H. (1991). *J. Surg. Res.* **50,** 469–474.

Poli, G., Bressler, P., Kinter, A., *et al.* (1990a). *J. Exp. Med.* **172,** 151–158.

Poli, G., Kinter, A., Justement, J. S. *et al.* (1990b). *Proc. Natl. Acad. Sci. USA* **87,** 782–785.

Porteu, F., and Nathan, C. (1990). *J. Exp. Med.* **172,** 599–607.

Powell, R. J., Machiedo, G. W., Rush, B. F., Jr., and Dikdan, G. S. (1991). *Ann. Surg.* **57,** 86–88.

Price, G., Brenner, M. K., Prentice, G. H., Hoffbrand, A. V., and Newland, A. C. (1987). *Br. J. Cancer* **55,** 287–290.

Pullman, W. E., Hapel, A. J., and Doe, W. F. (1991). *Gastroenterology* **100,** A608. (Abstract)

Rabinovitch, A. (1991). Immune cell and cytokine-mediated islet β-cell injury. *In* "Diabetes 1991" (H. Rifkin, J. A., Colwell, and S. I., Taylor, eds.), pp. 301–304. Exerpta Medica, The Netherlands.

Ramadori, G., Van Damme, J., Reider, H., Meyer zum Buschenfelde, K-H. (1988). *Eur. J. Immunol.* **18,** 1259–1264.

Reddy, M. M., Sorrell, S. J., Lange, M., and Grieco, M. H. (1988). *J. Acquired Immune Defic. Syndr.* **1,** 436–440.

Reed S. G., Nathan, C. F., Pihl, D. L., *et al.* (1987). *J. Exp. Med.* **166,** 1734–1746.

Reimund, J. M., Dumont, S., Sapin, R., and Chamouard, P. (1991). *Gastroenterology* **100,** A576. (Abstract)

Reka, S., and Kotler, D. P. (1991). *Gastroenterology* **100,** A609. (Abstract)

Renz, H., Gong, J. H., Schmidt, A., *et al.* (1988). *J. Immunol.* **141,** 2388–2393.

Rinaldo, J. E., and Christman, J. W. (1990). *Clin. Chest Med.* **11,** 621–632.

Roberts, D. J., Davies, J. M., Evans, C. C., Bell, M., and Mostafa, S. M. (1989). *Lancet* **ii,** 1043–1044.

Rook, G. A. W., and Attiyah, R. A. (1991). *Tubercule* **72,** 13–20.

Rosenberg, Z. F., and Fauci, A. S. (1990). *Immunol. Today* **11,** 176–180.

Roux-Lombard, P., Modoux, C., Cruchaud, A., and Dayer, J. M. (1989). *Clin. Immunol. Immunopathol.* **50,** 374–384.

Ruggiero, V., Johnson, S. E., and Baglioni, C. (1987). *Cell Immunol.* **107,** 317–325.

Sampaio, E. P., Sarno, E. N., Galilly, R., Cohn, Z. A., and Kaplan, G. (1991). *J. Exp. Med.* **173,** 699–703.

Sariben, E., Imamura, K., Luebbers, R., and Kufe, D. (1988). *J. Clin. Invest.* **81,** 1506–1510.

Saukkonen, K., Sande, S., Cioffe, C., *et al.* (1990). *J. Exp. Med.* **171,** 439–448.

Schade, U. F., Burmeister, I., Engel, R., Reinke, M., and Wolter, D. (1989). *Lymphokine Res.* **8,** 245–250.

Schattner, A., Lachmi, M., Livneh, A., Pras, M., and Hahn, T. (1991). *Am. J. Med.* **90,** 434–438.

Schiller, J. H., Bittner, G., Storer, B., and Willson, J. K. V. (1987). *Cancer Res.* **47,** 2809–2813.

Schilling, R. F. (1991). *Ann. Intern. Med.* **115,** 572–573.

Schleimer, R. P., Benenati, S. V., Friedman, B., and Bochner, B. S. (1991). *Am. Rev. Resp. Dis.* **143,** 1169–1174.

Schleunig, M. J., Dugan, A., and Reem, G. H. (1989). *Eur. J. Immunol.* **19,** 1491–1496.

Schmiegel, W., Roeder, C., Schmielau, J., *et al.* (1992). *Gastroenterology* **100,** A666. (Abstract)

Schoenfeld, H-J., Poeschi, B., Frey, J. R., *et al.* (1990). *J. Biol. Chem.* **266,** 3863–3869.

Schönharting, M. M., and Schade, U. F. (1989). *J. Med.* **20,** 97–105.

Schulman, K. A., Glick, H. A., Rubin, H., and Eisenberg, J. M. (1991). *J. Am. Med. Assoc.* **266,** 3466–3471.

Schultz, R. M., and Kleinschmidt, W. J. (1983). *Nature (London)* **305,** 239–240.

Schürer-Maly, C-G., Halter, F., Fiers, W., Urwyler, A., and Maly, F-E. (1991). *Gastroenterology* **100,** A546. (Abstract)

Scuderi, P., Lam, K. S., Ryan, K. J., *et al.* (1986). *Lancet* **ii,** 1364–1365.

Scuderi, P., Sterling, K. E., Raitano, A. B., Grogan, T. M., and Rippe, R. A. (1987). *J. Interferon Res.* **7,** 155–164.

Seckinger, P., Isaaz, S., and Dayer, J. M. (1989). *J. Biol. Chem.* **264,** 11966–11973.

Shakov, A. N., Collart, M. A., Vassalli, P., Nedospasov, S. A., and Jongeneel, C. V. (1990). *J. Exp. Med.* **171,** 35–47.

Shaffer, N., Gran, G. E., Hedberg, K., *et al.* (1991). *J. Infect. Dis.* **163,** 96–101.

Shalaby, M. R., Aggarwal, B. B., Rinderknecht, E., Svederly, L. P., Finkle, B. S., and Palladino, M. R. (1985). *J. Immunol.* **135,** 2069–2073.

Shalaby, M. R., Waage, A., Aarden, L., and Espevik, T. (1989). *Clin. Immunol. Immunopathol.* **53,** 488–498.

Shalaby, M. R., Sundan, A., Loetscher, H., Brockhaus, M., Lesslauer, W., and Espevik, T. (1990). *J. Exp. Med.* **172,** 1517–1520.

Sharief, M., and Hentges, R. (1991). *N. Engl. J. Med.* **325,** 467–472.

Sharp, B. M., Keone, W. F., Suh, H. J., Gekker, G., Tsukayama, D., and Peterson, P. K. (1985). *Endocrinology* **117,** 793–795.

Shaw, G., and Kamen, R. (1986). *Cell* **46,** 659–667.

Shenep, J. L., and Mogan, K. A. (1984). *J. Infect. Dis.* **150,** 380–388.

Shenep, J. L., Barton, R. P., and Mogan, K. A. (1985). *J. Infect. Dis.* **151,** 1012–1018.

Shepherd, V. L., and Abdolrasulnia, R. (1989). *Cytokine* **1,** 96. (Abstract)

Sherman, M. L., Spriggs, D. R., Arthur, K. A., Imamura, K., Frei, E., III, and Kufe, D. W. (1988). *J. Clin. Oncol.* **6,** 344–348.

Silva, C. L., and Figueiredo, F. (1991). *J. Infect. Dis.* **164,** 1033–1034.

Silva, C. L., Faccioli, L. H., and Rocha, G. M. (1988). *Braz. J. Med. Biol. Res.* **21,** 489–492.

Simon, J. M., Koenig, G., and Trenholme, G. M. (1991). *J. Infect. Dis.* **164,** 800–802.

Smith, E. F., Slivjak, M. J., Bartus, J. O., and Esser, K. M. (1991). *J. Cardiovasc. Pharmacol.* **18,** 721–728.

Smith, E. M., Hughes, T. K., Hashemi, F., and Stefano, G. B. (1992). *Proc. Natl. Acad. Sci. USA* **89,** 782–786.

Spies, T., Marton, C. C., Nedospasov, S. A., Fiers, W., Pious, D., and Strominger, J. L. (1986). *Proc. Natl. Acad. Sci. USA* **83,** 8699–8702.

Spies, T., Blanck, G., Bresnahan, M., Sands, J., and Strominger, J. L. (1989). *Science* **243,** 214–216.

Spinas, G., Bloesch, D., Keller, U., Zimmerli, W., and Cammisuli, S. (1991). *J. Infect. Dis.* **163,** 89–95.

Spriggs, D. R., Sherman, M. L., Michie, H., *et al.* (1988). *J. Natl. Cancer Inst.* **80,** 1039–1044.

Stephens, K. E., Ishizaka, A., Larrick, J. W., and Raffin, T. A. (1988). *Am. Rev. Resp. Dis.* **137,** 1364–1370.

Stolpen, A. H., Guinan, E. C., Fiers, W., and Pober, J. S. (1986). *Am. J. Pathol.* **123,** 16–24.

Suffredini, A. F., Harpel, P. C., and Parrillo, J. E. (1989a). *N. Engl. J. Med.* **320,** 1165–1172.

Suffredini, A. F., Fromm, R. E., Parker, M. M., *et al.* (1989b). *N. Engl. J. Med.* **321,** 280–287.

Sung, S.-S. J., Walters, J. A., Hudson, J., and Gimble, J. M. (1991). *J. Immunol.* **147,** 2047–2054.

Suputtamongkol, Y., Kwaitkowski, D., Dance, D. A. B., Chaowagul, W., and White, N. J. (1992). *J. Infect. Dis.* **165,** 561–564.

Sverdsky, L. P., Benton, V. V., Berger, W. H., Rinderknecht, E., Harkins, R. N., and Palladino, M. A. (1984). *J. Exp. Med.* **159,** 812–827.

Swartz, M. N. (1984). *N. Engl. J. Med.* **311,** 912–914.

Tabor, D. R., Burchett, S. K., and Jacobs, R. F. (1988). *Proc. Soc. Exp. Biol. Med.* **187,** 408–415.

Takasuka, N., Tokunaga, T., and Akagawa, K. S. (1991). *J. Immunol.* **146,** 3824–3830.

Talmadge, J. E., Tribble, H. R., Pennington, R. W., Phillips, H., and Wiltrant, R. H. (1987). *Cancer Res.* **47,** 2563–2570.

Täuber, M. G., Shibl, A. M., Hackbath, C. J., Larrick, J. W., and Sande, M. A. (1987). *J. Infect. Dis.* **156,** 456–462.

Thivierge, M., and Rola-Pleszczynski, M. (1991). *Am. Rev. Resp. Dis.* **144,** 272–277.

Torti, F. M., Dieckman, B., Beutler, B., Cerami, A., and Ringold, G. M. (1985). *Science* **229,** 867–869.

Tracey, K. J. (1989). *Lancet* **8647,** 1122–1125.

Tracey, K. J., Beutler, B., Lowry, S., *et al.* (1986). *Science* **234,** 470–474.

Tracey, K. J., Fong, Y., Hesse, D. G., *et al.* (1987a). *Nature (London)* **330,** 662–664.

Tracey, K. J., Lowry, S. F., Fahey, T. J., *et al.* (1987b). *Surg. Gynecol. Obstet.* **164,** 415–422.

Tracey, K. J., Wei, H., Manogue, K. R. *et al.* (1988a). *J. Exp. Med.* **167,** 1211–1227.

Tracey, K. J., Lowry, S. F., and Cerami, A., (1988b). *Am. Rev. Respir. Dis.* **138,** 1377–1379.

Treon, S. P., Dienstag, J. L., and Broitman, S. A. (1991). *Gastroenterology* **100,** A845. (Abstract)

Tsuchida, A., Salem, H., Thompson, N., and Hancock, W. W. (1992). *J. Exp. Med.* **175,** 81–90.

Tuomanen, E., Liu, H., Hengstler, B., Zak, O., and Tomasz, A. (1985a). *J. Infect. Dis.* **151,** 859–868.

Tuomanen, E., Tomasz, A., Hengstler, B., and Zak, O. (1985b). *J. Infect. Dis.* **151,** 535–540.

Tureen, J. H., Stella, F. B., Clyman, R. I., Mauroy, F., and Sande, M. A. (1987). *Pediatr. Infect. Dis. J.* **6,** 1151–1153.

Unanue, E. R., and Allen, P. R. (1987). *Science* **236,** 551–557.

Vaisman, N., Schattner, A., and Hahn, T. (1989). *Am. J. Med.* **87,** 115.

van der Poll, T., Büller, H. R., ten Cate, H., *et al.* (1990). *N. Engl. J. Med.* **322,** 1622–1627.

van der Poll, T., van Deventer, S. J. H., Büller, H. R., Sturk, A., and ten Cate, J. W. (1991). *J. Infect. Dis.* **164,** 599–601.

Vannier, E., Miller, L. C., and Dinarello, C. A. (1991). *J. Exp. Med.* **173,** 281–284.

Vayakarnam, A., McKeating, J., Meager, A., and Beverley, P. C. (1990). *AIDS* **4,** 21–27.

Veterans Administration Systemic Sepsis Cooperative Study Group (1987). *N. Engl. J. Med.* **317,** 659–665.

Vilcek, J., and Lee, T. H. (1991). *J. Biol. Chem.* **266,** 7313–7316.

Vincent, J-L., Bakker, J., Maricaux, G., Schandene, L., Kahn, R. J., and Dupont, E. (1992). Results of a pilot study. *Chest* **101,** 810–815.

Virelizer, J. L. (1991). *Curr. Opin. Immunol.* **2,** 409–413.

Waage, A., and Espevik, T. (1988). *J. Exp. Med.* **167,** 1987–1992.

Waage, A., Halstensen, A., and Espevik, T. (1987). *Lancet* **i,** 355–357.

Waage, A., Brandtzaeg, P., Halstensen, A., Kierulf, P., and Espevik, T. (1989a). *J. Exp. Med.* **169,** 333–338.

Waage, A., Halstensen, A., Shalaby, R., Brandtzaeg, P., Kierulf, P., and Espevik, T. (1989b). *J. Exp. Med.* **170,** 1859–1867.

Wakabayashi, G., Gelfand, J. A., Burke, J. F., Thompson, R. C., and Dinarello, C. A. (1991a). *FASEB J.* **5,** 338–343.

Wakabayashi, G., Gelfand, J. A., Burke, J. F., Thompson, R. C., and Dinarello, C. A. (1991b). *FASEB J.* **6,** 338–341.

Warner, S. J. C., and Libby, P. (1989). *J. Immunol.* **142,** 100–109.

Warrell, D. A. (1987). *Parasitology* **94,** 853–876.

Warren, R. S., Starnes, H. S., Gabrilove, J. L., Oettgen, H. F., and Brennan, M. F. (1987). *Arch. Surg.* **122,** 1396–1400.

Watanabe-Fukunaga, R., Brannan, C. I., Copeland, N. G., Jenkins, N. A., and Nagata, S. (1992). *Nature (London)* **356,** 314–317.

Weiss, S. J. (1989). *N. Engl. J. Med.* **320,** 365–375.

Westacott, C. I., Whicher, J. T., Barnes, I. C., Thompson, D., Swan, A. J., and Dieppe, P. A. (1990). *Ann. Rheum. Dis.* **49,** 676–681.

Whiting, J. F., Rosenbluth, A. B., Narciso, J. P., and Gollan, J. L. (1991). *Gastroenterology* **100,** A811. (Abstract)

Wilson, M. E., and Morrison, D. C. (1982). *Eur. J. Biochem.* **128,** 137–141.

Wing, E. J., Ampel, N. M., Waheed, A., and Shadduck, R. K. (1985). *J. Immunol.* **135,** 2052–2056.

Wong, G. H. W., and Goeddel, D. V. (1986). *Nature (London)* **323,** 819–822.

Wong, G. V., and Goeddel, D. V. (1988). *Science* **242,** 941–944.

Wright, S. C., Jewett, A., Mitsuyasu, R., and Bonavida, B. (1988). *J. Immunol.* **141,** 99–104.

Wright, S. D. (1991). *Curr. Opin. Immunol.* **3,** 83–90.

Wyle, F. A. (1991). *J. Clin. Gastroenterol. (Suppl. 1)* **13,** S114–S124.

Wyler, D. J. (1988). *J. Infect. Dis.* **158,** 320–324.

Yochum, D. E., Esparza, L., Dubry, S., Benjamin, J. B., Volz, R., and Scideri, P. (1989). *Cell. Immunol.* **121,** 131–145.

Yuhas, Y., Holtmann, H., Shemer-Avni, Y., Sarov, I., and Wallich, D. (1990). *Eur. Cytokine Net.* **1,** 35–40.

Zeni, F., Tardy, B., Vindimian, M., Comtet, C., Page, Y., and Bertrand, J. C. (1991). *J. Infect. Dis.* **164,** 1242–1243.

Zhang, J., Ye, Z. H., Zhou, T., Mountz, J. D., and Edwards, C. K., III (1991). *Arthritis Rheum.* **34,** 5117. (Abstract)

Zhang, J., Baker, T. J., De, M., Zhou, T., Mountz, J. D., and Edwards, C. K., III (1992). *FASEB J.* **6,** A1969. (Abstract #5982)

Zhang, J., Zhou, T., Baker, T. J., Long, R. E., Bluethmann, H., Mountz, J. D., and Edwards, III, C. K. (1994). *J. Immunol.,* In press.

Zhou, T., Blüthmann, H., Gay, R. E., Edwards, C. K. III, and Mountz, J. D. (1991). *J. Cell Biochem.* **15E,** 145. (Abstract)

Zuckerman, S. H., Evans, G. F., Snyder, Y. M., and Roeder, W. D. (1989). *J. Immunol.* **143,** 1223–1227.

Zuckerman, S. H., Evans, G. F., and Guthrie, L. (1991). *Immunology* **73,** 460–465.

6

Bone Marrow Phagocytes, Inflammatory Mediators, and Benzene Toxicity

Laureen MacEachern and Debra L. Laskin

I. Introduction

Hematopoiesis is the ordered process of proliferation and differentiation of blood cells that begins with pluripotent stem cells and terminates with the production of mature end-stage leukocytes and erythrocytes. As stem cells mature, they become irreversibly committed to develop along the lymphoid pathway, resulting in T and B lymphocytes, or along the myeloid pathway, leading to the production of megakaryocytes, erythrocytes, monocytes, and granulocytes including neutrophils, basophils, and eosinophils. The primary site of hematopoiesis is the bone marrow. In a normal healthy adult human, approximately 1×10^{10} erythrocytes and 4×10^8 leukocytes are produced per hour in the bone marrow (Metcalf, 1988). The production of these cells is regulated by cytokines and growth factors released from stromal cells and mature leukocytes within the bone marrow (Lord and Testa, 1988).

Benzene is a widely used organic compound that is known to induce hematotoxicity in chronically exposed humans and experimental animals (reviewed by Laskin and Goldstein, 1977; Kalf, 1987; Goldstein, 1988). Acute treatment of experimental animals with benzene or its metabolites results in a decrease in bone marrow cellularity as well as impaired host resistance to pathogens such as *Listeria monocytogenes* and engrafted tumor cells (Rosenthal and Snyder, 1985,1987; Laskin *et al.*, 1989; Renz and Kalf, 1991). The mechanism underlying the development of bone marrow toxicity in response to benzene exposure is unknown. Benzene has been reported to be cytotoxic to proliferating progenitor cells of lymphocytic, granulocytic, monocytic, and erythrocytic origin (Irons *et al.*, 1979, 1992; Tunek *et al.*, 1981; Wierda and Irons, 1982; Pfeiffer and Irons, 1983; Seidel *et al.*, 1989a,b), as well as to mature cells that constitute the bone marrow stroma (Garnett *et al.*, 1983; Gaido and Wierda, 1985,1987). These cells—which include macrophages, endothelial cells, and fibroblasts—release cytokines and growth factors that regulate hematopoiesis. Thus, altered production of these mediators after benzene exposure may contribute to hematoxicity.

A. Microenvironment of the Bone Marrow

The bone marrow consists of stem cells, rapidly dividing populations of progenitor cells that give rise to the formed elements of blood, and mature leukocytes and erythrocytes. Also found in the bone marrow are stromal cells that include endothelial cells, fibroblasts, adipocytes, and macrophages. Stromal cells provide a supporting matrix for hematopoietic cell growth and release cytokines, including granulocyte–macrophage colony stimulating factor (GM-CSF), granulocyte CSF (G-CSF), macrophage CSF (CSF-1), interleukin 3 (IL-3 or multi-CSF), Steel factor, leukemia inhibitory factor (LIF), interleukin 1 (IL-1), interleukin 6 (IL-6), and interleukin 7 (IL-7), all of which regulate the development of progenitor cells (Metcalf, 1988; Metcalf and Nicola, 1985; Nathan, 1990; Watson and McKenna, 1992). In addition, stromal cells produce extracellular matrix proteins such as collagens, fibronectin, and proteoglycans that bind to and sequester growth factors, thus concentrating these factors in the hematopoietic microenvironment (Gordon, 1987; Roberts *et al.*, 1988; Dorschkind, 1990). Several studies have demonstrated that, in the absence of stromal cells, hematopoiesis is impaired (Dexter *et al.*, 1977; Reimann and Burgrer, 1979; Bently, 1981; Dexter, 1982). For example, Dexter (1982) reported that progenitor cell proliferation is not sustained in cultures lacking an adherent stromal layer. In addition, Tavassoli and Friedenstein (1983) showed that stromal regeneration precedes the resumption of hematopoiesis after mechanical evacuation of the bone marrow cavity, or when bits of marrow are implanted into ectopic sites. Erschler *et al.* (1980) also described a defective hematopoietic microenvironment in a case of congenital hypoplastic anemia.

Macrophages constitute a major component of the bone marrow stroma. These cells support the development of erythroblasts, lymphoblasts, and developing eosinophils (Bessis, 1973; Lichtman, 1981) and have been identified in close proximity to islands of developing erythrocytes (Bessis, 1973; LaPushin and Trentin, 1977). Macrophages are thought to be the primary cells involved in the regulation of hematopoiesis (Kurland, 1978; Wright *et al.*, 1980, 1982; Simmons and Lord, 1985). These cells release IL-1, IL-6, and CSFs, which enhance proliferation and differentiation of progenitor cells (Metcalf, 1988; Nathan, 1990), as well as prostaglandins, which are negative regulators of myelopoiesis (Kurland and Moore, 1977; Schlick *et al.*, 1984; Moore *et al.*, 1985).

B. Developing Cells within the Bone Marrow

Mature blood cells are derived from pluripotent bone marrow stem cells (Katz et al., 1979; Ash et al., 1980; Lord and Testa, 1988). Stem cells are distinguished by their unique capacity for self-renewal and account for about 0.4% of the cells in the bone marrow. Stem cells progress through a series of proliferation and differentiation steps that result in irreversible commitment to develop along a specific pathway. Committed progenitor cells retain a residual capacity for self-replication. Thus, specific cell populations may be amplified during development. Committed progenitor cells constitute approximately 3% of the total bone marrow cell population (Lord and Testa, 1988).

Approximately 95% of hematopoietic cells in the bone marrow consist of maturing blood cells that express distinct morphological characteristics. Whereas early precursor cells maintain the capacity to replicate, the more mature differentiated cells do not. Erythrocytes, megakaryocytes, and granulocytes differentiate and mature exclusively in the bone marrow. In contrast, monocytes and lymphocytes terminally differentiate and mature in the blood and secondary lymphatic organs.

II. Regulation of Hematopoiesis

A. Stem Cell Development and Myelopoiesis

The development and maturation of stem cells and progenitor cells is regulated by cytokines and growth factors released from stromal cells and mature leukocytes within the bone marrow (Metcalf, 1988; Nathan, 1990). The major cytokines involved in hematopoietic regulation are CSF-1, G-CSF, GM-CSF, and IL-3 (Metcalf, 1988; Nathan, 1990). IL-3 is thought to contribute to the development of all cell types within the bone marrow by initiating stem cell differentiation (Lord and Testa, 1988; Ogawa, 1989). In addition, although IL-3 stimulates proliferation of early multipotent progenitor cells, terminal differentiation of precursor cells appears to be independent of IL-3 (Sonada et al., 1988). GM-CSF supports the development of neutrophils, eosinophils, basophils, macrophages, mast cells, megakaryocytes, and erythrocytes at intermediate stages (Broxmeyer et al., 1988; Nathan, 1990), and enhances functional maturation of granulocytes and macrophages (Heidenreich et al., 1989; Wirthmueller et al., 1989). G-CSF and CSF-1 are lineage-specific cytokines that act on maturing granulocytes and monocyte/macrophages (Eliason, 1986; Welte et al., 1987; Ogawa, 1989). G-CSF also augments IL-3-induced proliferation of stem cells (Ikebuchi et al., 1988).

Several other cytokines have also been identified that play a role in hematopoiesis, including IL-1, IL-6, and IL-8. IL-1 stimulates the proliferation of early hematopoietic progenitors by enhancing the responsiveness of these cells to IL-3 (Stanley *et al.*, 1986; Zhou *et al.*, 1988). IL-1 also enhances hematopoiesis by stimulating the production of GM-CSF, G-CSF, and IL-6 (Fibbe *et al.*, 1986; Rennick *et al.*, 1987; Helle *et al.*, 1989; Sironi *et al.*, 1989). In addition, IL-1 induces the production of prostaglandin E_2 (PGE_2) by stromal fibroblasts, resulting in decreased progenitor cell proliferation (Zucali *et al.*, 1986). IL-6, like IL-1, participates in hematopoiesis by augmenting IL-1- and IL-3-dependent growth and differentiation of multipotent hematopoietic progenitors (Ikebuchi *et al.*, 1987; Onozaki *et al.*, 1989). IL-6 also induces maturation of megakaryocytes, increases platelet counts, and enhances myeloid cell development (Ishibashi *et al.*, 1989; Akira *et al.*, 1990). IL-8 has been shown to be involved in the terminal differentiation and functional activation of neutrophils (Schroder, 1989; Djeu *et al.*, 1990).

B. Lymphopoiesis

Proliferation and differentiation of stem cells along the lymphocyte lineage is dependent on IL-1, IL-3, and IL-6, as described already. IL-2, which is primarily derived from T cells, also participates in lymphopoiesis by inducing the proliferation and differentiation of progenitor T and B lymphocytes (Watson, 1979; Gordon and Guy, 1987). Other cytokines, including IL-4, IL-5, and IL-7, have also been reported to contribute to proliferation and/or differentiation of lymphocytes (Leary *et al.*, 1988; Sieff, 1988; Sonada *et al.*, 1988; Clutterbuck *et al.*, 1989; Suda *et al.*, 1989; Welch *et al.*, 1989). IL-4 enhances the development of erythrocytes, macrophages, megakaryocytes, and mast cells (Mossman *et al.*, 1986; Smith and Rennick, 1986; Crawford *et al.*, 1987; Peschel *et al.*, 1987). Several studies have described another bone marrow stromal cell derived cytokine, IL-11, that participates in hematopoiesis. This cytokine stimulates T cell-dependent development of B cells, as well as megakaryocyte colony formation (Paul *et al.*, 1990).

III. Effects of Benzene on Bone Marrow

A. Hematopoietic Progenitor Cells

The clinical manifestations of benzene-induced hematotoxicity include aplastic anemia (Santesson, 1897), pancytopenia (Kipen *et al.*, 1989), and leukemia (Aksoy *et al.*, 1974; Aksoy, 1985). These effects suggest that benzene interferes with hematopoiesis. In this regard, benzene has been shown to be cytotoxic to hematopoietic progenitor cells at intermediate stages of development of almost all cell lineages. For example, Irons et al. (1979) evaluated bone marrow smears from rats exposed to benzene and found that myeloid and erythroid cells of intermediate stages of differentiation were most sensitive to the cytotoxic effects of benzene, whereas blast cells and mature nondividing cells were spared. In vivo and in vitro exposure of bone marrow lymphocytes to the benzene metabolites hydroquinone and catechol has also been shown to reduce proliferation and differentiation of lymphopoietic progenitors (King et al., 1987; Wierda and Irons, 1982). Benzene, as well as three of its metabolites—phenol, hydroquinone, and 1,2-dihydro-1,2-dihydroxy benzene—have also been reported to reduce the number of granulopoietic precursors in treated mice (Tunek et al., 1981). Similarly, erythrocyte production was impaired in mice exposed to benzene, as determined by reduced incorporation of ^{59}Fe into circulating erythrocytes (Lee et al., 1974). These investigators suggested that benzene interfered with the proliferation of erythrocyte precursors rather than with mature erythrocytes. Injury to the hematopoietic stem cell has also been described by Harigaya et al. (1981) in long-term bone marrow cultures established from benzene-treated mice. In these cultures, a progressive reduction in the number of spleen colony forming cells was observed.

B. Bone Marrow Stromal Cells

Several studies have suggested that the effects of benzene on progenitor cells are caused by alterations in stromal cell function. Bone marrow stromal cells form an adherent monolayer in culture dishes (Zipori and Bol, 1979; Tavassoli and Friedenstein, 1983). Because of this unique property, a system has been developed as a model of the hematopoietic microenvironment that involves culturing hematopoietic precursor cells with adherent stromal cells (Dexter et al., 1977; Dexter, 1982). Using this system, Garnett et al. (1983) showed that bone marrow stromal cells from mice exposed to benzene were unable to sustain hematopoiesis in vitro. In addition, the number of adherent bone marrow stromal cells was decreased and morphological alterations were noted in the adherent stromal layer. Harigaya et al. (1981) also reported a reduced capacity of bone marrow stromal cells from benzene-treated mice to maintain stem cell proliferation. Similarly, Gaido and Wierda (1985,1987) demonstrated that the ability of adherent stromal cells from benzene- or phenol-treated mice to support granulocyte/monocyte development in co-culture was depressed. Studies performed on stromal cells exposed in vitro to benzene metabolites such as hydroquinone, benzoquinone catechol, and benzenetriol also revealed a reduced capacity of these cells to regulate hematopoiesis (Gaido and Wierda, 1984,1987). These studies suggest that injury to bone marrow stroma of the hematopoietic microenvironment is a significant factor in benzene-induced toxicity.

C. Stromal Macrophages

As described earlier, mature bone marrow macrophages play a critical role in hematopoietic regulation. Thus, alterations in the functions of these cells by benzene may contribute to hematoxicity. These alterations may include inhibition of macrophage function leading to decreased production of growth regulatory cytokines, or activation of these cells in association with increased cytokine or reactive mediator production. Numerous studies have described depressed macrophage function after benzene treatment. For example, Lewis *et al.* (1988a) reported that *in vitro* exposure of peritoneal macrophages to catechol, hydroquinone, or benzoquinone, but not to benzene, inhibited production of hydrogen peroxide and reduced priming of these cells for cytotoxicity. King *et al.* (1987) also described inhibition of IL-1 production by bone marrow macrophages, leading to impaired B cell development. Similarly, Thomas and Wierda (1988) found that macrophage production of IL-1 was inhibited by hydroquinone and benzoquinone. These inhibitory effects appeared to be specific for bone marrow stromal macrophages (Thomas *et al.*, 1989). In contrast to these studies, Laskin and co-workers have found that benzene treatment of mice leads to increased maturation and/or activation of phagocytes in the bone marrow (Laskin *et al.*, 1989; MacEachern and Laskin, 1992; MacEachern *et al.*, 1992). These activated granulocytes and macrophages are thought to produce immune mediators, as well as cytotoxic products that directly contribute to hematotoxicity.

1. Morphological and Functional Activation of Bone Marrow Macrophages

In initial studies to test the possibility of macrophage involvement in benzene toxicity, techniques in flow cytometry and cell sorting were used to identify mature phagocytes in murine bone marrow. Based on laser light scattering properties, three distinct populations of cells in the bone marrow were identified that differed with respect to size and density (Figure 1): (1) a large dense population of cells (population 1, 41%), (2) a small, less dense population (population 3, 33%), and (3) a population of intermediate size and density (population 2, 23%). Using highly specific monoclonal antibodies, cells in population 1 were found to consist primarily of granulocytes, population 2 was identified as mononuclear phagocytes and precursor cells, and population 3 as B lymphocytes and precursors. The identity of the bone marrow populations was confirmed by cell sorting and microscopic examination. Treatment of mice with benzene (600–800 mg/kg, 1–2 times/day for 2–3 days) had no effect on the size, density, or antibody-binding profile of bone marrow leukocytes (MacEachern *et al.*, 1992).

Benzene treatment of mice is hypothesized to lead to increased maturation and/or activation of bone marrow macrophages (Laskin *et al.*, 1989). One characteristic of activated macrophages is altered morphology. Elec-

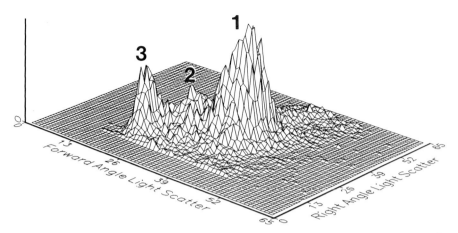

Fig. 1 Identification of bone marrow cell populations by flow cytometry. Bone marrow cells were analyzed by flow cytometry according to their laser light scattering properties. Cells scatter light in the forward angle direction according to size and in the right angle direction according to density or granularity. Note the identification of subpopulation 1, 2, and 3 which differed with respect to size and density.

tronic gating and sorting the macrophage-containing bone marrow cell population identified by flow cytometry (population 2) revealed that the mononuclear phagocytes from the bone marrow of benzene-treated mice exhibited characteristic morphology of activated macrophages, including increased cytoplasm-to-nucleus ratio and vacuolization (MacEachern et al., 1992). In addition, a 2-fold increase in the number of these cells was observed in the bone marrow of benzene-treated mice relative to control animals. These data indicate that benzene treatment of mice induces morphological maturation and/or activation of macrophages in the bone marrow.

In addition to alterations in morphology, activated phagocytes are characterized by enhanced functional capacity including increased chemotactic activity and elevated production of reactive intermediates. Mature bone marrow granulocytes and macrophages isolated from benzene-treated mice were found to display increased chemotactic activity relative to cells from control animals (MacEachern et al., 1992). Macrophages also displayed increased chemotaxis after treatment of mice with the combination of hydroquinone and phenol, two benzene metabolites. In contrast, the chemotactic activity of bone marrow granulocytes isolated from hydroquinone–phenol-treated mice was significantly depressed (MacEachern et al., 1992). These data demonstrate that benzene treatment of mice functionally activates bone marrow phagocytes. Investigators have suggested that the myeloperoxidase system of bone marrow granulocytes has the capacity to activate benzene metabolites to toxic intermediates (Eastmond et al., 1987). Higher levels of hydroquinone and phenol may accumulate on the bone marrow after their combined administration when compared with benzene, and these metabolites may be bioactivated by granulocytes, resulting in impaired functional capacity. Alternatively, granulocytes may be maximally activated *in vivo* by hydroquinone and phenol, resulting in an abrogated response to *in vitro* stimulation.

Activated phagocytes are also characterized by enhanced production of reactive oxygen intermediates, including superoxide anion and hydrogen peroxide (Adams and Hamilton, 1984; Glasser and Fiederlein, 1987). These products are nonspecific oxidants that induce lipid peroxidation reactions (Claster *et al.*, 1984; Lewis *et al.*, 1986), membrane and DNA damage (Fridovich, 1978; Birnboim, 1986; Lewis *et al.*, 1988b; Kawanishi *et al.*, 1989), tumor promotion (Kensler and Taffe, 1986; Kehrer *et al.*, 1988; Robertson *et al.*, 1990), carcinogenisis (Weitzman *et al.*, 1985; Lewis and Adams, 1987), and cytotoxicity (Clark and Klebanoff, 1975,1977). In additional experiments, the effects of benzene treatment of mice on the production of reactive oxygen intermediates by bone marrow phagocytes were analyzed using techniques in flow cytometry. In these experiments, an electronic map or gate was set around the three different bone marrow cell populations (Figure 1). Hydrogen peroxide production by each of these subpopulations was analyzed using the fluorescent indicator dye dichlorofluorescein diacetate (DCFH-DA; Bass *et al.*, 1983; Laskin *et al.*, 1989). In the absence of stimulation, hydrogen peroxide production was noted to be similar in all three populations (MacEachern *et al.*, 1992). Treatment of the cells with 12-*O*-tetradecanoyl-phorbol-13-acetate (TPA), which is known to induce a respiratory burst in granulocytes and macrophages (Bass *et al.*, 1983; Laskin and Pilaro, 1986), resulted in a significant increase in production of hydrogen peroxide by cells in populations 1 and 2, but not in population 3 (Table I; not shown). To determine which of the cells in population 2 produced hydrogen peroxide, anti-macrophage antibody binding and DCFH fluorescence were analyzed simultaneously. The majority (approximately 75%) of the cells in this population producing hydrogen peroxide was found to consist of mononuclear phagocytes (MacEachern *et al.*, 1992). Although benzene treatment of mice resulted in increased production of hydrogen peroxide by bone marrow granulocytes (population 1) in the absence of stimulation, basal levels of oxidative metabolism by macrophages (population 2) from control and benzene-treated mice were similar (MacEachern *et al.*, 1992). After treatment of the bone marrow cells with TPA, both granulocytes and mononuclear phagocytes from benzene-treated mice produced significantly more hydrogen peroxide than did cells from control animals (Table I).

In additional studies, the effects of benzene treatment of mice on nitric oxide production by bone marrow cells was analyzed. Nitric oxide is a potent vasodilator formed from L-arginine by the NADPH-dependent enzyme nitric oxide synthase and its activity is augmented after macrophage and neutrophil activation (Moncada *et al.*, 1991). Nitric oxide has been implicated in macrophage-mediated cytotoxicity and in inhibition of DNA synthesis in target cells (Moncada *et al.*, 1991). Studies revealed that benzene treatment of mice caused a significant increase in nitric oxide production by bone marrow macrophages and granulocytes relative to cells from control mice (Table I). These results are interesting since nitric oxide is also a potent antiproliferative agent in the bone marrow (Punjabi *et al.*, 1992). Increases in nitric oxide production by bone marrow phagocytes may account, at least in part, for the hematoxic effects of benzene.

Previous studies demonstrated that treatment of rats with hepatotoxicants such as acetaminophen or lipopolysaccharide (LPS) causes an accumulation of activated macrophages in the liver, and that these cells release increased levels of reactive oxygen intermediates (Laskin and Pilaro, 1986; McCloskey *et al.*, 1992). The release of these mediators from activated phagocytes may contribute to hepatic necrosis induced by these agents (Laskin *et al.*, 1986). Similarly, studies with benzene demonstrate that bone marrow macrophages and granulocytes from treated mice produce significantly more reactive oxygen intermediates, as well as reactive nitrogen intermediates, than do cells from control animals. Cytotoxic reactive oxygen and nitrogen intermediates released by bone marrow phagocytes may con-

Table I Effects of Benzene Treatment of Mice on Hydrogen Peroxide and Nitric Oxide Production by Bone Marrow Phagocytes[a]

	H_2O_2 (mean channel number)		Nitric oxide (nmol/10^6 cells)
Control	pop 1	325	6.4 ± 0.7
	pop 2	266	
Benzene	pop 1	495	19.5 ± 1.2
	pop 2	525	

[a] For measurement of hydrogen peroxide production, bone marrow cells from control or benzene-treated mice were incubated with $5\mu M$ dichlorofluorescin diacetate (DCFH-DA) for 20 min and then stimulated with 170 nM 12-O-tetradecanoyl-phorbol-13-acetate (TPA). After 20 min, hydrogen peroxide produced by cells in populations 1 and 2 (see Figure 1) was quantified by flow cytometry. The data are presented as mean fluorescence channel number. On the flow cytometer, data are presented on a four decade log scale that is divided into 1024 channels. Nitric oxide production by adherent bone marrow leukocytes was quantified by the accumulation of nitrite in the culture medium 3 days after treatment of cells with 10 μg/ml lipopolysaccharide, as previously described (Punjabi *et al.*, 1992).

tribute to the decrease in bone marrow cellularity and aberrant progenitor cell development that are observed after benzene exposure (Laskin et al., 1989; Kalf et al., 1989; Harigaya et al., 1981). In support of this possibility, Lewis et al. (1988b) reported that oxygen radicals such as superoxide anion are involved in the DNA damage that is induced by benzene metabolites. Reactive oxygen intermediates released by activated bone marrow granulocytes and macrophages may also augment activation of benzene and its metabolites to toxic intermediates. In this regard, researchers have reported that the enzyme systems involved in this activation process are dependent on hydrogen peroxide (Eastmond et al., 1987; Schlosser et al., 1990). Thus, production of hydrogen peroxide by bone marrow phagocytes from benzene-treated mice may lead to increased bioactivation of benzene metabolites, resulting in hematotoxicity.

2. *Increased Production of Immune Mediators by Bone Marrow Phagocytes*
Another characteristic of activated macrophages is production of immune mediators and pro-inflammatory cytokines such as tumor necrosis factor α (TNFα), IL-1, and IL-6. TNFα mediates of a number of diverse processes including cachexia (Beutler and Cerami, 1989), endotoxic shock (Beutler et al., 1985; Tracey et al., 1986), and hematopoiesis (Eliason and Vassalli, 1988). Although TNFα has been reported to inhibit hematopoiesis in murine bone marrow cell cultures directly (Eliason and Vassalii, 1988), this cytokine also stimulates production of G-CSF, CSF-1, and GM-CSF by mononuclear phagocytes and endothelial cells (Broudy et al., 1986; Munker et al., 1986). This stimulation may augment progenitor cell development. Thus, alterations in levels of TNFα in the bone marrow could have profound effects on hematopoiesis. Studies have revealed that isolated bone marrow phagocytes produce significant levels of TNFα in response to LPS stimulation (MacEachern and Laskin, 1992). Release of TNFα by these cells was time dependent, reaching maximal levels 4 hr after inoculation of the cells into the culture dishes. At this time, bone marrow cells from mice treated with benzene produced 40–50% more TNFα than did cells from control mice (Table II). Production of TNFα by bone marrow cells from both control and benzene-treated mice was also found to increase when the macrophage growth factor CSF-1 was added to the cultures. In fact, the stimulatory effect of benzene treatment of mice on TNFα production by bone marrow leukocytes appeared to be dependent on the presence of CSF-1. This macrophage-specific growth factor is known to induce morphological changes in mononuclear phagocytes that are characteristic of mature activated macrophages (Metcalf, 1988; Falk and Vogel, 1990), and to stimulate antigen presentation (Falk et al., 1988a), phagocytosis (Falk and Vogel, 1988), and tumor cytotoxicity (Falk et al., 1988b), as well as production of IL-1 (Moore et al., 1980), G-CSF (Metcalf, 1985), TNFα (Warren and Ralph, 1986), and reactive oxygen intermediates (Wing et al., 1985). Increased

Table II Effects of Benzene Treatment of Mice on
Cytokine Production by Bone Marrow Leukocytes[a]

Cytokine	Control	Benzene
TNFα (U/ml)	2.8± 0.4	4.0 ± 0.3
IL-1 (cpm × 10^{-3})	9.1 ± 0.4	11.4 ± 0.6
IL-6 (cpm × 10^{-3})	5.8 ± 0.5	5.8 ± 0.2

[a] Bone marrow from control or benzene treated mice were
cultured in the presence of lipopolysaccharide (0.1-1 μg/ml)
and, for the measurement of tumor necrosis factor (TNFα),
10% L-cell conditioned medium containing colony stimulating factor 1 (CSF-1). Supernatants were collected 2 hr later
for analysis of interleukin 1 (IL-1) and IL-6, and 4 hr later
for analysis of TNFα. IL-1 activity was quantified by proliferation of D10.G4.1 cells (Hopkins and Humphreys, 1989). IL-
6 activity was assayed by proliferation of B9 cells (Helle et
al., 1989). TNFα activity was determined by cytotoxicity to
actinomycin D-sensitized L929 fibroblasts (Satoh et al., 1987).
The data are presented as mean cpm × 10^{-3} ± SE of IL-1
and IL-6 or mean units of TNFα/ml ± SE of three samples
from one representative experiment.

production of TNFα by bone marrow cells cultured in the presence of CSF-
1 correlates with reports that have identified mature activated macrophages
as the predominant source of this cytokine (Mannel et al., 1980; Bloksma
et al., 1984; Kornbluth and Edgington, 1986).

TNFα is a potent inflammatory mediator that activates both granulocytes
and macrophages (Mace et al., 1988; Philip and Epstein, 1986; Tenneberg
and Solomkin, 1990; Berkow and Dodson, 1988). These activated phagocytes produce increased levels of hydrogen peroxide, superoxide anion, and
hydrolytic enzymes, and have been implicated in tissue injury (Klebanoff et
al., 1986; Tennenberg and Solomkin, 1990). Reactive oxygen species, such
as those produced by activated phagocytes, have also been shown to facilitate the release of TNFα (Chaudhri and Clark, 1989). Thus, TNFα may
contribute to benzene-induced hematotoxicity by amplifying the activation
of bone marrow phagocytes. TNFα may also exert a direct cytotoxic action
on developing cells. In this regard, chronic administration of TNFα to mice,
as well as to humans, has been reported to result in anemia (Tracey et al.,
1988; Blick et al., 1987).

Activated macrophages are also characterized by increased production
of IL-1 (Ogawa, 1989; Ogawa et al., 1989). This cytokine enhances the
proliferation of both uncommitted and committed hematopoietic progenitor
cells (Lord and Testa, 1988; Ogawa et al., 1989), and also induces bone
marrow stromal cells to produce growth factors that stimulate blood cell
development (Lee et al., 1987; Fibbe et al., 1989). In studies of bone marrow

cells from both control and benzene-treated mice, these cells were found to produce significant quantities of IL-1 (MacEachern and Laskin, 1992). Production of IL-1 was time dependent, reaching a maximum 6 hr after isolation of the cells, and remained detectable for up to 48 hr. In addition, bone marrow cells from benzene-treated mice were found to produce significantly more IL-1 than did cells from control mice (Table II). This increased production of IL-1 was rapid, reaching a maximum 2 hr after inoculation of the cells into culture, and transient. IL-1 has been hypothesized to initiate hematopoiesis by decreasing the time that stem cells reside in the G_0 phase of the cell cycle (Ogawa, 1989). The rapid and transient increase in IL-1 production in the bone marrow after benzene exposure may act to stimulate progenitor cell proliferation by initiating cell cycle traverse.

IL-6 is a pleiotropic cytokine released by a variety of cells. This cytokine participates in hematopoiesis indirectly by augmenting IL-1- and IL-3-dependent growth and differentiation of multipotent hematopoietic progenitors (Ikebuchi et al., 1987; Onozaki et al., 1989), by inducing maturation of megakaryocytes, and by enhancing myeloid and B cell development (Bot et al., 1989; Kunimoto et al., 1989; Ishibashi et al., 1989; Akira et al., 1990). Studies have demonstrated that mature bone marrow leukocytes release IL-6 in a time-dependent manner, reaching a maximum 2 hr after inoculation of the cells into culture (MacEachern and Laskin, 1992). However, in contrast to results with IL-1 and TNFα, cells from control and benzene-treated mice produce similar amounts of IL-6 (Table II), suggesting that IL-6 may not play a role in benzene-induced hematotoxicity. Previous studies demonstrated that activated macrophages from livers of rats treated with hepatotoxicants produce levels of IL-6 that are similar to those in cells from untreated animals (Feder et al., 1993). These data suggest that IL-6 is not involved in pathophysiological responses that are associated with macrophage activation.

IV. Benzene-Induced Alterations in Bone Marrow Cell Proliferation

As described earlier, stromal cells and mature leukocytes play critical roles in the regulation of hematopoiesis. Thus, alterations in the functioning of these cells by hematotoxicants such as benzene may contribute to toxicity. Several investigators have reported aberrant stromal regulation of hematopoiesis after in vivo exposure of mice to benzene (Harigaya et al., 1981) or in vitro exposure of bone marrow stromal cells to hydroquinone–phenol (Thomas et al., 1989). These effects may be the result of altered release of mediators from activated bone marrow macrophages that modify progenitor cell growth. To analyze this possibility, culture supernatants were collected from bone marrow phagocytes after benzene treatment of mice and were analyzed for their effects on progenitor cell proliferation. Isolated bone marrow cells from mice treated with benzene were found to exhibit a 25–30% decrease in growth relative to cells from control animals (MacEachern et al., 1991). Similar decreases in bone marrow cell growth were observed when the cells were incubated with conditioned medium from bone marrow phagocytes from benzene-treated mice. Growth depression induced by conditioned medium was apparent in cultures incubated with supernatants collected as early as 2 hr after isolation of the bone marrow cells from benzene-treated mice, and was maintained for up to 24 hr. These results suggest that benzene treatment of mice induces bone marrow phagocytes to release soluble factors that alter the proliferation of blood cells. These soluble factors may contribute to the early clinical manifestations of benzene exposure that include decreased red and white blood cell counts.

V. Effects of Modifying Macrophage Function on Benzene Toxicity

Treatment of mice with benzene is hypothesized to lead to activation of phagocytes in the bone marrow that release mediators that contribute to toxicity (Laskin et al., 1989). If macrophages play a role in benzene-induced hematotoxicity, modulating the activity of these cells should modify the toxicity of benzene. In preliminary in vitro studies to test this possibility, LPS and interferon (IFNγ), two agents known to activate macrophages (Pace and Russell, 1981; Pace et al., 1983; Schreiber et al., 1983), were used. Addition of LPS to cultures of bone marrow cells from both control and benzene-treated mice resulted in a decrease in cellular proliferation (Table III). In contrast to LPS, IFNγ, which primes macrophages for activation, had no detectable effect on bone marrow cell growth. However, the combination of LPS and IFNγ was markedly synergistic (Table III). Cells from benzene-treated mice were more sensitive to the effects of LPS alone and in combination with IFNγ than were cells from control mice. Benzene treatment may result in partial activation of macrophages in the bone marrow, which is augmented by LPS and IFNγ. This possibility is consistent with studies that have reported that macrophages can be primed and/or activated to varying degrees (Weinberg et al., 1978; Adams and Hamilton, 1984). The mechanism underlying the effects of LPS and IFNγ on bone marrow cell proliferation is unknown. LPS and IFNγ have previously been reported to stimulate bone marrow cell nitric oxide production (Punjabi et al., 1992). These data, in conjunction with the findings that the inhibitory effects of LPS and IFNγ on bone marrow cell growth can be blocked by the addition of the nitric oxide synthase inhibitor N^G-monomethyl-L-arginine to the cultures, suggest that nitric oxide is involved in the response.

In additional studies, the effects of the macrophage inhibitor dextran sulfate (Souhani and Bradfield, 1974; Laskin, 1990) on bone marrow cell

Table III Effects of Modifying Macrophage Function on Bone Marrow Cell Proliferation[a]

| | Percentage growth | |
Treatment	Control	Benzene
None	100	100
LPS	62.5 ± 11.9*	37.2 ± 1.8*
IFNγ	101.8 ± 5.8	103.2 ± 6.8
IFNγ + LPS	45.8 ± 7.8*	9.6 ± 2.6*
DS	133.6 ± 1.6*	101.0 ± 2.0
DS + LPS	73.2 ± 4.1*	65.0 ± 7.7*

[a] Bone marrow cells from control or benzene-treated mice were incubated in 96-well dishes (5 × 10^5 cells/well) in the presence of lipopolysaccharide (LPS; 10 μg/ml), dextran sulfate (DS; 100 μg/ml), interferon γ (IFNγ; 100 U/ml), the combination of LPS and DS, or medium control for 19 hr at 37°C. ³H-TdR (1 μCi/ml) was then added. After 5 hr, the cells were harvested and counted for radioactivity. Each value represents the average ± SE of three samples from one representative experiment. The data are presented as percentage growth of cells from either untreated or treated mice cultured in medium alone; these were normalized to 100%.
* Statistically significant ($p \leq 0.02$) difference between untreated and treated cells.

proliferation was analyzed. In contrast to the results observed with the macrophage activator LPS, incubation of the bone marrow cells with dextran sulfate resulted in a 30–40% increase in proliferation, but only in cells from control mice (Table III). Further, dextran sulfate abrogated the growth suppression induced by LPS. Interestingly, despite the fact that cells from benzene-treated mice did not respond to dextran sulfate alone, they were more responsive to the combination of dextran sulfate and LPS than were cells from control mice (Table III). Collectively, these data suggest that activating macrophages augments benzene-induced decreases in bone marrow cell proliferation, whereas inhibiting macrophage activation ameliorates these effects.

VI. Model for Benzene-Induced Hematotoxicity

Based on the results of the studies described here, a model for benzene-induced hematotoxicity has been developed (Figure 2). According to this model, benzene treatment of mice leads to increased maturation and/or activation of granulocytes and macrophages in the bone marrow. These cells display altered morphology and release increased amounts of inflammatory mediators and cytokines—including reactive oxygen and nitrogen intermediates, TNFα, and IL-1—which can alter stromal regulation of hematopoiesis. Inflammatory mediators and cytokines may also directly modify stem cell or progenitor cell proliferation and differentiation. This phenomenon can lead to decreased proliferation of bone marrow cells, resulting in bone marrow depression, or increased proliferation, which is characteristic of leukemia.

VII. Summary and Conclusions

Studies done over the past several years demonstrate that phagocytes in the bone marrow are morphologically and functionally activated after benzene treatment of mice. These cells display increased chemotaxis, as well as production of reactive oxygen and nitrogen intermediates and release of

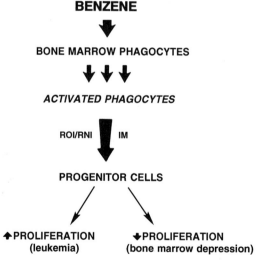

Fig. 2 Model for the potential role of bone marrow phagocytes in benzene-induced hematotoxicity. Toxic doses of benzene induce activation of bone marrow phagocytes. These activated phagocytes release reactive oxygen intermediates (ROI) and reactive nitrogen intermediates (RNI) that are cytotoxic to stem cells and other stromal cells, resulting in bone marrow depression. Activated phagocytes also can produce elevated levels of immune mediators (IM) and pro-inflammatory cytokines, including interleukin 1 (IL-1) and tumor necrosis factor α (TNFα) that alter the proliferation of subpopulations of bone marrow cells. This effect may be important in leukemogenesis.

IL-1 and TNFα. These mediators are known to have profound effects on hematopoiesis. These results, in conjunction with the findings that benzene-induced alterations in bone cell proliferation can be modified by modulating macrophage functioning, suggest that phagocytes play a role in hematotoxicity. Additional studies are necessary to define the precise contribution of bone marrow phagocytes and their mediators to benzene-induced hematotoxicity.

References

Adams, D. O., and Hamilton, T. A. (1984). The cell biology of macrophage activation. *Annu. Rev. Immunol.* **2**, 283–318.

Akira, S., Hirano, T., Taga, T., and Kishimoto, T. (1990). Biology of multifunctional cytokines: IL-6 and related molecules (IL-1 and TNF). *FASEB J.* **4**, 2860–2867.

Aksoy, M. (1985). Malignancies due to occupational exposure to benzene. *Am. J. Ind. Med.* **7**, 395–402.

Aksoy, M., Erdem, S., and Dincol, G. (1974). Leukemia in shoe workers exposed chronically to benzene. *Blood* **44**, 837–841.

Ash, P., Loutit, J. F., and Townsend, K. M. S. (1980). Osteoclasts derived from haemopoietic stem cells. *Nature (London)* **283**, 669–670.

Austyn, J. M., and Gordon, S. (1981). F4/80: A monoclonal antibody directed specifically against the mouse macrophage. *Eur. J. Immunol.* **11**, 805–813.

Bass, D. A., Parce, J. W., Dechatelet, L. R., Szejda, P., Seeds, M. C., and Thomas, M. (1983). Flow cytometric studies of oxidative product formation by neutrophils: A graded response to membrane stimulation. *J. Immunol.* **130**, 1910–1917.

Bently, S. A. (1981). Close range cell : cell interaction required for stem cell maintenance in continuous bone marrow culture. *Exp. Hematol.* **9**, 308–312.

Berkow, R. L., and Dodson, M. R. (1988). Biochemical mechanisms involved in the priming of neutrophils by tumor necrosis factor. *J. Leukocyte Biol.* **44**, 345–352.

Bessis, M. (1973). "Living Blood Cells and Their Ultrastructure." Springer-Verlag, New York.

Beutler, B., and Cerami, A. (1989). The biology of cachectin/TNF-α primary mediator of the host response. *Annu. Rev. Immunol.* **7**, 625–655.

Beutler, B., Milsark, I. W., and Cerami, A. (1985). Passive immunization against cachectin/ tumor necrosis factor (TNF) protects mice from the lethal effect of endotoxin. *Science* **229**, 869–871.

Birnboim, H. C. (1986). DNA strand breaks in human leukocytes induced by superoxide anion, hydrogen peroxide and tumor promoters are repaired slowly compared to breaks induced by ionizing radiation. *Carcinogenesis* **7**, 1511–1517.

Blick, M., Sherwin, S. A., Ronsenblum, M., and Gutterman, J. (1987). Phase I study of recombinant tumor necrosis factor in cancer patients. *Cancer Res.* **47**, 2986–2989.

Bloksma, N., Hofhuis, F. M., and Willers, J. M. (1984). Role of mononuclear phagocyte function in endotoxin-induced tumor necrosis. *Eur. J. Cancer Clin. Oncol.* **20**, 397–403.

Bot, F. J., van Eijk, L., Broeders, L., Aarden, L. A., and Lowenberg, B. (1989). Interleukin-6 synergizes with M-CSF in the formation of macrophage colonies from purified human marrow progenitor cells. *Blood* **73**, 435–437.

Broudy, V. C., Kaushansky, D., Segal, G. M., Harlan, J. M., and Adamson, J. W. (1986). Tumor necrosis factor type alpha stimulates human endothelial cells to produce granulocyte/ macrophage colony-stimulating factor. *Proc. Natl. Acad. Sci. USA* **83**, 7467–7471.

Broxmeyer, H. E., Williams, D. E., Hangoc, G., and Ralph, P. (1988). Recombinant human granulocyte-colony stimulating factor and recombinant human macrophage-colony stimulating factor synergize in vivo to enhance proliferation of granulocyte-macrophage, erythroid, and multipotential progenitor cells in mice. *J. Cell. Biochem.* **38**, 127–136.

Chaudhri, G., and Clark, I. A. (1989). Reactive oxygen species facilitate the *in vitro* and *in vivo* lipopolysaccharide-induced release of tumor necrosis factor. *J. Immunol.* **143**, 1290–1294.

Clark, R. A., and Klebanoff, S. J. (1975). Neutrophil-mediated cytotoxicity: Role of the peroxidase system. *J. Exp. Med.* **141**, 1442–1447.

Clark, R. A., and Klebanoff, S. J. (1977). Myeloperoxidase–H_2O_2–halide system: Cytotoxic effect on human blood leukocytes. *Blood* **50**, 65–70.

Claster, S., Chiu, D. T., Quintanilha, A., and Lubin, B. (1984). Neutrophils mediate lipid peroxidation in human red cells. *Blood* **64**, 1079–1084.

Clutterbuck, E. J., Hirst, E. M., and Sanderson, C. J. (1989). Human interleukin-5 (IL-5) regulates the production of eosinophils in human bone marrow cultures: Comparison and interaction with IL-1, IL-3, IL-6 and GMCSF. *Blood* **73**, 1504–1512.

Crawford, R. M., Finbloodm, D. S., Ohara, J., Paul, W. E., and Meltzer, M. S. (1987). B cell stimulatory factor-1 (interleukin 4) activates macrophages for increased tumoricidal activity and expression of Ia antigens. *J. Immunol.* **139**, 135–141.

Dexter, T. M. (1982). Stromal cell associated haemopoiesis. *J. Cell. Physiol.* **1**, 87–94.

Dexter, T. M., Allen, T. D., and Lajtha, L. G. (1977). Conditions controlling the proliferation of haemopoietic stem cells in vitro. *J. Cell. Physiol.* **91**, 335–344.

Djeu, J. Y., Matsushima, K., Oppenheim, J. J., Shiotsuki, K., and Blanchard, D. K. (1990). Functional activation of human neutrophils by recombinant monocyte-derived neutrophil chemotactic factor/IL-8. *J. Immunol.* **144**, 2205–2210.

Dorshkind, K. (1990). Regulation of hemopoiesis by bone marrow stromal cells and their products. *Annu. Rev. Immunol.* **8**, 111–137.

Eastmond, D. A., Smith, M. T., and Irons, R. D. (1987). An interaction of benzene metabolites reproduces the myelotoxicity observed with benzene exposure. *Toxicol. Appl. Pharmacol.* **91**, 85–95.

Eliason, J. F. (1986). Granulocyte-macrophage colony formation in serum-free culture: Effects of purified colony-stimulating factors and modulation by hydrocortisone. *J. Cell. Physiol.* **128**, 231–238.

Eliason, J. F., and Vassalli, P. (1988). Inhibition of hemopoiesis in murine marrow cell cultures by recombinant murine tumor necrosis factor alpha: Evidence for long-term effects on stromal cells. *Blood Cells* **14**, 339–354.

Ershler, W. B., Ross, J., Finlay, J. L., and Shahidi, N. T. (1980). Bone marrow microenvironment defect in congenital hypoplastic anemia. *N. Engl. J. Med.* **302**, 1321–1322.

Falk, L. A., and Vogel, S. N. (1988). Comparison of bone marrow progenitors responsive to granulocyte-macrophage colony stimulating factor and macrophage colony stimulating factor-1. *J. Leuk. Biol.* **43**, 148–157.

Falk, L. A., and Vogel, S. N. (1990). Differential production of IFN-a/b by CSF-1 and GM-CSF-derived macrophages. *J. Leukocyte Biol.* **48**, 43–49.

Falk, L. A., Wahl, L. M., and Vogel S. N. (1988a). Analysis of Ia antigen expression in macrophages derived from bone marrow cells cultured in granulocyte-macrophage colony stimulating factor or macrophage colony-stimulating factor. *J. Immunol.* **140**, 2652–2660.

Falk, L. A., Hogan, M. M., and Vogel, S. N. (1988b). Bone marrow progenitors cultured in the presence of granulocyte-macrophage colony-stimulating factor versus macrophage colony-stimulating factor differentiate into macrophages with distinct tumoricidal capacities. *J. Leukocyte Biol.* **43**, 471–476.

Feder, L. S., Todaro, J. A., and Laskin, D. L. (1993). Characterization of interleukin-1 (IL-1) and interleukin-6 (IL-6) production by hepatic endothelial cells and macrophages. *J. Leukocyte Biol.* **53**, 126–132.

Fibbe, W. E., van Damme, J., Billiau, A., Voogt, P. J., Duinkerken, J., Kluck, P. M. C., and Falkenburg, J. H. F. (1986). Interleukin-1 (22-K Factor) induces release of granulocyte-macrophage colony-stimulating activity from human mononuclear phagocytes. *Blood* **68**, 1316–1321.

Fibbe, W. E., Daha, M. R., Hiemstra, P. S., Duinkerken, M., Lurvink, E., Ralph, P., Altrock, B. W., Kaushansky, K., Willemze, R., and Falkenburg, J. H. F. (1989). Interleukin 1 and ploy(rI)-poly(rC) induce production of granulocyte CSF, macrophage CSF, and granulocyte-macrophage CSF by human endothelial cells. *Exp. Hematol.* **17**, 229–234.

Fridovich, I. (1978). The biology of oxygen radicals. *Science* **201**, 875–880.

Gaido, K., and Wierda, D. (1984). *In vitro* effects of benzene metabolites on mouse bone marrow stromal cells. *Toxicol. Appl. Pharmacol.* **76**, 45–55.

Gaido, K. W., and Wierda, D. (1985). Modulation of stromal cell function in DBA/2J and B6C3F1 mice exposed to benzene or phenol. *Toxicol. Appl. Pharmacol.* **81**, 469–475.

Gaido, K. W., and Wierda, D. (1987). Suppression of bone marrow stromal cell function by benzene and hydroquinone is ameliorated by indomethacin. *Toxicol. Appl. Pharmacol.* **89**, 378–390.

Garnett, H. M., Cronkite, E. P., and Drew, R. T. (1983). Effect of *in vivo* exposure to benzene on the characteristics of bone marrow adherent cells. *Leuk. Res.* **7**, 803–810.

Glasser, L., and Fiederlein, R. L. (1987). Functional differentiation of normal human neutrophils. *Blood* **69**, 937–944.

Goldstein, B. D. (1988). Benzene toxicity. *Occup. Med. State of the Art Rev.* **3**, 541–554.

Gordon, M. Y., and Guy, G. R. (1987). The molecules controlling B lymphocytes. *Immunol. Today* **8**, 339–344.

Gordon, M. Y., Riley, G. P., Watt, S. M., and Greaves, M. F. (1987). Compartmentalisation of a haemopoietic growth factor (GM-CSF) by glycosaminoglycans in the bone marrow microenvironment. *Nature (London)* **326**, 403–405.

Harigaya, K., Miller, M. E., and Cronkite, E. P. (1981). The detection of *in vivo* hematotoxicity of benzene by *in vitro* liquid bone marrow cultures. *Toxicol. Appl. Pharmacol.* **60**, 346–353.

Heidenreich, S., Gong, J. H., Schmidt, A., Nain, M., and Gemsa, D. (1989). Macrophage activation by granulocyte/macrophage colony stimulating factor: Priming for enhanced release of tumor necrosis factor-alpha and prostaglandin E_2. *J. Immunol.* **143**, 1198–1205.

Helle, M., Boeije, L., and Aarden, L. A. (1989). IL-6 is an intermediate in IL-1 induced thymocyte proliferation. *J. Immunol.* **142**, 4335–4338.

Hopkins, S. J., and Humphreys, M. (1989). Simple, sensitive and specific bioassay of interleukin-1. *J. Immunol. Meth.* **120**, 271–276.

Ikebuchi, K., Wong, G. G., Clark, S. C., Ihle, J. N., Hirai, Y., and Ogawa, M. (1987). Interleukin 6 enhancement of interleukin 3-dependent proliferation of multipotential hemopoietic progenitors. *Proc. Natl. Acad. Sci. USA* **84**, 9035–9039.

Ikebuchi, K., Clark, S. C., Ihle, J. N., Souza, L. M., and Ogawa, M. (1988). Granulocyte colony stimulating factor enhances interleukin-3-dependent proliferation of multipotential hemopoietic progenitors. *Proc. Natl. Acad. Sci. USA* **85**, 3445–3449.

Irons, R. D., Heck, H. D., Moore, B. J., and Muirhead, K. A. (1979). Effects of short-term benzene administration on bone marrow cell cycle kinetics in the rat. *Toxicol. Appl. Pharmacol.* **51**, 399–409.

Irons, R. D., Stillman, W. S., Colagiovanni, D. B., and Henry, V. A. (1992). Synergistic action of the benzene metabolite hydroquinone on myelopoietic stimulating activity of granulocyte/macrophage colony-stimulating factor in vitro. *Proc. Natl. Acad. Sci. USA* **89**, 3691–3695.

Ishibashi, T., Kimura, H., Shikama, Y., Uchida, T., Kariyone, S., Hirano, T., Kishimoto, T., Takatsuki, T., and Akiyama, A. (1989). Interleukin-6 is a potent thrombopoietic factor in vivo in mice. *Blood* **74**, 1241–1244.

Kalf, G. F. (1987). Recent advances in the metabolism and toxicity of benzene. *CRC Crit. Rev. Toxicol.* **18**, 141–159.

Kalf, G. F., Schlosser, M. J., Renz, J. F., and Pirozzi, S. J. (1989). Prevention of benzene-induced myelotoxicity by nonsteroidal anti-inflammatory drugs. *Environ. Health Perspect.* **82**, 57–64.

Katz, S. I., Tamaki, D., and Sachs, D. H. (1979). Epidermal Langerhans cells are derived from cells originating in bone marrow. *Nature (London)* **282**, 324–325.

Kawanishi, S., Inoue, S., and Kawanishi, M. (1989). Human DNA damage induced by 1,2,4-benzenetriol, a benzene metabolite. *Cancer Res.* **49**, 164–168.

Kehrer, J. P., Mossman, B. T., Sevanian, A., Trush, M. A., and Smith, M. T. (1988). Contemporary issues in toxicology. Free radical mechanisms in chemical pathogenesis. *Toxicol. Appl. Pharmacol.* **95**, 349–362.

Kensler, T. W., and Taffe, B. G. (1986). Free radicals in tumor promotion. *Adv. Free Rad. Biol. Med.* **2**, 347–387.

King, A. G., Landreth, K. S., and Wierda, D. (1987). Hydroquinone inhibits bone marrow pre-B cell maturation in vitro. *Mol. Pharmacol.* **32**, 807–812.

Kipen, H. M., Cody, R. P., and Goldstein, B. D. (1989). Use of longitudinal analysis of peripheral blood counts to validate historical reconstructions of benzene exposure. *Environ. Health Perspect.* **82**, 199–206.

Klebanoff, S. J., Vadas, M. A., Harlan, J. M., Sparks, L. H., Gamble, J. R., Agosti, J. M., and Waltersdorph, A. M. (1986). Stimulation of neutrophils by tumor necrosis factor. *J. Immunol.* **136**, 4220–4225.

Kornbluth, R. S., and Edgington, T. S. (1986). Tumor necrosis factor production by human monocytes is a regulated event: Induction of TNF-α mediated cellular cytotoxicity by endotoxin. *J. Immunol.* **137**, 2585–2591.

Kunimoto, D. Y., Nordan, R. P., and Strober, W. (1989). IL-6 is a potent cofactor of IL-1 in IgM synthesis and of IL-5 in IgA synthesis. *J. Immunol.* **143**, 2230–2235.

Kurland, J. I. (1978). The mononuclear phagocyte and its regulatory interactions in hemopoiesis. In "Experimental Hematology Today" (S. J. Baum and G. D. Ledney, eds., pp. 47–60. Springer-Verlag, New York.

Kurland, J. I., and Moore, M. A. S. (1977). Modulation of hemopoiesis by prostaglandins. *Exp. Hematol.* **5**, 357–373.

LaPushin, R. W., and Trentin, J. J. (1977). Identification of distinctive stromal elements in erythroid and neutrophil granuloid spleen colonies: Light and electron microscopic studies. *Exp. Hematol.* **5**, 505–522.

Laskin, D. L. (1990). Nonparenchymal cells in hepatotoxicity. *Sem. Liver Dis.* **10**, 293–304.

Laskin, D. L., and Pilaro, A. M. (1986). Potential role of activated macrophages in acetaminophen hepatotoxicity. I. Isolation and characterization of activated macrophages from rat liver. *Toxicol. Appl. Pharmacol.* **86**, 204–215.

Laskin, D. L., Pilaro, A. M., and Sungchul, J. (1986). Potential role of activated macrophages in acetaminophen hepatotoxicity. II. Mechanism of macrophage accumulation and activation. *Toxicol. Appl. Pharmacol.* **86**, 216–226.

Laskin, D. L., MacEachern, L., and Snyder, R. (1989). Activation of bone marrow phagocytes following benzene treatment of mice. *Environ. Health Perspect.* **82**, 75–79.

Laskin, S., and Goldstein, B. D. (1977). Benzene Toxicity: A Critical Evaluation. Hemisphere Publishing Corp., Washington, D.C.

Leary, A. G., Ikebuchi, K., Hirai, Y., Wong, G. G., Yang, Y. C., Clark, S. C., and Ogawa, M. (1988). Synergism between interleukin-6 and interleukin-3 in supporting proliferation of human hematopoietic stem cells: Comparison with interleukin-1 alpha. *Blood* **71**, 1759–1763.

Lee, E. W., Kocsis, J. J., and Snyder, R. (1974). Acute effect of benzene on ^{59}Fe incorporation into circulating erythrocytes. *Toxicol. Appl. Pharmacol.* **27**, 431–436.

Lee, M., Segal, G. M., and Bagby, G. C. (1987). Interleukin-1 induces human bone marrow-derived fibroblasts to produce multilineage hematopoietic growth factors. *Exp. Hematol.* **15**, 983–988.

Lewis, J. G., and Adams, D. O. (1987). Inflammation, oxidative DNA damage, and carcinogenesis. *Environ. Health Perspect.* **76**, 19–27.

Lewis, J. G., Hamilton, T., and Adams, D. O. (1986). The effect of macrophage development on the release of reactive oxygen intermediates and lipid oxidation products, and their ability to induce oxidative DNA damage in mammalian cells. *Carcinogenesis* **7**, 813–818.

Lewis, J. G., Odom, B., and Adams, D. O. (1988a). Toxic effects of benzene and benzene metabolites on mononuclear phagocytes. *Toxicol. Appl. Pharmacol.* **92**, 246–254.

Lewis, J. G., Steward, W., and Adams, D. O. (1988b). Role of oxygen radicals in induction of DNA damage by metabolites of benzene. *Cancer Res.* **48**, 4762–4765.

Lichtman, M. A. (1981). The ultrastructure of the hemopoietic environment of the marrow: A review. *Exp. Hematol.* **9**, 391–410.

Lord, B. I., and Testa, N. G. (1988). The hemopoietic system. *In* "Hematopoiesis. Long-Term Effects of Chemotherapy and Radiation." (N. G. Testa and R. P. Gale, eds.), pp. 1–26. Marcel Dekker, New York.

Mace, K. F., Ehrke, M. J., Hori, K., Maccubbin, D. L., and Mihich, E. (1988). Role of tumor necrosis factor in macrophage activation and tumoricidal activity. *Cancer Res.* **48**, 5427–5432.

MacEachern, L., and Laskin, D. L. (1992). Increased production of tumor necrosis factor-alpha by bone marrow leukocytes following benzene treatment of mice. *Toxicol. Appl. Pharmacol.* **113**, 260–266.

MacEachern, L., Snyder, R., and Laskin, D. L. (1991). Benzene-induce phagocyte activation alters mouse bone marrow progenitor cell development. *Toxicologist* **11**, 77.

MacEachern, L., Snyder, R., and Laskin, D. L. (1992). Alterations in the morphology and functional activity of bone marrow phagocytes following benzene treatment of mice. *Toxicol. Appl. Pharmacol.* **117**, 147–154.

Mannel, D. N., Moore, R. N., and Mergenhagen, S. E. (1980). Macrophages as a source of tumoricidal activity (tumor necrotizing factor). *Infect. Immun.* **30**, 523–530.

McCloskey, T. W., Todaro, J. A., and Laskin, D. L. (1992). Lipopolysaccharide treatment of rats alters antigen expression and oxidative metabolism in hepatic macrophages and endothelial cells. *Hepatology* **16**, 191–203.

McGarry, M., and Stewart, C. C. (1991). Murine eosinophil granulocytes bind the macrophage-monocyte specific monoclonal antibody F4/80 positive. *J. Leukocyte Biol.* **50**, 471–478.

Metcalf, D. (1985). The granulocyte-macrophage colony-stimulating factors. *Science* **229**, 16–22.

Metcalf, D. (1988). "The Molecular Control of Blood Cells." Harvard University Press, Cambridge, MA.

Metcalf, D., and Nicola, N. A. (1985). Proliferative effects of purified granulocyte colony-stimulating factor (G-CSF) on normal mouse hemopoietic cells. *J. Cell. Physiol.* **116**, 198–206.

Moncada, S. R., Palmer, M. J., and Higgs, E. A. (1991). Nitric oxide: physiology, pathophysiology and pharmacology. *Pharmacol. Rev.* **43**, 109–142.

Moore, R. N., Oppenheim, J. J., Farrar, J. J., Carter, C. S., Waheed, A., and Shadduck, R. K. (1980). Production of lymphocyte-activating factors (interleukin 1) by macrophages activated with colony-stimulating factors. *J. Immunol.* **125**, 1302–1305.

Moore, R. N., Pitruzello, F. J., Deana, F. J., and Rouse, B. T. (1985). Endogenous regulation of macrophage proliferation and differentiation by E prostaglandins and interferon alpha/beta. *Lymphokine Res.* **4**, 43–50.

Mossmann, T. R., Bond, M. W., Coffman, R. L., Ohara, J., and Paul, W. E. (1986). T cell and mast cell lines respond to B cell stimulatory factor-1. *Proc. Natl. Acad. Sci. USA* **83**, 5654–5658.

Munker, R., Gasson, J., Ogawa, M., and Koeffler, H. P. (1986). Recombinant human TNF induces production of granulocyte-monocyte colony-stimulating factor. *Nature (London)* **323**, 79–82.

Nathan, D. G. (1990). Regulation of Hematopoiesis. *Pediatr. Res.* **27**, 423–431.

Ogawa, M. (1989). Hemopoietic stem cells: Stochastic differentiation and humoral control of proliferation. *Environ. Health Perspect.* **80**, 199–207.

Ogawa, M., Ikebuchi, K., and Leary, A. G. (1989). Humoral regulation of stem cell proliferation. *Ann. N.Y. Acad. Sci.* **554**, 185–191.

Onozaki, K., Akiyama, Y., Okano, A., Hirano, T., Kishimoto, T., Hashimoto, T., Yoshizawa, K., and Taniyama, T. (1989). Synergistic regulatory effects of interleukin-6 and interleukin 1 on the growth and differentiation of human and mouse myeloid leukemic cell lines. *Cancer Res.* **49**, 3602–3607.

Pace, J. L., and Russell, S. W. (1981). Activation of mouse macrophages for tumor cell killing. I. Quantitative analysis of interactions between lymphokine and lipopolysaccharide. *J. Immunol.* **126**, 1863–1867.

Pace, J. L., Russell, S. W., Schreiber, R. D., Altman, A., and Katz, D. H. (1983). Macrophage activation: Priming activity from a T-cell hybridoma is attributable to interferon-gamma. *Proc. Natl. Acad. Sci. USA* **80**, 3782–3786.

Paul, S. R., Bennett, F., Calvetti, J. A., Kelleher, K., Wood, C. R., O'Hara, R. M., Jr., Leary, A. C., Sibley, B., Clark, S. C., Williams, D. A., and Yang, Y. C. (1990). Molecular cloning of a cDNA encoding interleukin 11, a stromal cell-derived lymphopoietic and hematopoietic cytokine. *Proc. Natl. Acad. Sci. USA* **87**, 7512–7516.

Peschel, C., Paul, W. E., Ohara, J., and Green, I. (1987). Effects of B cell stimulatory factor-1/interleukin 4 on hematopoietic progenitor cells. *Blood* **70**, 254–263.

Pfeifer, R. W., and Irons, R. D. (1983). Alteration of lymphocyte function by quinones through a sulfhydryl-dependent disruption of microtubule assembly. *J. Immunopharmacol.* **5**, 463–470.

Philip, R., and Epstein, L. B. (1986). Tumour necrosis factor as immunomodulator and mediator of monocyte cytotoxicity induced by itself, gamma-interferon, and interleukin-1. *Nature (London)* **323**, 86–89.

Punjabi, C. J., Laskin, D. L., Heck, D. E., and Laskin, J. D. (1992). Production of nitric oxide by murine bone marrow cells: Inverse correlation with cellular proliferation. *J. Immunol.* **149**, 2179–2184.

Reimann, J., and Burgrer, H. (1979). In vitro proliferation of hematopoietic cells in the presence of adherent cell layers. *Exp. Hematol.* **7**, 45–51.

Rennick, D., Yang, G., Gemmell, L., and Lee, F. (1987). Control of hemopoiesis by a bone marrow stromal cell clone: Lipopolysaccharide and interleukin-1 inducible production of colony stimulating factors. *Blood* **69**, 682–691.

Renz, J. F., and Kalf, G. (1991). Role for interleukin-1 in benzene induced hematotoxicity: Inhibition of conversion of pre-IL-1α to mature cytokine in mure macrophages by hydroquinone and prevention of benzene-induced hematotoxicity in mice by IL-1α. *Blood* **78**, 938–944.

Roberts, R., Gallagher, J., Spooncer, E., Allen, T. D., Bloomfield, F., and Dexter, T. M. (1988). Heparin sulphate bound growth factors: A mechanism for stromal cell mediated haemopoiesis. *Nature (London)* **332**, 376–378.

Robertson, F. M., Beavis, A. J., Oberyszyn, T. M., O'Connell, S. M., Dokidos, A., Laskin, D. L., Laskin, J. D., and Reiners, J. J. (1990). Production of hydrogen peroxide by murine epidermal keratinocytes following treatment with the tumor promoter 12-O-tetradecanoylphorbol-13 acetate. *Cancer Res.* **50**, 6062–6067.

Rosenthal, G. J., and Snyder, C. A. (1985). Modulation of the immune response to Listeria monocytogenes by benzene inhalation. *Toxicol. Appl. Pharmacol.* **80**, 502–510.

Rosenthal, G. J., and Snyder, C. A. (1987). Inhaled benzene reduces aspects of cell-mediated tumor surveillance in mice. *Toxicol. Appl. Pharmacol.* **88**, 35–43.

Santesson, C. (1897). Chronic poisoning with coal tar benzene; four deaths. Clinical and path-anatomical observations of several colleges and illustrating animal experiments. *Arch. Hyg.* **31**, 336–376.

Satoh, M., Oshima, H., Abe, S., Yamazaki, M., and Mizuno, D. (1987). Role of in vivo scavenger function of macrophages in priming for endogenous production of tumor necrosis factor. *J. Biol. Response Modif.* **6**, 499–511.

Schlick, E., Hartung, K., and Chirigos, M. A. (1984). Role of prostaglandin E and interferon in secretion of colony-stimulating factor by murine macrophages after *in vitro* treatment with biological response modifiers. *Int. J. Immunopharmacol.* **6**, 407–418.

Schlosser, M. J., Shurina, R. D., and Kalf, G. F. (1990). Prostaglandin H synthase catalyzed oxidation of hydroquinone to a sulfhydryl-binding and DNA damaging metabolite. *Chem. Res. Toxicol.* **3**, 333–339.

Schreiber, R. D., Pace, J. L., Russell, S. W., Altman, A., and Katz, D. H. (1983). Macrophage-activating factor produced by a T cell hybridoma: Physiochemical and biosynthetic resemblance to gamma-interferon. *J. Immunol.* **131**, 826–832.

Schroder, J. M. (1989). The monocyte-derived neutrophil activating peptide (NAP/interleukin-8) stimulates human neutrophil arachidonate-5-lipoxygenase, but not the release of cellular arachidonate. *J. Exp. Med.* **170**, 847–863.

Seidel, H. J., Barthel, E., and Zinser, D. (1989a). The hematopoietic stem cell compartments in mice during and after long-term inhalation of three doses of benzene. *Exp. Hematol.* **17**, 300–303.

Seidel, H. J., Beyvers, G., Pape, M., and Barthel, E. (1989b). The influence of benzene on the erythroid cell system in mice. *Exp. Hematol.* **17**, 760–764.

Sieff, C. A. (1988). Hemopoietic growth factors: *In vivo* and *in vitro* studies. *In* "Recent Advances in Haematology" (A. V. Hoffbrand, ed.), Vol. V, pp. 1–18. Churchill Livingstone, Edinburgh.

Simmons, P. J., and Lord, B. I. (1985). Enrichment of CFU-S proliferation inhibitor producing cells based on their identification by the monoclonal antibody F4/80. *J. Cell Sci.* **78**, 117–131.

Sironi, M., Breviario, F., Proserpio, P., Biondi, A., Vecchi, A., van Damme, J., Dejana, E., and Mantovani, A. (1989). IL-1 stimulates IL-6 production in endothelial cells. *J. Immunol.* **142**, 549–553.

Smith, C. A., and Rennick, D. M. (1986). Characterization of a murine lymphokine distinct from interleukin 2 and interleukin 3 (IL-3) possessing a T-cell growth factor activity and a mast-cell growth factor activity that synergizes with IL-3. *Proc. Natl. Acad. Sci. USA* **83**, 1857–1861.

Sonada, Y., Yang, Y. C., Wong, G. G., Clark, S. C., and Ogawa, M. (1988). Analysis in serum-free culture of the targets of recombinant human hemopoietic growth factors: Interleukin 3 and granulocyte/macrophage-colony stimulating factor are specific for early developmental stages. *Proc. Natl. Acad. Sci. USA* **85**, 4360–4364.

Souhami, R. L., and Bradfield, J. W. (1974). The recovery of hepatic phagocytosis after blockade of Kupffer cells. *J. Reticuloendothel. Soc.* **16**, 75–86.

Stanley, E. R., Bartocci, A., Patinkin, D., Rosendaal, M., and Bradley, T. R. (1986). Regulation of very primitive, multipotent, hemopoietic cells by hemopoietin-1. *Cell* **45**, 667–674.

Suda, T., Okada, S., Suda, J., Miura, Y., Ito, M., Sudo, T., Hayashi, S., Nishikawa, S., and Nakauchi, H. (1989). A stimulatory effect of recombinant murine interleukin-7 (IL-7) on B-cell colony formation and an inhibitory effect of IL-1a. *Blood* **74**, 1936–1941.

Tavassoli, M., and Friedenstein, A. (1983). Hematopoietic stromal microenvironment. *Am. J. Hematol.* **15**, 195–203.

Tennenberg, S. D., and Solomkin, J. S. (1990). Activation of neutrophils by cachectin/tumor necrosis factor: Priming of N-formyl-methionyl-leucyl-phenylalanine-induced oxidative responsiveness via receptor mobilization without degranulation. *J. Leukocyte Biol.* **47**, 217–223.

Thomas, D. J., and Wierda, D. (1988). Bone marrow stromal macrophage production of interleukin-1 activity is altered by benzene metabolites. *Toxicologist* **8**, 72.

Thomas, D. J., Reasor, M. J., and Wierda, D. (1989). Macrophage regulation of myelopoiesis is altered by exposure to the benzene metabolite hydroquinone. *Toxicol. Appl. Pharmacol.* **97**, 440–453.

Tracey, K. J., Beutler, B., Lowry, S. F., Merryweather, J., Wolpe, S., Milsark, I. W., Hariri, R. J., Fahey, T. J., Zentella, A., Albert, J. D., Shires, G. T., and Cerami, A. (1986). Shock and tissue injury induced by recombinant human cachectin. *Science* **234**, 470–474.

Tracey, K. J., Wei, H., Manogue, K. R., Fony, Y., Hesse, D. G., Nguyen, H. T., Kuo, G. C., Beutler, B., Cotran, R. A., Cerami, A., and Lowry, S. F. (1988). Cachectin/tumor necrosis factor induces cachexia, anemia and inflammation. *J. Exp. Med.* **167,** 1222–1227.

Tunek, A., Olofsson, T., and Berlin, M. (1981). Toxic effects of benzene and benzene metabolites on granulopoietic stem cells and bone marrow cellularity in mice. *Toxicol. Appl. Pharmacol.* **59,** 149–156.

Warren, M. K., and Ralph, P. (1986). Macrophage growth factor CSF-1 stimulates human monocyte production of interferon, tumor necrosis factor, and colony stimulating activity. *J. Immunol.* **137,** 2281–2285.

Watson, J. (1979). Continuous proliferation of murine antigen specific helper T lymphocytes in culture. *J. Exp. Med.* **150,** 1510–1519.

Watson, T., and McKenna, H. J. (1992). Novel factors from stromal cells: Bone marrow and thymus microenvironments. *Int. J. Cell Cloning* **10,** 144–152.

Weinberg, J. B., Chapman, H. A., and Hibbs, J. B. (1978). Characterization of the effects of endotoxin on macrophage tumor cell killing. *J. Immunol.* **121,** 72–80.

Weitzman, S. A., Weitberg, A. B., Clark, E. P., and Stossel, T. P. (1985). Phagocytes as carcinogens: Malignant transformation produced by human neutrophils. *Science* **227,** 1231–1233.

Welch, P. A., Namen, A. E., Goodwin, R. G., Armitage, R., and Cooper, M. D. (1989). Human IL-7: A novel T cell growth factor. *J. Immunol.* **143,** 3562–3567.

Welte, K., Bonilla, A. M., Gillio, A. P., Boone, T. C., Potter, G. K., Gabrilove, J. L., Moore, M. A. S., O'Reilly, R. J., and Souza, L. M. (1987). Recombinant human granulocyte colony-stimulating factor: Effects on hematopoiesis in normal and cyclophosphamide-treated primates. *J. Exp. Med.* **165,** 941–948.

Wierda, D., and Irons, R. D. (1982). Hydroquinone and catechol reduce the frequency of progenitor B lymphocytes in mouse spleen and bone marrow. *Immunopharmacol.* **4,** 41–54.

Wing, E. J., Ampel, N. M., Waheed, A., and Shadduck, R. K. (1985). Macrophage colony stimulating factor (M-CSF) enhances the capacity of murine macrophages to secrete oxygen reduction products. *J. Immunol.* **135,** 2052–2056.

Wirthmueller, U., De Weck, A. L., and Dahinden, C. A. (1989). Platelet-activating factor production in human neutrophils by sequential stimulation with granulocyte-macrophage colony-stimulating factor and the chemotactic factors C5A or formyl-methionyl-leucyl-phenylalanine. *J. Immunol.* **142,** 3213–3218.

Wright, E. G., Ali, A. M., Riches, A. C., and Lord, B. I. (1980). Stimulation of haemopoietic stem cell proliferation: Characteristics of the stimulator producing cells. *Leuk. Res.* **6,** 531–539.

Wright, E. G., Garland, J. M., and Lord, B. I. (1982). Specific inhibition of haemopoietic stem cell proliferation: Characteristics of the inhibitor producing cells. *Leuk. Res.* **4,** 537–545.

Zhou B. Y., Stanley, E. R., Clark, S. C., Hatzfeld, J. A., Levesque, J. P., Federici, C., Watt, S. M., and Hatzfeld, A. (1988). Interleukin-3 and interleukin-1-alpha allow earlier bone marrow progenitors to respond to human colony-stimulating factor 1. *Blood* **72,** 1870–1874.

Zipori, D., and Bol, S. (1979). The role of fibroblastoid cells and macrophages from mouse bone marrow in the *in vitro* growth promotion of haemopoietic tumour cells. *Exp. Hematol.* **7,** 6–218.

Zucali, J. R., Dinarello, C. A., Oblon, D. J., Gross, M. A., Anderson, L., and Weiner, R. S. (1986). Interleukin 1 stimulates granulocyte macrophage colony-stimulating activity and prostaglandin E_2. *J. Clin. Invest.* **77,** 1857–1863.

7

Dimethylnitrosamine-Associated Inflammation: Induction of Cytokines Affecting Macrophage Differentiation and Functions

Lawrence B. Schook, Alice L. Witsell,
John F. Lockwood, and Michael J. Myers

I. Introduction

The process of wound healing begins immediately after chemical and radiation damage (ten Dijke and Iwata, 1989, Figure 1). This process involves the release of cytokines from damaged cells (epithelial, endothelial, and parenchymal); these proteins promote the migration of cells to the injured site, the stimulation of fibroblast and epithelial growth, angiogenesis, and the repair of the affected area (Laskin and Pilaro, 1986; Laskin *et al.*, 1986; ten Dijke and Iwata, 1989). Growth factors (cytokines) released at the site of injury include epidermal growth factor (EGF), fibroblast growth factor (FGF), platelet-derived growth factor (PDGF), transforming growth factor α (TGFα), transforming growth factor β (TGFβ), and hematopoietic growth factors (CSF-1 and GM-CSF) (Mantovani and Dejana, 1989; Wahl *et al.*, 1989). Recruitment of mononuclear phagocytes to the inflammatory site has also been well documented (Laskin, 1990). On recruitment to the site of inflammation, monocytes contribute to the inflammatory process through the release of eicosanoid metabolites and cytokines (Morley, 1981; Khalil *et al.*, 1989; Schreiner *et al.*, 1989).

The organic nitroso compounds comprise the nitrosamines, nitrosamides, and C-nitroso compounds. Nitrosamines are readily formed by the reaction of secondary amines with nitrous acid (nitrite under acid conditions) and are relatively stable. Nitrosamides are unstable in alkaline environments, yielding the corresponding dialkanes, and are extensively used as alkylating reagents in synthetic organic reactions. This chapter focuses on nitrosamines, specifically, *N*-nitrosodimethylamine (dimethylnitrosamine,

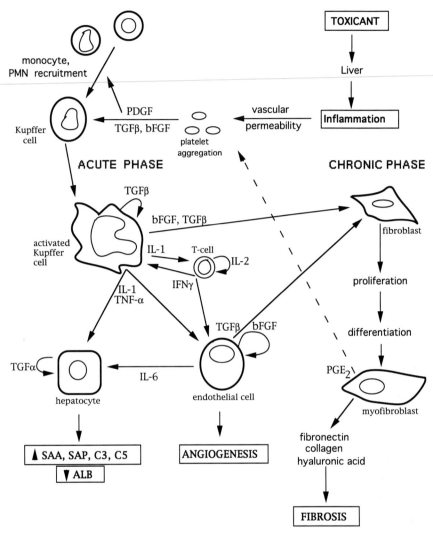

Fig. 1 Chemical-induced inflammation. Abbreviations: TGFα,β, transforming growth factor α,β; PDGF, platelet derived growth factor; TNFα, tumor necrosis factor α; IL-1, IL-6, interleukins 1 and 6; α2-M, α₂-macroglobulin; SAA, serum amyloid A; SAP, serum amyloid P; IFNγ, interferon gamma; PGE₂, prostaglandin E₂; C3, complement 3; C5, complement 5; ALB, albumin; bFGF, basic fibroblast growth factor.

DMN) and the mechanisms by which exposure to this compound alters cellular immunity.

Several studies have demonstrated that, after exposure to DMN, many parameters associated with T cell function and cell-mediated immunity are affected. These events have included changes in the delayed type hypersensitivity response to keyhole limpet hemocyanin (KLH), allogeneic mixed lymphocyte reactions (MLRs), phytohemagglutinin (PHA)- and concanavalin A (Con-A)-induced T cell mitogenesis, and *in vitro* and *in vivo* antitumor activity (Duke *et al.*, 1985; Holsapple *et al.*, 1985; Myers *et al.*, 1987a; Schook and Bick, 1991). These studies have, for the most part, utilized a chronic exposure regimen of varying doses of DMN (1.5, 3.0, and 5.0 mg/kg) given by daily ip injections for 2 wk. Controls have included sham injections or vehicle (phosphate buffered saline) using the same injection schedule. Moreover, these studies have also demonstrated that changes in hematopoiesis and macrophage influx into inflammatory sites are affected. DMN exposure results in a paradox of changes in cell-mediated immunity. On the one hand, T cell responses are diminished whereas, on the other hand, macrophage functions are increased. Thus, a series of experiments has been performed to resolve the mechanism(s) that may be responsible for these immune dysfunctions resulting from DMN exposure.

The liver is the principle target organ for DMN-induced toxicity. Several hepatotoxicants including acetaminophen, carbon tetrachloride, galactosamine, endotoxin, and DMN have been shown to modify macrophage activities *in situ* (Myers *et al.*, 1986; Myers and Schook, 1987; Laskin, 1990). Recruited monocytes are activated locally and/or systemically by cytokines and, thus, play an important role in the inflammatory response to xenobiotic-induced tissue damage. These activated macrophages release multifunctional cytokines such as interleukin 1β (IL-1β) and tumor necrosis factor α (TNFα), which regulate the inflammatory response, hematopoiesis, and immune responses (Akira *et al.*, 1990). The pleiotropic cytokine IL-6 also plays an important role in controlling macrophage functions, as well as in the induction of acute-phase and C-reactive proteins during liver tissue damage (Zahedi and Whitehead, 1989; Akira *et al.*, 1990).

The inflammatory reaction of tissues is a common manifestation of chemical- and radiation-induced toxicity (Chapter 1). Common features of organ inflammation, whether involving the kidneys, lungs, or liver, include the induction of nonspecific and/or specific immune responses. These responses may be directed toward the xenobiotic itself, toward the tissue damage caused by the xenobiotic, or both. Although these overall immune responses are very complex, a primary immunological response shared by xenobiotics is the induction of inflammatory cytokines. Examples of xenobiotics that modulate cytokine production are environmental/occupational agents [ozone, asbestos, benzo(*a*)pyrene, benzene, carbon tetrachloride, and nitrosamines], drugs (cyclosporin A, corticosteroids, bleomycin, and acetaminophen), and naturally occurring agents [ultraviolet (UV) light, dust, nitrogen dioxide; see Chapter 1].

Historical approaches to monitoring immunotoxicity have included pathological, humoral, cellular, host-resistance, and hypersensitivity assays. These tests have provided important insights into target organ sensitivities and possible mechanisms of action. However, such end point tests fall short of developing approaches that are adequate for making risk assessments following chemical exposure. Tests that monitor individuals prior to, during, and after exposure to xenobiotics are needed more than ones that measure end point changes. Cytokines are "sensitive indicators" not only of tissue damage but also of the immune system status. As such, cytokines serve as coordinators of both immune and nonimmune inflammatory responses (Arai *et al.*, 1990). Approaches to monitoring the process rather than the end point after DMN exposure are the focus of this chapter.

The original interest in DMN was based on the premise that daily subchronic exposure to chemicals might permit identification of regulatory factors that are produced in response to primary toxicological changes that subsequently affect immune function. A model linking changes in granulocyte–macrophage colony stimulating factor (GM-CSF) and TNFα gene expression with altered immune function and a new methodology to predict changes in immune status have been developed (Myers *et al.*, 1989a; Lockwood *et al.*, 1991; Witsell and Schook, 1991,1992; Schook *et al.*, 1992).

Lassalle *et al.* (1990) have previously used this approach demonstrating that IL-1 and TNFα secretion can be used to monitor early events that follow mineral dust exposure. This result is significant for studying not only the mechanisms leading to coal worker's pneumoconiosis, but also the progression from simple to massive fibrosis. Further, a "cytokine hypothesis" for chemical-induced changes is supported by research demonstrating a requirement of TNFα for the development of silica-induced pulmonary fibrosis (Piguet *et al.*, 1990), the reversal of acute toxicity by 2,3,7,8-tetrachlorodibenzo-*p*-dioxin (TCDD) following treatment with anti-TNFα antibodies *in vivo* (Clark *et al.*, 1991), altered macrophage cytokine production by TCDD (Steppan and Kerkvliet, 1991), and cytokine involvement in pulmonary asbestosis (Bissonnette and Rola-Pleszczynski, 1989).

An important strategy for understanding immune dysfunction following chemical exposure is reviewing the known mechanisms leading to autoimmunity and chronic inflammatory diseases. Such a strategy can be productive, since autoimmunity results from the loss of normal regulation and many chemicals may cause immune dysfunction via the induction of autoimmunity. Evidence in systemic lupus erythematosus (SLE) suggests that elevated levels of endogenous IL-6 and TNFα (Linker-Israeli *et al.*, 1991) may play a role in pathogenesis. Additional evidence for the role of cytokines is provided by Beyaert *et al.* (1991a), who induced an inflammatory response in mice by a combined treatment *in vivo* with TNFα and lithium chloride, demonstrating that lithium chloride potentiated not only TNFα and IL-1 production by macrophages, but also expression of their respective receptors (Beyaert *et al.*, 1991b). Additional support for characterizing "cytokine networks" is furnished by studies conducted by Piguet *et al.* (1990,1991; Chapter 12), who demonstrated that such cytokine networks have evolved to protect the body against injury but can also cause disease when their regulation goes awry (psoriasis and bleomycin models, respectively). Finally, the DMN model that has been developed appears to be very similar in nature to cytokine-associated inflammation observed in rheumatoid arthritis (Alvaro-Gracia *et al.*, 1991).

This chapter describes the balance between tissue destruction and healing after chemical exposure. The working hypothesis has been that the difference between chemical- and infection-stimulated inflammatory responses is the lack of adequate down-regulation of the inflammatory response, resulting in inappropriate cytokine expression which affects regulation of immune responses. The DMN model has several advantages (e.g., heptotoxicity separate from immunotoxicity) for developing molecular and cellular approaches to understanding chemical-induced immunotoxicity. Further, experiments presented in this chapter provide important information and experimental approaches that are not restricted to DMN immunotoxicity, but provide biomarkers of general toxicity (Figure 2).

II. Effects on Cytokine Production, Macrophage Differentiation, and Immune Responses

A. DMN-Induced Alteration of Stem Cell Response to Hematopoietic Growth Factors

Since alterations in cellular immunity resulting from DMN exposure were associated with changes in myelopoiesis, studies were performed to determine the response of bone marrow precursor cells to hematopoietic growth factors (Myers and Schook, 1987). Bone marrow obtained after DMN or vehicle exposure demonstrated no alterations in the capacity to generate CFU-S (colony forming units; pluripotent stem cells) as monitored using the splenic foci assay, nor were any changes noted in the number of CFU-mix colonies [interleukin 3 (IL-3)-responsive stem cells] among treatment groups.

However, the generation of granulocyte/macrophage (GM)-CFU and macrophage (M)-CFU were altered, resulting in an increased number of both colony types from marrow obtained from DMN-exposed animals. GM-CFU generated from the bone marrow obtained from DMN-exposed mice also had increased numbers of cells produced by each colony. Indirect immunofluorescence studies demonstrated no changes in the percentages of granulocytes and macrophages following GM-CSF stimulation. Moreover, no change was seen in the total number of CSF-1-generated macrophages/10^6 bone marrow cells in DMN and vehicle treatment groups.

Marrow cells obtained from DMN-exposed mice when cultured *in vitro* with GM-CSF demonstrated both a shift in kinetics and an increase in the

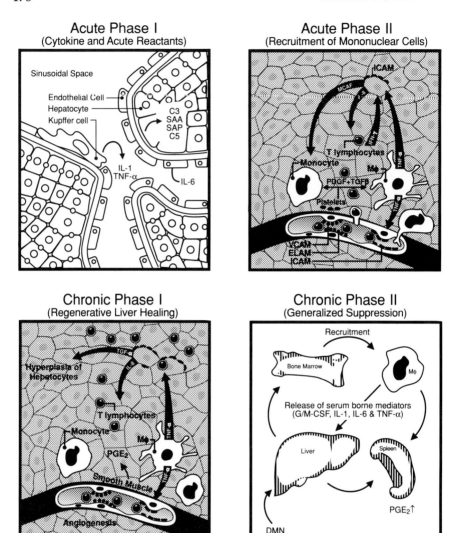

Fig. 2 Dimethylnitrosamine (DMN)-induced inflammation. Effects on cytokine production, macrophage differentiation, and immune responses. The disease model system includes two acute phases and two chronic phases. See text for abbreviations of cytokines.

peak proliferative responses. In contrast, these same marrow cells showed no shift in their kinetics but a decrease in their proliferative response to CSF-1 (M-CSF). Examination of the sera from DMN-exposed mice demonstrated a net decrease in CSF-1 activity but no changes in the concentrations of two inhibitory factors controlling myelopoiesis (transferrin and lactoferrin). These results suggest that DMN exposure affected macrophage differentiation at the level of the GM-CSF-responsive stem cell.

B. Induction of Serum GM-CSF Activity after DMN Exposure

The findings discussed in the previous section suggest that DMN exposure *in vivo* affects hematopoiesis at the level of the CFU-GM and CFU-M precursor cells. Since this effect on hematopoiesis is an indirect consequence of DMN exposure, studies were performed to examine the serum from animals exposed to DMN *in vivo* for the presence of hematopoietic growth factor activity (Myers *et al.*, 1989b). Serum obtained from animals exposed to DMN *in vivo* supported colony formation in normal bone marrow cells, whereas serum obtained from untreated or vehicle-exposed animals failed to support colony growth.

Differential staining of the colonies demonstrated the presence of cells of both monocytic and granulocytic lineages. Pretreatment of serum from DMN-exposed animals with anti-CSF-1 antibodies had no effect on cell number, cell phenotype, or colony-stimulating activity, thus supporting the hypothesis that GM-CSF was present in the serum of DMN-exposed animals. The addition of serum from DMN-exposed animals to naive recipient animals resulted in increased percentages of blood-borne monocytes and neutrophils, mimicking the profile observed in DMN-exposed animals.

Since several studies have demonstrated the role of GM-CSF in the induction of acute inflammatory responses, experiments were conducted to determine whether GM-CSF could be detected in the liver after DMN exposure. Studies using oligonucleotide-directed DNA amplification did demonstrate the presence of GM-CSF transcripts in the livers of animals after DMN exposure (Myers *et al.*, 1989b). These results provided further support for the model, demonstrating that DMN exposure in part results in the induction of inflammatory cytokines produced in the liver and released into the blood. The ability to measure GM-CSF activity in the serum of DMN-exposed animals and the ability of this cytokine to mimic hematopoietic profiles associated with DMN exposure clearly implicate this cytokine in DMN-induced alterations in macrophage differentiation and activation.

C. DMN-Induced IL-1β, TNFα, and IL-6 Inflammatory Cytokine Expression

To increase current understanding of the role that pro-inflammatory cytokines play in DMN-induced immune dysfunction, experiments were performed to monitor the release of cytokines into the serum following DMN exposure (Schook *et al.*, 1992). Further, researchers had to demonstrate that the induction of such cytokines occurs, in part, within the liver after DMN exposure. Animals were exposed daily to either vehicle or DMN for 14 days. Serum and liver samples were obtained from individual mice at 0, 1, 2, 3, 6, 12, and 24 hr after the first exposure; additional samples were collected every 24 hr preceding the daily DMN exposure. Sera then were analyzed for IL-1β, IL-3, IL-6, CSF-1, GM-CSF, and TNFα activities using either biological or immunological assays. Total liver cellular RNA was also examined for the induction of IL-1β transcripts using the solution hybridization/RNase protection assay.

IL-1β, IL-6, and TNFα serum activities were observed within 2 hr of DMN exposure and returned to control levels by 72 hr, although DMN exposure was maintained. No IL-3 was detected, nor was any change in CSF-1 activity noted after DMN exposure. Chronic expression of cytokine activity (after 72 hr) was only observed for GM-CSF, confirming the results of previous studies (Myers *et al.*, 1989b). A rapid induction of IL-1β transcripts (within 1 hr) was observed in liver tissue by solution hybridization in both vehicle and DMN-treated animals. However, by 3 hr postexposure, transcript levels decreased in the vehicle-treated animals whereas IL-1β transcript levels remained elevated in the DMN-treated animals for over 6 hr. These results demonstrate that DMN exposure *in vivo* induced the expression of serum-borne cytokine activities that included rapid IL-1β transcription in liver tissue.

D. Transcriptional Changes in TNFα Expression after DMN Exposure

Since DMN exposure increases macrophage cytotoxic activity against tumor targets both *in vitro* and *in vivo*, additional studies were performed to determine whether changes in TNFα gene transcription and biosynthesis resulted from DMN exposure. Thioglycollate-elicited macrophages obtained from DMN-exposed animals displayed enhanced levels of constitutively expressed TNFα transcripts relative to vehicle-treated controls (Lockwood *et al.*, 1991). Northern blot analysis of the time course of TNFα expression after endotoxin stimulation *in vitro* showed a significantly greater induction of TNFα transcripts in macrophages from DMN-exposed animals than in those from control animals. Peak levels of transcripts were observed between 30 and 120 min after stimulation. Maximum endotoxin-induced TNFα secretion occurred later than the accumulation of the transcripts, with greater secretion occurring between 120 and 360 min poststimulation.

TNFα activity was measured by testing supernatants from medium and endotoxin-stimulated thioglycollate-stimulated macrophages against the WEHI-164 cell line. Supernatants of macrophages obtained from DMN-exposed animals cultured in medium alone demonstrated a 5-fold increase in TNFα activity relative to supernatants from control macrophages. Treatments with either superoxide dismutase or catalase to remove reactive oxygen products did not alter bioactivity. However, the addition of anti-TNFα antibody reduced the lytic activity by 90%. Accumulation of IL-1β transcripts and activity did not differ among macrophages from DMN and vehicle treatment groups. These findings demonstrate that DMN exposure enhances the expression of TNFα in peripheral macrophages via transcriptional regulatory mechanisms, but does not affect the transcription and synthesis of another monokine IL-1β.

E. Alteration of Macrophage Antitumor Activity after DMN Exposure

Macrophages obtained by the *in vitro* culture of bone marrow-derived macrophages from animals exposed to DMN *in vivo* demonstrated enhanced cytotoxicity against tumor cells (Myers *et al.*, 1987a). The enhanced cytotoxicity was also present in Con A- and *Corynebacterium parvum*-elicited peritoneal exudate cells obtained from DMN-exposed animals. Thioglycollate-elicited macrophages from DMN-exposed animals displayed no increase in their cytotoxic activity relative to vehicle-exposed animals. However, treatment of the thioglycollate-elicited macrophage with interferon γ (IFN-γ) induced cytotoxic activity in macrophages obtained from DMN-exposed animals, but not in those from control animals. The expression of the transferrin-binding receptor, a marker of the activational status of macrophages, was observed earlier during *in vitro* macrophage differentiation and at higher levels in cultures using bone marrow from DMN-exposed animals. Thus, DMN exposure induced changes in macrophage differentiation, resulting in an altered activational status associated with enhanced cytotoxicity against tumor cells.

F. Differential Immunocompetence of Macrophages Derived Using CSF-1 or GM-CSF

Because a functional link is formed between hematopoietic progenitors and peripheral cells through the production of cytokines, distinguishing between normal or "steady-state" hematopoiesis occurring in the absence of an inflammatory response and "induced" hematopoiesis associated with such a response becomes important. Thus, additional studies were performed to test the hypothesis that DMN exposure leads to an alteration of macrophage differentiation and activation through the presence of elevated GM-CSF activity. Hence, changes in macrophage functions associated with DMN exposure may result from the shift in macrophage production from constitutive generation in response to CSF-1 to peripheral populations generated by GM-CSF.

Macrophages were derived *in vitro* from bone marrow progenitors using either CSF-1 or GM-CSF as the myelopoietic stimulus (Rutherford and Schook, 1992a). These studies confirmed the hypothesis that different hematopoietic growth factors produce macrophage populations that display different functional, morphological, and mRNA transcriptional phenotypes. GM-CSF-derived macrophages, compared with CSF-1-derived macrophages, demonstrated greater cytolytic activity against tumor cells. This phenomenon is illustrated by the killing of K562 cells (TNFα resistant). GM-CSF-derived macrophages required only an endotoxin signal to kill K562 cells effectively whereas CSF-1-derived macrophages required the classical IFNγ priming prior to endotoxin exposure to become tumoricidal.

The two populations also demonstrated differential sensitivities to endotoxin induction of TNFα. The CSF-1-derived cells were more sensitive to endotoxin induction (100-fold) whereas the GM-CSF-derived macrophages were refractory to prostaglandin E_2 (PGE_2) down-regulation of TNFα synthesis. No differences between these two macrophage populations could be demonstrated for the induction of PGE_2. These results show that the functional heterogeneity of CSF-1- and GM-CSF-derived macrophages resulted from differences in the activational signals required by each population to elicit a given function.

Further, these results strengthen the hypothesis that changes in immune functions following *in vivo* DMN exposure are caused in part by increased production of GM-CSF. Increased antitumoricidal activity by fully activated macrophages, the need for only IFNγ to induce cytotoxicity in thioglycollate-elicited (responsive) macrophages, and increased PGE_2 production by macrophages in all stages of activation are features that are consistent with the hypothesis of GM-CSF as the inducer of many of the immune alterations observed after DMN exposure. Results demonstrating the presence of serum-borne GM-CSF in conjunction with these observations provide compelling evidence for the role of GM-CSF in DMN-induced immune modulation.

G. Enhanced Macrophage Antimicrobial Activity after DMN Exposure: Augmented Production of Reactive Oxygen Intermediates

Since prior studies had demonstrated that mice exposed to DMN *in vivo* were more resistant to both bacterial (*L. monocytogenes*) and tumor (melanoma) challenges (Duke *et al.*, 1985; Thomas *et al.*, 1985), experiments were conducted to resolve the mechanisms responsible for increased host resistance (Edwards *et al.*, 1991). Since reactive oxygen intermediates (ROI) represent a key mechanism of antimicrobial action, determining whether macrophage ROI levels were related to augmented antimicrobial action in animals exposed to DMN *in vivo* was deemed important.

Peritoneal exudate macrophages were elicited with thioglycollate, Con A, or *C. parvum* and were examined for their production of ROIs. Macrophages obtained from DMN-exposed animals by any of these methods demonstrated increased superoxide anion (O_2^-) production following stimulation *in vivo* with either phorbol myristate acetate (PMA) or opsonized zymosan relative to macrophages obtained from vehicle-treated animals. ROI production was also determined for macrophages derived using either GM-CSF or CSF-1. Results from these studies demonstrated that bone marrow-derived macrophages (BMDM), derived using either growth factor from marrow of DMN-exposed animals, had increased ROI activity relative to BMDM obtained from vehicle-exposed animals.

Analysis of extracellular antilistericidal activity of thioglycollate- and Con

A-elicited macrophages revealed that only the thioglycollate-elicited macrophages had enhanced killing capacity. Also, no difference was seen in the intracellular killing capability of macrophage obtained from DMN- and vehicle-exposed animals. Thioglycollate-elicited macrophages from either vehicle- or DMN-exposed animals were also examined for antimicrobial activity and H_2O_2 production following *in vitro* PMA activation. PMA activation demonstrated that the thioglycollate-elicited macrophages from DMN-exposed animals produced significantly higher levels of H_2O_2 and cell killing than PMA-treated vehicle control groups. These results suggest that observed differences in antimicrobial activity by macrophages following DMN exposure are the results of enhanced ROI production by "activated" macrophages that are present *in vivo* after DMN exposure.

H. Role of Acute Phase Reactants in DMN-Induced Inflammatory Responses

A cascade of events (acute-phase response) is initiated immediately following injury or infection. These events (cognitive/activation phase) involve the induction of inflammatory cytokines and acute-phase protein responses by hepatocytes (see Figures 1, 2, 3). Positive acute-phase proteins (α_1-acid glycoprotein, α_2-macroglobulin, the β chain of fibrinogen, transferrin, and major acute-phase α_1-protein) increase in concentration in the bloodstream during inflammation, whereas negative acute-phase proteins (albumin, transthyretin, and α_{2a}-globulin) decrease during inflammation (Birch and Schreiber, 1986).

A series of experiments has been initiated to determine the nature of the acute-phase reactant response to DMN exposure. The strategy is similar to that used by Mackiewicz *et al.* (1991) for evaluating the effects of cytokines on hepatocyte cell lines for the induction of acute-phase proteins. Note that fibrinogen, C3, serum amyloid A (SAA), serum amyloid P (SAP), and the complement factor B are regulated by IL-1 and IL-6, and that mice, unlike humans, do not express C-reactive protein but produce SAP (Standyk and Gauldie, 1991). Goldberger *et al.* (1987) have demonstrated the induction of a sterile inflammatory reaction induced by exposure to turpentine in rabbits. This reaction was characterized by an increase in the hepatocellular content of C-reactive protein, SAA, C3, and factor B mRNA. Additional work by Zahedi and Whitehead (1989) correlated the induction of acute-phase hepatic mRNA levels with other parameters of inflammation. These researchers exposed mice to thioglycollate or azocasein and monitored the induction of acute-phase reactant mRNA synthesis using labeled oligonucleotides in liver samples after various times of exposure. SAP mRNA levels were correlated with other parameters of inflammation, including increased numbers of peritoneal exudate cells and elevated SAP serum concentrations.

Total liver RNA was obtained from mice after DMN or vehicle exposure (Figure 3). RNA samples were collected at various time points following exposure and were probed with radiolabeled oligonucleotides for the acute-phase proteins (see Figure 3), as described by Zahedi and Whitehead (1989). Within 3 hr of DMN exposure, changes in the expression of acute-phase protein transcription in hepatocytes is observed. The positive acute-phase proteins SAA and SAP demonstrated enhanced transcription after DMN exposure. SAA was elevated over 100-fold 6 hr after DMN exposure and was quickly down-regulated after 12 hr. SAP also was up-regulated at 6 hr, but to a lesser extent. In contrast, transcription of the negative acute-phase protein, albumin, was shut off by 3 hr in the DMN treatment groups and was depressed throughout the 24-hr period. These results demonstrate that the acute-phase proteins are involved in DMN-induced inflammatory responses.

I. Augmented Macrophage PGE_2 Production after DMN Exposure: Relevance to Suppressed T Cell Responses

Prior observations had demonstrated that DMN exposure results in suppressed T cell responses (Duke *et al.*, 1985; Holsapple *et al.*, 1985). Efforts thus were focused on determining the mechanism(s) responsible for DMN-induced suppression of T cell responses (Myers *et al.*, 1989a). Accordingly, the production of PGE_2, a potent inhibitor of T cell activation, was examined in macrophages obtained from animals exposed to DMN or vehicle *in vivo*. The production of PGE_2 was determined in peripheral macrophages representing various stages of activation (responsive, primed, and fully activated) and various stages of differentiation (CSF-1- or GM-CSF-derived macrophages).

All peritoneal macrophages obtained from DMN-exposed animals demonstrated enhanced production of PGE_2 after stimulation with either endotoxin or IFNγ relative to macrophages obtained from vehicle-exposed mice. Moreover, the enhanced levels of PGE_2 were caused by increased PGE_2 production rather than by shifts in the kinetics of PGE_2 production and utilization. CSF-1- or GM-CSF-derived macrophages produced minimal levels of PGE_2 regardless of the *in vitro* stimulation or treatment group. Splenic macrophages obtained from DMN-exposed animals produced significantly higher levels of PGE_2 after endotoxin stimulation than did vehicle controls.

Splenocytes from DMN-exposed animals exhibited suppressed proliferative responses to the mitogen Con A (Myers *et al.*, 1989a). However, when splenocytes from DMN-exposed animals were co-cultured with the PGE_2 synthesis inhibitor indomethacin, they demonstrated Con A-stimulated proliferation similar to that observed in vehicle control splenocyte cultures. These results demonstrate that DMN exposure results in populations of macrophages with the potential to produce increased PGE_2 when induced

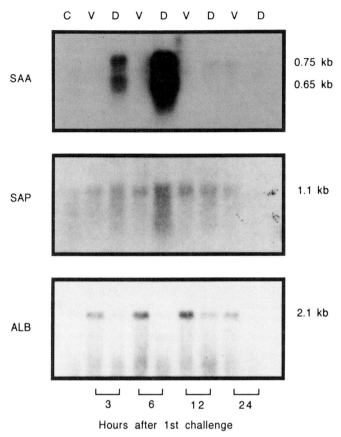

Fig. 3 Expression of acute phase protein transcripts in liver after DMN exposure *in vivo*. Livers were isolated from (B6C3)F$_1$ mice at 3, 6, 12, and 24 hr after ip treatment with nothing (sham control, C), phosphate buffered saline (vehicle, V), or 5.0 mg/kg dimethylnitrosamine (DMN, D). Total cellular RNA was isolated, separated by agarose gel electrophoresis, blotted and probed with ^{32}P-labeled oligonucleotides specific for serum amyloid A (SAA), serum amyloid P (SAP) and albumin (ALB). The sizes of the expected transcripts are provided. SAA has two species of transcripts that are detectable, as shown.

by either endotoxin or T cell-derived cytokines. Therefore, this increased production of PGE$_2$ may be responsible for the suppressed T cell responses observed *in vivo* after DMN exposure.

III. Role of Hematopoietic Growth Factors and Developmental Mechanisms in Macrophage Heterogeneity

The versatility and importance of macrophages in host defense and homeostasis have long been recognized. To determine the mechanisms responsible for generating macrophage heterogeneity, the reverse transcriptase–polymerase chain reaction was used to determine the molecular phenotype of macrophages during their differentiation from bone marrow (Witsell and Schook, 1990,1991). Colonies of BMDM were selected during various stages of differentiation and analyzed for the expression of genes associated with macrophage function and differentiation (e.g., IL-1α, IL-1β, GM-CSF, TNFα, major histocompatability complex class II Aα, myeloperoxidase, and C4). The results of this method revealed a hierarchical expression of macrophage-associated genes. TNFα was expressed in all colonies that were analyzed, suggesting an important role for this molecule during macrophage differentiation. Predominant colony phenotypes were unique for their period of differentiation and the growth factor with which they were derived (either CSF-1 or GM-CSF). Thus, changes in GM-CSF production associated with DMN exposure would affect clonal phenotypes in differentiating macrophages.

Exogenous stimulation of the bone marrow cultures with either endotoxin or IFNγ led to predictable phenotypic transitions. Thus, the expression of genes associated with macrophage function is regulated by the hematopoietic growth factor used to derive the macrophage populations. These results suggest that changes in macrophage functions associated with DMN exposure occur through differentiation-related mechanisms, and that generated macrophage populations are then maintained by systemic environmental constraints (e.g., the presence of elevated levels of GM-CSF in the serum of animals exposed to DMN).

Since these experiments also revealed the expression of TNFα in all bone marrow-derived macrophage colonies isolated on days 5–9 of differentiation *in vitro*, additional studies were performed to determine the role of TNFα expression during macrophage differentiation. Two approaches were used to assess the function of TNFα during differentiation (Witsell and Schook, 1992). First, antisense oligomers to the initiation region of the TNFα message were used to inhibit its translation and expression. Results demonstrated that TNFα controlled the proliferation of macrophages during differentiation. Cells isolated on day 3 of differentiation were exclusively vulnerable to the effects of blocking TNFα expression, displaying a 30% increase in proliferation over control or sense oligomer-treated cells. Thus, in the absence of TNFα, cells maintained proliferation instead of undergoing terminal differentiation. Exogenous TNFα was capable of rescuing day 3 antisense-treated cells, thereby maintaining normal levels of proliferation. In contrast, blocking IL-1β gene expression by antisense oligonucleotide treatment had no effect on proliferation.

Also, the addition of exogenous recombinant murine or human TNFα to bone marrow cultures decreased total cell number by 25–50%, whether cells were derived in CSF-1 or GM-CSF. These results suggest that exogenous TNFα suppresses proliferation of early hematopoietic progenitors, whereas endogenous TNFα regulates proliferation of macrophage progenitors. Although the total number of cells was decreased after TNFα treatment of marrow cultures, the total number of differentiated adherent macrophages obtained after differentiation induced by GM-CSF *in vitro* was increased by TNFα treatment. In contrast, treatment of CSF-1 derived macrophages with TNFα suppressed the number of adherent macrophages. In addition, both murine and human TNFα were able to produce this effect. Since human TNFα can only bind the p60 receptor and not the p80 receptor, the signaling associated with the TNFα autocrine growth regulation of macrophages must be via the p60 receptor and not the p80 receptor (Witsell and Schook, 1992).

In summary, these results demonstrate that macrophages generated by either CSF-1 or GM-CSF have unique patterns of gene expression. Further, the role of TNFα in the autocrine regulation of macrophage differentiation is confined to the GM-CSF-derived macrophage population. Thus, signaling mechanisms differ between these two macrophage populations. This point is supported further by other work in which macrophage functions in response to PGE$_2$ and activation by CSFs were determined (Rutherford and Schook, 1992b). Macrophages derived *in vitro* using CSF-1 displayed greater sensitivity to PGE$_2$-induced suppression of TNFα production than did macrophages derived using GM-CSF. Differential signaling mechanisms were also supported by studies to determine the role of cyclic AMP (cAMP) in controlling macrophage functions. The addition of exogenous cAMP inhibited TNFα production in both populations, but GM-CSF-derived macrophages accumulated less cAMP after PGE$_2$ treatment than did CSF-1-derived cells. The treatment of fully differentiated macrophages, derived with either growth factor, with additional growth factors did not activate the cells to produce TNFα. However, GM-CSF efficiently primed the BMDM for augmented TNFα secretion in response to secondary stimuli. These results demonstrate the potential for differential macrophage functions within inflammatory sites based on the combination of macrophage hematopoietic stimuli and the specific conditions present in the lesion.

IV. Paradox of Enhanced Macrophage Functions and Suppressed T Cell Responses

Experimental findings have demonstrated that alterations in cell-mediated immunity are associated with changes in macrophage function (Myers *et al.*, 1986). These alterations are attributed to augmented myelopoietic activity (Myers and Schook, 1987) and changes in TNFα transcriptional activity (Lockwood *et al.*, 1991). The paradox of depressed T cell responses following DMN exposure is that, although the macrophages demonstrate increased tumor cell killing, these cells are also responsible for inducing depressed T cell responses (Myers *et al.*, 1986, 1987a).

The augmented levels of PGE_2 in the supernatants of peritoneal macrophages elicited from DMN-exposed animals are in accordance with current understanding of the underlying mechanisms responsible for alterations in cell-mediated immunity. The demonstration that serum from mice exposed to DMN *in vivo* contains GM-CSF (Myers *et al.*, 1989b) suggests that this cytokine enhances the production of PGE_2 in peripheral macrophages found in the spleen and lymph nodes. This notion is supported by results obtained by other investigators, who demonstrated that the addition of GM-CSF to macrophages increases PGE_2 synthesis (Kurland *et al.*, 1979; Falk *et al.*, 1988a,b).

GM-CSF also enhances the tumoricidal and antimicrobial activities of the macrophage (Hundman and Burgess, 1979; Grabstein *et al.*, 1986). Thus, these findings provide not only a central mechanism by which DMN exposure affects cell-mediated immunity, but also a rationale capable of explaining the underlying alterations in the cellular and molecular events that occur as a consequence of DMN exposure.

Subsequent to the demonstration that macrophages produce and secrete numerous pro-inflammatory cytokines (GM-CSF, IL-1β, and TNFα) was the observation of a hierarchy governing the induction of these agents. Activation of macrophages results in the production of GM-CSF, which in turn induces the production of TNFα and IL-1β (Thorens *et al.*, 1987). The induction of IL-1β may be either a direct effect of GM-CSF or may be the result of the ability of TNFα to induce IL-1 (Philip and Epstein, 1986). Nonetheless, both TNFα and IL-1β induce the synthesis and secretion of PGE_2, whereas PGE_2 down-regulates the production of both TNFα and IL-1 (Kunkel *et al.*, 1986).

In addition to its up-regulatory effects on macrophage effector activities, GM-CSF also enhances the role of the macrophage in the afferent limb of the cell-mediated response. GM-CSF increases the expression of membrane IL-1, Fc receptors, and Mac-1 cell surface antigen (Morrissey *et al.*, 1988). Macrophages exposed to GM-CSF also produce greater levels of secreted IL-1 (Morrissey *et al.*, 1987,1988). Splenic macrophages and GM-CSF-derived macrophages exhibit high levels of major histocompatibility complex class II expression (Falk *et al.*, 1988b; Morrissey *et al.*, 1987). Heterogeneity exists in the response of macrophage populations to GM-CSF, since peritoneal macrophage class II is unaffected by exposure to GM-CSF (Morrissey *et al.*, 1988).

Investigators anticipated that macrophages obtained from DMN-exposed animals would display similar changes in function. Surprisingly, the opposite result was observed with peritoneal macrophages from DMN-exposed animals, which demonstrated increased expression of class II cell surface products (Myers *et al.*, 1986). No changes in the expression of membrane IL-1 were noted following DMN exposure.

Thus, if GM-CSF is the principle agent mediating the immune alterations in DMN-exposed animals, how can it selectively alter macrophage effector functions (TNFα production and tumor and bacterial killing)? The augmented production of PGE$_2$, as previously noted, is sufficient to induce depressed T cell responses, but should also depress TNFα production (Kunkel et al., 1986). This paradox suggests that additional factors (i.e., cytokines), sustained systemic exposure to GM-CSF, or both are involved in selectively inducing the differentiation of unique macrophage populations.

Acknowledgments

Research presented in this chapter was supported in part by the National Institutes of Health (ES04348). The authors also express their appreciation to Helen Gawthorp for her excellent secretarial assistance.

References

Akira, S., Hirano, T., Taga, T., and Kishimoto, T. (1990). Biology of multifunctional cytokines: IL 6 and related molecules (IL-1 and TNF). FASEB J. **4**, 2860–2867.

Alvaro-Gracia, J.-M., Zvaifler, N. J., Brown, C. B., Kaushansky, K., and Firestein, G. S. (1991). Cytokines in chronic inflammatory arthritis. VI. Analysis of the synovial cells involved in granulocyte-colony-stimulating factor production and gene expression in rheumatoid arthritis and its regulation by IL-1 and tumor necrosis factor-α. J. Immunol. **146**, 3365–3371.

Arai, K.-I., Lee, F., Miyajima, A., Miyatake, S., Arai, N., and Yokota, T. (1990). Cytokines: Coordinators of immune and inflammatory responses. Annu. Rev. Biochem. **59**, 783–836.

Beyaert, R., de Potter, C., Vanhaesebroeck, B., van Roy, F., and Fiers, W. (1991a). Induction of inflammatory cell infiltration and necrosis in normal mouse skin by the combine treatment with tumor necrosis factor and lithium chloride. Am. J. Pathol. **138**, 727–739.

Beyaert, R., Schulze-Osthoff, K., van Roy, F., and Fiers, W. (1991b). Lithium chloride potentiates tumor necrosis factor- and interleukin-1-induced cytokine and cytokine receptor expression. Cytokine **3**, 284–291.

Birch, H. E., and Schreiber, G. (1986). Transcriptional regulation of plasma protein synthesis during inflammation. J. Biol. Chem. **261**, 8077–8080.

Bissonnette, E., and Rola-Pleszczynski, M. (1989). Pulmonary inflammation and fibrosis in a murine model of asbestosis and silicosis—Possible role of tumor necrosis factor. Inflammation **13**, 329–339.

Clark, G., Lucier, G., Luster, M., Thompson, M., Mahler, J., and Taylor, M. (1991). Tumor necrosis factor (TNF) antibodies and dexamethasone (DEX) treatment reverse the acute toxicity of 2,3,7,8-tetrachlorodibenzo-p-dioxin (TCDD). Toxicologist **11**, 53.

Duke, S. S., Schook, L. B., and Holsapple, M. P. (1985). Effects of N-nitrosodimethylamine on tumor susceptibility. J. Leuk. Biol. **37**, 383–394.

Edwards, C. F., III, Myers, M. J., Rutherford, M. S., and Schook, L. B. (1991). Enhanced macrophage anti-microbial activity following dimethylnitrosamine exposure in vivo is related to augmented production of reactive oxygen metabolites. Immunopharmacol. Immunotoxicol. **13**, 359–411.

Falk, L. A., Hogan, M. M., and Vogel, S. N. (1988a). Bone marrow progenitors cultured in the presence of granulocyte-macrophage colony-stimulating factor versus macrophage colony-stimulating factor differentiate into macrophages with distinct tumoricidal capacities. *J. Leuk. Biol.* **43**, 471–476.

Falk, L. A., Wahl, L. M., and Vogel, S. N. (1988b). Analysis of Ia antigen expression in macrophages derived from bone marrow cells cultured in granulocyte-macrophage colony-stimulating factor or macrophage colony-stimulating factor. *J. Immunol* **140**, 2652 2660.

Goldberger, G., Bing, D. H., Sipe, J. D., Rits, M., and Colten, H. R. (1987). Transcriptional regulation of genes encoding the acute-phase proteins CRP, SAA, and C3. *J. Immunol.* **138**, 3967–3971.

Grabstein, K. H., Urdal, D. L., Tushinski, R. J., Mochizuki, D. T., Price, V. L., Cantrell, M. A., Gillis, S., and Conlon, P. J. (1986). Induction of macrophage tumoricidal activity by granulocyte-macrophage colony-stimulating factor. *Science* **232**, 506–508.

Holsapple, M. P., Bick, P. H., and Duke, S. S. (1985). Effects of N-nitrosodimethylamine on cell-mediated immunity. *J. Leuk. Biol.* **37**, 367–381.

Hundman, E., and Burgess, A. W. (1979). Stimulation by granulocyte-macrophage colony stimulating factor of *Leishmania tropica* killing by macrophages. *J. Immunol.* **122**, 1134–1137.

Khalil, N., Bereznay, O., Sporn, M., and Greenberg, A. H. (1989). Macrophage production of transforming growth factor-beta and fibroblast collagen synthesis in chronic pulmonary inflammation. *J. Exp. Med.* **170**, 727–737.

Kunkel, S. L., Chensue, S. W., and Phan, S. H. (1986). Prostaglandins as endogenous mediators of interleukin-1 production. *J. Immunol.* **136**, 186–192.

Kurland, J. I., Bockman, R. S., Broxmeyer, H. E., and Moore, M. A. S. (1979). Induction of prostaglandin E synthesis in normal and neoplastic macrophages: Role for colony-stimulating factor(s) distinct from effects on myeloid progenitor cell proliferation. *Proc. Natl. Acad. Sci. USA* **76**, 2326–2330.

Laskin, D. L. (1990). Nonparenchymal cells and hepatotoxicity. *Sem. Liver Dis.* **10**, 293–304.

Laskin, D. L., and Pilaro, A. M. (1986). Potential role of activated macrophages in acetaminophen hepatotoxicity. I. Isolation and characterization of activated macrophages from liver. *Toxicol. Appl. Pharmacol.* **86**, 204–215.

Laskin, D. L., Pilaro, A. M., and Ji, S. (1986). Potential role of activated macrophages in acetaminophen hepatotoxicity. II. Mechanism of macrophage accumulation and activation. *Toxicol. Appl. Pharmacol.* **86**, 216–226.

Lassalle, P., Gosset, P., Aerts, C., Fournier, E., Lafitte, J. J., Degreet, J. M., Wallaert, B., Tonnel, A. B., and Voisin, C. (1990). Abnormal secretion of interleukin-1 and tumor necrosis factor α by alveolar macrophages in coal worker's pneumoconiosis: Comparison between simple pneumoconiosis and progressive massive fibrosis. *Exp. Lung Res.* **16**, 73–80.

Linker-Israeli, M., Deans, R. J., Wallace, D. J., Prehn, J., Ozeri-Chen, T., and Klinenberg, J. R. (1991). Elevated levels of endogenous IL-6 in systemic lupus erythematosus. *J. Immunol.* **147**, 117–123.

Lockwood, J. F., Myers, M. J., Rutherford, M. S., and Schook, L. B. (1991). Transcriptional changes in macrophage TNF-α expression following dimethylnitrosamine exposure *in vivo*. *Immunopharmacol* **22**, 27–37.

Mackiewicz, A., Speroff, T., Ganapathi, M. K., and Kushner, I. (1991). Effects of cytokine combinations on acute phase protein production in two human hepatoma cell lines. *J. Immunol.* **146**, 3032–3037.

Mantovani, A., and Dejana, E. (1989). Cytokines as communcation signals between leukocytes and endothelial cells. *Immunol. Today* **10**, 370–375.

Morrissey, P. J., Bressler, L., Park, L. S., Alpert, A., and Gillis, S. (1987). Granulocyte-macrophage colony-stimulating factor augments the primary antibody response by enhancing the function of antigen-presenting cells. *J. Immunol.* **139**, 1113–1119.

Morrissey, P. J., Bressler, L., Charrier, K., and Alpert, A. (1988). Response of resident murine peritoneal macrophages to *in vivo* administration of granulocyte-macrophage colony-stimulating factor. *J. Immunol.* **140**, 1910–1915.

Morley, J. (1981). Role of prostaglandins secreted by macrophages in the inflammatory process. *Lymphokine* **4**, 377–394.

Myers, M. J., and Schook, L. B. (1987). Modification of macrophage differentiation: Dimethylnitrosamine-induced alteration in the response towards the regulatory signals controlling myelopoiesis. *Int. J. Immunopharmacol.* **9**, 817–825.

Myers, M. J., Pullen, J. K., and Schook, L. B. (1986). Alteration of macrophage differentiation into accessory and effector cells from exposure to dimethylnitrosamine *in vivo*. *Immunopharmacol.* **12**, 105–115.

Myers, M., Dickens, C., and Schook, L. B. (1987a). Alteration of macrophage anti-tumor activity and transferrin receptor expression by exposure to dimethylnitrosamine *in vivo*. *Immunopharmacol.* **13**, 195–205.

Myers, M. J., Schook, L. B., and Bick, P. H. (1987b). Mechanisms of benzo(*a*)pyrene-induced modulation of antigen presentation. *J. Pharmacol. Exp. Therapeut.* **242**, 399–404.

Myers, M. J., Hanafin, W. P., and Schook, L. B. (1989a). Augmented macrophage PGE$_2$ production following exposure to dimethylnitrosamine *in vivo*: Relevance to suppressed T cell responses. *Immunopharmacol.* **18**, 115–124.

Myers, M. J., Witsell, A. L., and Schook, L. B. (1989b). Induction of serum colony stimulating activity (CSA) following dimethylnitrosamine (DMN) exposure: Effects on macrophage differentiation. *Immunopharmacol.* **18**, 125–134.

Philip, R., and Epstein, L. B. (1986). Tumor necrosis factor as immunomodulator and mediator of monocyte cytotoxicity induced by itself, to interferon and interleukin-1. *Nature (London)* **323**, 86–89.

Piguet, P. F., Collart, M. A., Grau, G. E., Sappino, A.-P., and Vassalli, P. (1990). Requirement of tumor necrosis factor for development of silica-induced pulmonary fibrosis. *Nature (London)* **344**, 245–247.

Piguet, P. F., Grau, G. E., and Vassalli, P. (1991). Tumor necrosis factor (TNF) and immunopathology. *Immunol. Res.* **10**, 122–140.

Rutherford, M. S., and Schook, L. B. (1992a). Differential immunocompetence of macrophages derived using macrophage or granulocyte-macrophage colony-stimulating factor. *J. Leuk. Biol.* **51**, 69–76.

Rutherford, M. S., and Schook, L. B. (1992b). Macrophage function in response to PGE$_2$, L-arginine depravation, and activation by colony-stimulating factors is dependent on hematopoietic stimulus. *J. Leuk. Biol.* **52**, 228–235.

Schook, L. B., and Bick, P. H. (1991). Symposium on "Macrophage-xenobiotic interactions: Modulation of toxicity and macrophage functions." *Fund. Appl. Toxicol.* **17**, 1–6.

Schook, L. B., Lockwood, J. F., Yang, S.-D., and Myers, M. J. (1992). Dimethylnitrosamine (DMN)-induced IL-1β, TNF-α and IL-6 inflammatory cytokine expression. *Toxicol. Appl. Pharmacol.* **116**, 110–116.

Schreiner, G. F., Rovin, B., and Lefkowith, J. B. (1989). The antiinflammatory effects of essential fatty acid deficiency in experimental glomerulonephritis. The modulation of macrophage migration and eicosanoid metabolism. *J. Immunol.* **143**, 3192–3199.

Stadnyk, A. W., and Gauldie, J. (1991). The acute phase protein response during parasitic infection. *Immunol. Today* **12**, A7–A12.

Steppan, L. B., and Kerkvliet, N. I. (1991). Influence of 2,3,7,8-tetrachlorodibenzo-*p*-dioxin (TCDD) on the production of inflammatory cytokine mRNA by C57B1/6 macrophages. *Toxicologist* **11**, 35.

ten Dijke, P., and Iwata, K. K. (1989). Growth factors for wound healing. *BioTechnology* **7**, 793–798.

Thomas, P., Fugmann, R., Arany, C., Barbera, P., Gibbons, R., and Fenters, J. (1985). The effect of dimethylnitrosamine on host resistance and immunity. *Toxicol. Appl. Pharmacol.* **77**, 219–229.

Thorens, B., Mermod, J.-J., and Vassalli, P. (1987). Phagocytosis and inflammatory stimuli induce GM-CSF mRNA in macrophages through posttranscriptional regulation. *Cell* **28,** 671.

Wahl, S. M., Wong H., and McCartney-Francis N. (1989). Role of growth factors in inflammation and repair. *J. Cell. Biochem.* **40,** 193–199.

Witsell, A. L., and Schook, L. B. (1990). Clonal analysis of gene expression by PCR. *BioTechniques* **9,** 318–322.

Witsell, A. L., and Schook, L. B. (1991). Macrophage heterogeneity occurs through a developmental pathway. *Proc. Natl. Acad. Sci. USA* **88,** 1963–1967.

Witsell, A. L., and Schook, L. B. (1992). Tumor necrosis factor α is an autocrine growth regulator during macrophage differentiation. *Proc. Natl. Acad. Sci. USA* **89,** 4754–4758.

Zahedi, K., and Whitehead, A. S. (1989). Acute phase induction of mouse serum amyloid P component. Correlation with other parameters of inflammation. *J. Immunol.* **143,** 2880–2886.

8

Effects of Metals on Lymphocyte Development and Function

Michael J. McCabe, Jr., and David A. Lawrence

I. Introduction

In adult mammals, most lymphocytes initiate their development in the bone marrow. The multipotent stem cells (which represents a minor population of bone marrow cells; <1%) give rise to a progenitor of the lymphoid lineage that can migrate to the thymus to become a thymus-derived lymphocyte (T cell) or develop further within the bone marrow compartment to become a conventional B cell (B-2 lineage). This same stem cell population also gives rise to all the other forms of blood cells. Some metals can modulate the cellularity of the bone marrow (Ringenberg *et al.*, 1988), but the mechanisms involved have not been studied to date. Significant changes in the subpopulations of mouse bone marrow cells were reported after a single ip injection of cadmium (Cd) acetate (0.9 mg/kg) or lead (Pb) acetate (12 mg/kg); these metals appeared to cause a general inhibition of the development of cells past the progenitor stage (Burchiel *et al.*, 1987). A higher dose of Pb acetate (10 mM drinking water for 2 wk, approximately 600 mg/kg/day), however, has been reported to have no effect on mouse bone marrow or spleen cellularity or on percentages of splenic lymphocytes (Kowolenko *et al.*, 1991). Likewise in rats, a high dose of Pb acetate (200 mg/kg/day for 13 wk) did not alter the blood leukocyte differential (Yagminas *et al.*, 1990). Doses of Pb acetate (0.01–1 mg/kg) for 1–10 days did not influence bone marrow cellularity; however, continued exposure to the 1 mg/kg dose for 1 mo caused a reversible (within 2 wk) loss of cellularity as well as of stem cells (Schlick and Friedberg, 1982). Although high Pb exposure for 2 wk did not appear to alter bone marrow cellularity, hematopoiesis was compromised on exposure to an infectious agent (*Listeria monocytogenes*; Kowolenko *et al.*, 1991). Long-term oral exposure to Cd (1.6 mM for 12 mo) produced a generalized bone marrow hypoplasia as well as increased

Xenobiotics and Inflammation

morbidity and mortality (Hays and Margaretten, 1985). For most metals, inhibition of the development of erythrocytes, neutrophils, and/or platelets from bone marrow stem cells is the most prevalent effect, especially for arsenic (As), gold (Au), copper (Cu) and Pb (Lutton et al., 1984; Ringenberg et al., 1988; Yan and Davis, 1990). Cu effects on bone marrow cells are somewhat controversial because similar exposures of mice to Cu sulfate (1.1–6.6 mg/kg) produced no influence on bone marrow cells based on a micronucleus assay (Tinwell and Ashby, 1990) or significantly altered bone marrow cells based on the analysis of chromosomal aberrations (Agarwal et al., 1990). In vitro, Cu actually caused an increase in the percentage of macrophages in rat stromal populations (Miszta, 1990). Heavy metal influences on hematopoiesis are likely to be influenced by the amount of calcium (Ca) and other nutrients available in the diet. A low Ca intake has been reported to enhance bone marrow cell intoxication by zinc (Zn), Pb, and Cd (Deknudt and Gerber, 1979); however, the administration of Pb to rabbits did not influence the amount of Zn, Cu, Ca, or iron (Fe) associated with bone marrow (Zareba and Chmielnicka, 1989). Although lymphocytes are derived from bone marrow cells, metal effects on early maturation have not been evaluated to date. As suggested by the brief preceding discussion of generalized metal effects on bone marrow, investigation of the specific bone marrow cell types modified by metals is needed. Even the direct influence of metals on stromal and progenitor populations is unknown, although a study with Cd (Stelzer and Pazdernik, 1983) stressed the need for research in this area.

This chapter focuses mainly on aspects of T cell and B cell development that could be detrimentally affected by metals. Metals that are known to be lymphotropic and/or cause lymphocytic dysplasia are discussed; however, substantial new investigations are still needed before the mechanisms by which metals can modulate lymphocyte development and functions will be understood.

The thymus gland is the site at which T cells develop, in conjunction with selection based on the T cells' antigen-specific receptor (TCR; Nikolic-Zugic, 1991). Environmental toxicants, such as some metals, that target the thymus gland may influence immune responses by modulating thymocyte development and/or the concomitant positive and negative selection of T cell clones with a specific TCR repertoire. In other words, if thymocytes expressing beneficial TCR specificities toward "non-self" epitopes (antigenic determinants) are not properly positively selected, decreased host resistance to pathogens could result. On the other hand, an increased propensity for autoimmune diseases can occur if thymocytes with TCR specificities for "self" epitopes are not properly negatively selected (deleted). In addition to directly affecting the selection of the TCR repertoire, other aspects of T cell function could be influenced by metals during the developmental stages within the thymic microenvironment. Since the thymic environment clearly influences the reactivity of mature T cells, a metal-intoxicated thymus could result in the alteration of the normal regulatory functions of mature T cells and T cell products. Also, metals could affect "self" epitopes directly by combining with cell surface molecules such as the major histocompatibility complex (MHC) molecules, damaging DNA or decreasing DNA repair processes, or altering the specificity of the TCR itself at the genetic level. Workers exposed to heavy metals are known to have reduced DNA repair processes (Chopikashvili et al., 1989).

Mechanistically, relatively little is known about how metals influence thymocyte development. Nonetheless, T cell development, which itself is not entirely understood, is an intensely studied area of immunobiology. Progress regarding metal modulation of thymopoiesis and its linkage to immune-related diseases is likely to be made in the near future.

Unlike the T cell, the B cell seems to undergo no, or at least very little, scrutiny in the development of its antigen-specific receptor, which is a plasma membrane-bound immunoglobulin or surface immunoglobulin (sIg). Selection of this receptor and the antibody secreted, which have the same antigen specificity, seems to be a random genetic event. B cells with specificities for self epitopes can become immunologically mature; however, most B cell development into active antibody-secreting cells is highly dependent on signals from selected T cells. Thus, regulation of antigen-specific immune responses is controlled more by the specificities of the available T cells.

II. Thymocytes and Mature T Cell Subpopulations

T cells play a central role in the regulation of most immune responses. Numerous phenotypic and functional subpopulations of T cells have been defined. For instance, helper and inflammatory T cells, which are generally restricted to recognizing antigen in association with MHC class II molecules, express the CD4 accessory molecule. In contrast, cytotoxic and suppressor T cells, which express the CD8 molecule, recognize antigen in association with MHC class I molecules. Most mature T cells express the $\alpha\beta$TcR in association with the CD3 complex. The CD3 complex is usually coexpressed with both TCR types ($\alpha\beta$ and $\gamma\delta$).

The most immature prothymocytes express none of these aforementioned T cell markers, that is, initially thymocytes are CD3$^-$CD4$^-$CD8$^-$. As thymocytes mature, these surface molecules are acquired progressively. First, the CD8 molecule is expressed, followed by the coexpression of CD4 and CD8 prior to the expression of the β and then α chains of the TCR, as well as the associated CD3 complex (composed of ε, γ, δ, ζ, and η chains), which functions as the signal transducing element for the TCR. Hence, most (65–80%) thymocytes are "double positive" with respect to CD4 and

CD8 expression. Many studies have shown that this population of cortical thymocytes is subjected to selection (Finkel *et al.*, 1991). Unlike the intra-thymic T cells, the double-positive population does not produce lympho-kines or proliferate in response to any of the known lymphokines.

III. Signal Transduction in Cells of the T Lineage

The engagement of the $\alpha\beta$TCR on mature T cells results in their prolifera-tion and differentiation into effector cells. In contrast, engagement of the $\alpha\beta$TCR on immature thymocytes by self antigens does not result in prolifera-tion or differentiation. Instead, interactions between the thymocyte $\alpha\beta$TCR and self MHC (presumably complexed with endogenous self peptides) nurtures the development of those cells bearing appropriate receptors that recognize foreign antigen plus self MHC, and prevents the development and expansion of potentially harmful self-reactive T cells. A major issue in T cell immunobiology is how a single receptor performs both positive and negative selection on immature thymocytes, as well as stimulates prolifera-tion and differentiation of mature T cells.

In mature T cells, ligation of the $\alpha\beta$TCR results in the activation of several interrelated second messenger pathways. This receptor–ligand interaction leads to the activation of a phospholipase C ($PLC_{\gamma 1}$), resulting in the hydro-lysis of polyphosphoinositides to yield diacylglycerol (DAG) and inositol 1,4,5-trisphosphate (IP_3). These second messengers respectively mediate the activation of protein kinase C (PKC) and the mobilization of intracellular Ca^{2+} followed by the influx of extracellular Ca^{2+}. In addition, ligand binding to the TCR complex results in the phosphorylation of tyrosine residues of several proteins including the TCR-associated ζ chain and $PLC_{\gamma 1}$. The identity of the tyrosine kinase responsible for this activity is not entirely known, but may be the $p59^{fyn}$ or the $p56^{lck}$ proto-oncogene product. Tyro-sine kinase activity is necessary for activation of the phosphoinositide pathway since inhibitors of tyrosine kinases have been shown to prevent IP_3 generation as well as proliferation and lymphokine production (Mustelin *et al.*, 1989,1990). Also, tyrosine kinase activity has been shown to precede the activation of $PLC_{\gamma 1}$ (June *et al.*, 1990). Hence, in mature T cells, the activation of an interrelated multifaceted signal transduction cascade after the ligation of the antigen-specific receptor and associated surface components results in cellular proliferation and differentiation to lympho-kine production. Since T cell activation via the antigen receptor complex can be bypassed by calcium ionophores and phorbol esters, agents that re-spectively elevate intracellular Ca^{2+} and activate PKC, these two second messengers are believed to play critical roles in T cell proliferation and differentiation.

In contrast to mature T cells, relatively little is known about the intricacies of signal transduction pathways that are active in the various thymocyte subsets. The immature thymocyte shows a much reduced increase in cytosolic Ca^{2+} on stimulation via the TCR–CD3 complex, indicating that, at this stage of development, the antigen receptor complex is inefficiently coupled to the signal transducing elements, the intracellular Ca^{2+} pools are reduced, or Ca^{2+} entry is prohibited. Treatment of thymocytes with intracellular Ca^{2+}-elevating agents including calcium ionophores, compounds that stimulate the release of the IP_3-sensitive endoplasmic reticular Ca^{2+} store (e.g., thapsigargin and 2,5-di-(tertbutyl)-1,4-benzohydroquinone), the environmental toxicants 2,3,7,8-tetrachlorodibenzo-p-dioxin (TCDD) and tributyltin, and antibodies to the CD3 complex results in cell death by the mechanism of apoptosis (McCabe et al., 1992). More detailed studies have indicated that the most immature double-negative thymocytes proliferate and produce cytokines on treatment with calcium ionophore in conjunction with phorbol ester (Fisher et al., 1991), whereas conflicting reports indicate that phorbol ester treatment either prevents (McConkey et al., 1989) or enhances (Kizaki et al., 1989; Suzuki et al., 1991) calcium ionophore-induced apoptosis in the double-positive population. Hence, at different stages of thymocyte maturation, signal transduction differs both quantitatively and qualitatively, perhaps because of the diverse coupling of the various receptor-linked signal transduction elements, and the interpretation (i.e., activation versus apoptosis) of these second messenger signals, especially Ca^{2+}, differs.

Current understanding of metal modulation of thymocyte maturation is not complete. Most of the reports discussed in the subsequent sections have dealt mainly with gross assessment of thymic structure after metal intoxication *in vivo*. Hence, when metal intoxication has been correlated with thymic dysplasia, whether the observed thymic atrophy is the result of direct action of the toxic metal on the thymus or of indirect action by general stress is not clear. This distinction is important since, under a stressed condition, serum glucocorticoids are elevated and glucocorticoids are well known to cause thymic atrophy by the mechanism of apoptosis (Wyllie, 1980; Cohen and Duke, 1984). Nutritional Zn deficiency (DePasquale-Jardieu and Fraker, 1979) and the administration of nickel (Ni; Benson et al., 1987) elevate serum corticosterone. Although all populations of thymocytes are either directly or indirectly affected by glucocorticoids, the double-positive subpopulation is most sensitive to the thymolytic action of glucocorticoids.

Metals could influence thymocyte maturation and TCR repertoire selection in a variety of ways. Distinct thymocyte subpopulations could be targeted or the effect could be more generalized, that is, could affect all subpopulations equally. For instance, evidence has indicated that Pb differentially affects the activation of mature T helper cell subsets (McCabe and Lawrence, 1991). Mercury (Hg) and Au also have been reported to modify

T cell subset activities differentially (Goldman *et al.*, 1991; Kosuda *et al.*, 1991). Mechanistically, these differential effects of metals on the T cell subsets are not well understood. Potential effects on thymic development of the T cell subsets have not been evaluated. Metals could influence signal transduction at various levels. Receptor–ligand interactions could be interfered with so the proper signaling event(s) is not properly initiated. These receptor–ligand interactions may involve cell-to-cell interactions between thymocytes and thymic stromal cells or interactions between thymocytes and soluble mediators such as cytokines and thymic factors. Another possibility is that metals can mimic the signals that are generated by these receptor–ligand interactions or modulate the intracellular generation of second messengers. For example, Cd has been reported to elicit IP_3 formation in fibroblasts (Smith *et al.*, 1989). Although Cd and Hg can inhibit Ca^{2+} influx, presumably via plasma membrane calcium channels (Blazka and Shaikh, 1991), Cd and Hg as well as Pb have been reported to mobilize calcium in various cell types (Pounds, 1984; Smith *et al.*, 1989). Ni is another metal known to block Ca^{2+} entry (Amigorena *et al.*, 1990). Pb can substitute for Ca in the activation of PKC (Markovac and Goldstein, 1988), and Zn may play a physiological role in the activation of PKC (Csermely *et al.*, 1988a), the tyrosine kinase $p56^{lck}$ (Pernelle *et al.*, 1991), and the phosphotyrosine phosphatase CD45 (Tonks *et al.*, 1990). Aside from the modulation of signal transduction that may occur in metal-exposed thymocytes, metals may modify the generation of appropriate T cell clones by direct cytotoxic effects as well as by energy depletion. A more extensive review of the modification of cell signaling in the cytotoxicity of metals has been published (Rossi *et al.*, 1991).

IV. Physiological Regulation of Thymocyte Maturation by Metal Ions

That endogenous metal ions play a part in thymocyte maturation , is an important consideration. Certainly Ca^{2+}, although not a metal ion per se, functions in the biochemical events that shape the selection of the TCR repertoire. The most important aspect of the role of Ca^{2+} with respect to metal toxicity is that Ca^{2+}-dependent events are most likely targeted in thymocytes, as they are in other tissues and cell types (Kass *et al.*, 1991).

Zn is an endogenous metal that functions in thymocyte development. Zn is an essential trace element, functioning in nearly 300 enzymes (Valle and Auld, 1990). Researchers recognize that faulty intestinal Zn adsorption leading to Zn deficiency can be immunocompromising. A syndrome known as acrodermatitis enteropathica that occurs in humans who have faultly Zn absorption has been associated with gross thymic deficiency and increased susceptibility to infection (Brummerstedt, 1977; Prasad, 1984). Also, a pronounced alteration in the development of the T cell subsets occurs in Down syndrome patients and has been linked with a Zn deficiency (Cossarizza *et al.*, 1990). Further, a relationship between diminished Zn status and immunosuppression during aging has been described (Winchurch *et al.*, 1984). Evidence from many laboratories has indicated that Zn deficiency decreases both the humoral and the cell-mediated immune responses. The parameters affected include antibody formation, cell-mediated cytotoxicity, natural killer cell function, macrophage phagocytosis, and intracellular killing, as well as the level of circulating thymic hormones (Luecke and Fraker, 1979; Wirth *et al.*, 1984; Prasad *et al.*, 1988). Zn acts as a cofactor for some thymic hormones, most notably thymulin. Zn itself is mitogenic for T lymphocytes (Warner and Lawrence, 1986) and thymocytes (Winchurch, 1988), and increases the production of interleukin 1 (IL-1) and IL-4 (Winchurch *et al.*, 1987). With respect to thymocyte proliferation, Zn has been shown to replace signals derived from the T cell mitogen phytohemagglutinin (PHA) in association with IL-1, suggesting that Zn mimics a proliferative signal that is normally delivered to thymocytes by PHA. Interestingly, PKC contains a Zn binding domain (Parker *et al.*, 1986) which, on binding Zn increases the affinity of the enzyme for phorbol esters (Csermely *et al.*, 1988b), regulatory ligands (Forbes *et al.*, 1990b), and the cytoskeleton (Zalewski *et al.*, 1990,1991; Forbes *et al.*, 1990a). Au and Cd also have been reported to enhance PKC binding, whereas Cu and Fe were inhibitory and Pb was without effect (Forbes *et al.*, 1990b). Many reports have indicated that Zn is necessary for the activation of PKC and that Zn influences the distribution of PKC within T cells. Conversely, the PKC activators phorbol myristic acetate (PMA) and phorbol dibutyrate (PDBu) have been shown to promote an intracellular redistribution of Zn from the nucleus and mitochondria to the cytosol and microsome in T cells (Csermely *et al.*, 1987). Zn appears to enhance membrane-interacting properties of PKC in cell extracts. Similarly, Csermely *et al.*, (1988a) showed an absolute requirement for endogenous Zn in the activation and translocation of PKC by using a membrane permeable metal chelator, tetrakis-(2-pyridylmethyl)ethylene-diamine (TPEN). Other investigators have shown that, for purified PKC at low concentrations of Ca^{2+} (about 50 μM), Zn enhances PKC activity, but at higher Ca^{2+} concentrations, Zn is inhibitory (Murakami *et al.*, 1987). In the absence of Ca^{2+}, Zn has no effect on PKC activity. Whereas Ca^{2+} controls the binding of PKC to the lipid component of the cell membrane, Zn controls the distribution of PKC to the cytoskeleton (Zalewski *et al.*, 1990,1991; Forbes *et al.*, 1990b). Interestingly, Pb also can stimulate PKC (Markovac and Goldstein, 1988).

In addition to PKC, many other Zn-binding proteins function in thymocyte maturation. The leukocyte common antigen CD45, which is a phosphotyrosine phosphatase, has been reported to be stimulated by divalent metal ions, including Zn and manganese (Mn) (Tonks *et al.*, 1990). CD45 functions to dephosphorylate and activate the CD4-associated tyrosine kinase p56[lck]

(Mustelin and Altman, 1990), which itself is directly regulated by Zn (Pernelle et al., 1991). Investigators have suggested that two cysteines within the N-terminal region of p56^{lck} associate with two cysteines in the C-terminal cytoplasmic domain of CD4 or CD8α via a Zn molecule (Turner et al., 1990).

The Ca^{2+}-dependent endonuclease that functions in the selection process is regulated by Zn. Studies have shown that activation of DNA fragmentation in thymocytes by a variety of agents including glucocorticoids (Cohen and Duke, 1984), irradiation (Sellins and Cohen, 1987), and DNA topoisomerase-II inhibitors (Shimizu et al., 1990) is blocked by Zn. Presumably, the endonuclease contains a Zn-binding site that inactivates its enzymatic activity. On the other hand, Zn increases the affinity of glucocorticoids (Freedman et al., 1988) and estrogen (Hutchens et al., 1989) for their receptors, so in this respect Zn is likely to facilitate DNA fragmentation. Based on Zn finger consensus sequences derived from cDNAs isolated from human T cell lines, investigators suggested that at least 27 nonoverlapping structures can be defined (Huebner et al., 1991). Numerous transcription factors have been shown to possess Zn finger domains (Berg, 1990) including GATA-3, a lineage-restricted transcription factor that regulates the expression of the T cell receptor genes (Ho et al., 1991; Marine and Winoto, 1991), and MBP-1, a protein binding to the enhancer region for the MHC class I and κ immunoglobulin genes (Baldwin et al., 1990). Although multiple, potentially regulatory proteins with Zn finger-like domains appear to be present in T cells as well as B cells (see subsequent discussion), proof of the actual binding of Zn still is needed for most of these proteins. Further, even if Zn can bind, evidence must be found that the Zn binding can modulate regulation. In addition, the possibility remains that cations other than Zn also bind and alter the normal endogenous functions. Thus, the quantitative subcellular distribution of various cations may be critical for appropriate T cell development and selective processes. These metals may function or induce dysfunction at different levels within the cell, from surface membrane signaling to the regulation of gene expression and DNA replication. Other work indicates that chelation of intracellular Zn by the membrane-permeable metal chelator TPEN selectively induces apoptosis in thymocytes that have a mature phenotype (i.e., CD4 or CD8 single positive) as well as in splenocytes and lymph node cells (M. J. McCabe, Jr., et al., unpublished observations). The effect of TPEN can be prevented by the simultaneous addition of Zn but not by Mn or Fe. TPEN has very low affinity for Ca^{2+} and treatment with TPEN does not result in an elevation of the cytosolic Ca^{2+}. Nonetheless, Ca^{2+} is required for TPEN-induced DNA fragmentation, since simultaneous chelation of intracellular Ca^{2+} prevents apoptosis by TPEN. Perhaps regulation of the endonuclease, like the regulation of PKC, is Ca^{2+} dependent.

As mentioned previously, glucocorticoids induce apoptosis in all thymocyte subpopulations, although the double-positive population is most sensitive (Mathieson and Fowlkes, 1984; Screpanti et al., 1989). Possibly, the protection afforded by the addition of exogenous Zn to glucocorticoid-treated thymocytes applies only to the more mature cells (i.e., medullary thymocytes); however, this possibility remains to be tested. Perhaps the metallothioneins (MT) regulate signaling in thymocytes by Zn ions by acting as Zn-delivery molecules or as endogenous Zn chelators. MTs can be induced by glucocorticoids (Karin et al., 1984a,b), IL-1 (Karin et al., 1985), interferon γ (Friedman et al., 1984), phorbol esters (Imbra and Karin, 1987), ionizing radiation (Shiraishi et al., 1986,1989), and heavy metals (Lynes et al., 1990; Yamada and Koizumi, 1991). Cd has been reported to induce MT expression, particularly in thymocytes (Maytin and Young, 1983). Presently, whether MT has a protective or stimulatory role in apoptosis or whether MT is expressed in distinct thymocyte subsets is unclear.

Note that a thymocyte surface molecule expressed on double-negative thymocytes (CD4$^-$CD8$^-$) has been discovered to induce apoptosis (Itoh et al., 1991). This molecule, referred to as Fas, is a 35-kDa molecule that has been classified in the family of receptor molecules with nerve growth factor receptor, tumor necrosis factor (TNF) receptors, CD40, and OX40; all these molecules have multiple cysteine-rich exofacial domains. Thus, the expression of these molecules could be influenced by cations, suggesting another possible link between cations and apoptosis. Interestingly, the Fas protein is mutated in lpr/lpr mice (Watanabe-Fukunaga, 1992) which have a lymphoproliferative disease (excess numbers of double-negative T cells). Thus, Fas may also influence the maturation of thymocytes from double-negative cells into double-positive cells, suggesting that Fas could play a role in negative and positive selection.

V. Toxic Effects of Metals on Thymocytes

A. Organotin Compounds

Organotin compounds are used as heat stabilizers for polyvinyl chloride (PVC)-containing plastics, as pesticides and fungicides for agriculture, and as components of antifoulant paints (Boyer, 1989; Subramanian, 1985). One of the most widely used organotin compounds, tributyltin (TBT), is the main active ingredient in antifoulant marine paints. Because of its extensive use on marine vessels, TBT has been reported to accumulate in coastal waters and, subsequently, in aquatic organisms to high levels (Coghlan, 1990).

The toxicity of organotin compounds has been studied extensively. Effects on many organ systems including the central nervous system and the reproductive system have been reviewed (Boyer, 1989). Notably, organotin cytotoxicity and tissue selectivity is strongly influenced by the chain length of the organic group bound to the tin (Blunden and Chapman, 1986). Cells of the immune system are particularly sensitive to TBT. At relatively low concentrations (0.5–5 ppm), TBT has been reported to cause severe depletion of cortical thymocytes and thymic involution in rats (Krajnc et al., 1984; Vos et al., 1984; Smialowicz et al., 1989; Snoeij et al., 1985; Seinen and Penninks, 1979). The organotin inhibition of T cell development appears to be limited to its effects on the thymus, because effects on bone marrow progenitors were not observed (Penninks et al., 1985). The immunotoxic effects of organotin compounds do not appear to be the result of a stress-related elevation of glucocorticoid hormones (Miller et al., 1984), although organotins (Penninks et al., 1985) like Cd (Yamada et al., 1981) selectively deplete cortical thymocytes. The thymic involution is reversible when TBT treatment is ended; however, inappropriate clones could escape from the thymus during this treatment period.

Many mechanisms have been postulated to account for the marked thymic atrophy following treatment with organotin compounds. For example, organotin compounds have been reported to inhibit thymocyte proliferation *in vitro* (Seinen et al., 1979), to disrupt protein synthesis and mitochondrial energy production (Snoeij et al., 1986; Powers and Beavis, 1991), to modify the cytoskeleton (Marinovich et al., 1990), and to trigger the apoptotic pathway (Aw et al., 1990; Raffray and Cohen, 1991). As discussed previously, DNA fragmentation characteristic of apoptosis is often mediated by sustained increases in cytosolic free Ca^{2+}. Consistent with this feature, TBT has been shown to elevate cytosolic Ca^{2+} rapidly in both rat and human thymocytes. Buffering the rise in intracellular Ca^{2+} concentration with Ca^{2+} chelators such as BAPTA, EGTA, or Quin2 prevents DNA fragmentation, and cell death requires the presence of extracellular Ca^{2+} (M. J. McCabe, Jr., et al., unpublished observations). TBT-increased cytosolic Ca^{2+} occurs by multiple mechanisms including release of intracellular Ca^{2+} stores from IP_3-sensitive storage pools, stimulation of a Ca^{2+}-entry pathway, and inhibition of Ca^{2+} efflux by the plasma membrane Ca^{2+}-ATPase (B. Chow et al., 1992; M. J. McCabe, Jr., unpublished data). The influx of Ca^{2+} from the extracellular pool plays the major role in elevating the cytosolic level. Although TBT can reduce thymocyte ATP pools as well, the induction of cell death as well as the reduction in cellular ATP content is linked to the presence of extracellular Ca^{2+} (M. J. McCabe, Jr., et al., unpublished data). In the absence of extracellular Ca^{2+}, the kinetics of ATP depletion by TBT are slowed, but eventually the ATP levels are reduced to the same extent seen with TBT in the presence of extracellular Ca^{2+}. Despite the reduced ATP pool, in the absence of extracellular Ca^{2+} the cells remain viable after TBT treatment, establishing a clear link between TBT-induced elevation of cytosolic Ca^{2+} and cell death.

B. Other Metals

In addition to studies concerning the organotin compounds, only a few isolated studies regarding modulation of thymocyte development or thymic function by metals have been published. A few examples may offer clues to the metals that should be studied in more detail and to the mechanisms by which they affect the thymus.

Inhalation of Ni compounds at relatively high doses has been reported to result in acute thymic involution (Benson et al., 1987; Knight et al., 1987; Milicevic and Milicevic, 1989; Haley et al., 1990), whereas conflicting reports have indicated that Cd administration results in thymic atrophy (Yamada et al., 1982; Xu et al., 1989) or has no effect on the thymus as measured by thymus weight (Cifone et al., 1989). Not surprisingly, a relationship appears to exist between Cd-induced thymocyte toxicity and Zn status, that is, Cd has been reported to decrease the content of Zn in the thymus (Huerta et al., 1988) and thymic atrophy associated with Cd administration can be prevented by the administration of Zn (Chowdhury et al., 1987; Herkovits and Perez-Coll, 1990). Whether Cd has a differential effect on thymocyte subpopulations similar to that postulated for Zn is unknown; however, in the periphery at low concentrations, Cd selectively decreases T cell mitogenesis (Otsuka and Ohsawa, 1991). Here, too, the effects of Cd can be prevented by the addition of exogenous Zn, but intracellular Cd content and the Cd-induced MT levels remain unchanged in these cells. Presumably, Cd antagonizes an intracellular Zn-dependent process required for T cell proliferation. Either MT is uninvolved or it plays a protective role against Cd toxicity. Importantly, the total cellular Cd content remains the same but is more efficiently complexed with MT on prior Zn induction.

Although the mechanism and the developmental phase influenced are not known, Fe^{3+}, Ni^{2+}, and Co^{2+} have been reported to block the ability of human T cells to rosette with sheep erythrocytes (Bravo et al., 1990). T cell rosetting with sheep erythrocytes is dependent on the expression of CD2 and functional microfilaments. In vitro treatment with Fe and Co interfered with the expression of CD2, whereas Ni inhibited the expression of CD2 and CD3. As suggested earlier, numerous cations can alter T cell development. However, the mechanisms of these actions are still unknown.

VI. B Lymphocytes

The B lymphocyte lineage is directly responsible for humoral immunity because the n-terminal cell (the plasma cell) is the main producer of antibodies, the effector molecules of humoral immunity. Intermediary cells in this lineage, however, also are capable of synthesizing and secreting antibody molecules. In fact, investigators have suggested that most serum IgM immunoglobulins, the so-called "natural IgM antibodies," are derived from CD5$^+$ B cells. The CD5$^+$ B cells appear to come from a separate B cell lineage (the B-1 lineage; Kantor, 1991) because their stem cells seem to be of non-bone marrow cell origin and, thus, are different from the bone marrow-derived stem cells (in the adult) that give rise to the B cells that participate in the conventional immune responses (for review, see Hayakawa and Hardy, 1988; Kipps, 1989). With respect to conventional B cell (B-2 lineage) and T cell development, clearly their lymphoid progenitors exist in the same fetal and adult sites (liver and bone marrow, respectively) as the myeloid progenitors discussed earlier. Unfortunately, almost no data directly address the influences of a metal on B cell development. Studies have reported a loss of cellularity of secondary lymphoid organs (spleen and/or lymph nodes) after *in vivo* exposure to a metal; however, the precise types of cells lost were not delineated. Indirect evidence suggests that few metals selectively block B cell development, because no reports to date show the absence of B cells in an otherwise normal animal or human after *in vivo* exposure to a metal. Ohsawa *et al.*, (1983) reported that Cd (3–300 ppm for 10 wk) can lower the number of B cells in the peripheral blood of mice (ICR strain), but a concomitant rise in the number of splenic B cells was seen, suggesting that Cd causes a redistribution of lymphocytes but not a blockage in B cell development. Likewise, Cd-exposed humans did not appear to have decreased numbers of peripheral blood T cells or B cells (Williams *et al.*, 1983). Cd (200 ng CdCl$_2$/day for 40 days) also has been reported to increase the number of B cells in the spleen (Bozelka *et al.*, 1978); however, a single injection of Cd did not affect the number of splenic B cells (Burchiel *et al.*, 1987) and inhibited the number of antibody-producing cells (Koller *et al.*, 1976). Although substantial changes in peripheral B cell numbers are not evident, researchers have reported that injection of mice with CdCl$_2$ causes a greater effect on immature B cells in the bone marrow than on mature B cells in the spleen (Stelzer and Pazdernik, 1983). Bone marrow cellularity was not affected, but cell phenotypes were changed. A single ip injection of Zn (12 mg/kg) into mice caused a decrease in bone marrow and spleen cellularity, splenic B cell progenitor development, and T cell and B cell responsiveness to mitogens (Murray *et al.*, 1983). In a human study, researchers also demonstrated that Au can induce maturational abnormalities in the B cell compartment (Guillemin *et al.*, 1987). Few metal studies have reported a decrease in the number of B cells or the amount of Ig in the serum after exposure. The amount of Ig in the serum is a measure of the existence of B cells but not of their ability to be involved in a specific antibody response. This condition is clearly evident in patients with acquired immunodeficiency syndrome (AIDS), who can have normal serum Ig concentrations with no ability to produce specific antibodies.

Pb acetate (10 mM drinking water for 8 wk) has been reported not to alter the serum Ig concentrations or the antibody response to sheep red blood cells, (Mudzinski et al., 1986), although a single injection of Pb acetate has been reported to increase the number of splenic B cells (Burchiel et al., 1987) and the number of antibody-producing cells (Koller et al., 1976). Similarly, Pb exposure of humans has been reported to increase the number of B cells (Yoshida et al., 1980); however, human serum Ig values do not seem to be affected by Pb (Reigart and Graber, 1976; Ewers et al., 1982; Ho et al., 1982; Kimber et al., 1986). In one study with extensive exposure of rats to Pb (prefertilization, throughout gestation, and until 5–6 wk of age) at a low dose (25–50 ppm), a decrease in serum IgG but not IgM or IgA (Luster et al., 1978) was seen. Workers occupationally exposed to Hg had elevated levels of serum IgA and IgM, but their serum IgG levels were normal (Bencko et al., 1990).

Although a deficiency of numerous metals can inhibit T cell development, little data suggests a similar effect on B cell development. Cu deficiency in rats leads to lower T cell numbers and functions, but B cells seem to be unaffected (Bala et al., 1991). In mice, Cu deficiency results in an increase in the number of B cells (Lukasewycz et al., 1985). The B cell deficit associated with Down syndrome has been suggested to be the result of a Zn deficiency in these patients (Cossarizza et al., 1990). Marginal Zn deprivation in infant rhesus monkeys led to decreased serum IgM levels but the serum IgA and IgG levels were normal (Haynes et al., 1985). Zn modulation of B cell development may be accomplished by a Zn-dependent metalloprotease (BP-1, Ramakrishnan et al., 1990; Wu et al., 1991; CD10, Shipp et al., 1990) on the surface of pre-B cells. Interestingly, IL-7, a lymphocyte-inducing factor from bone marrow stromal cells, can up-regulate BP-1 expression by B cell precursors (BP-1$^-$, B220$^-$, Ia$^-$) and concomitant cell growth (Welch et al., 1990).

Several reports do indicate that metals can modulate the phenotype and/or function of B cells at various stages of development and that metals can modulate T cell-dependent B cell differentiation into an antibody-producing cell. B cell development is discussed briefly in the following paragraphs, followed by a review of some metal influences on various aspects of B cell growth and differentiation.

The development of the human B-2 lineage initiates with a lymphoid progenitor in the bone marrow that lacks any known surface antigen (designated as a cluster of differentiation, CD) restricted to B cells; however, it does possess one form (DR) of the MHC class II molecules (DP, DQ, and DR), referred to herein as HLA-D. Cells of the B cell lineage do eventually acquire all three products of the MHC class II genes. The first evidence to suggest that the cell is in the B cell lineage is rearrangement of the D–J$_H$ genes. These cells are sometimes classified as early pro-B cells and express CD19 (a marker that is used to delineate cells in the B cell lineage, a pan-B cell marker), although some cells not of the B cell lineage (e.g., monocytic lineage cells) possess a low level of this marker. Early B cell progenitors also possess the enzyme terminal deoxynucleotide transferase (TdT), which plays a role in diversification of the variable (V) domains of antibody molecules. At a later stage of the pro-B cell, the V–D–J_H genes are rearranged. Once the heavy chain genes are expressed as the cytoplasmic μ chain (V–D–J–μ), the cell is referred to as a pre-B cell. The pre-B cell then rearranged the genes for light chain expression. The pre-B cell first attempts V–J_κ rearrangement but, if faulty rearrangements occur (both alleles), the cell goes on to rearrange V–J_λ. Lymphocytes are recognized and defined as B cells when they express sIg. The first isotype to appear is sIgM (μ and κ or λ); however, these early B cells are still immature functionally (more readily induced into a state of tolerance than activation). Mature B cells express sIgM and sIgD, which use common V–D–J genes (and, thus, have identical idiotypes). The sIgs serve as antigen-specific receptors (with identical antigen-binding specificities or paratopes). When a B cell is induced to secrete antibodies, the mRNA for its membrane form of Ig (sIg) is spliced to produce a message lacking a transmembrane sequence. Finally, the B cell is fully differentiated when it loses its sIg (as well as all previously expressed CD molecules) and becomes the plasma cell, an active secretor of one antibody isotype (IgA, IgG, IgM, IgE, or IgD). This differentiation is dependent on numerous cytokines (ILs) from stromal cells, macrophages, and T cells. Each stage of B cell development is responsive to different combinations of cytokines that influence cell growth and/or differentiation. IL-7, IL-1, IL-3, and IL-4 influence the early stages of pro-B cell development. IL-4, IL-5, IL-6, and interferon γ have multiple regulatory effects on mature B cells and, thus, can influence the amount of Ig produced as well as its isotypic form.

Numerous studies have assessed the influences of metals on humoral immunity, that is, on the production of antibodies induced by a specific antigen or polyclonal activator such as lipopolysaccharide (LPS). However, most of these studies are not able to differentiate a direct effect on the B cell from effects on a T cell subset or on another type of cell such as a macrophage, that may aid the immune response. The ability of metals to modify B cell reactivities, especially by altering T cell functions, has been reviewed (Kowolenko et al., 1992); therefore, studies that evaluate the direct effects of metals on B cells are discussed here.

Numerous studies address the terminal effect of metals on B cell proliferation and differentiation, that is, antibody production. However, the development of antibody-producing cells (plasmocytes, plasmoblasts, or plasma cells) is usually a T cell-dependent process. Metals have been shown to inhibit, enhance, or unmodify antibody production in vivo. A good example of the indirect effects of a metal on B cell activity (antibody production) was given in the study by Schuhmann et al. (1990): Au^{3+} but not Au^+ enhanced in vivo autoantibody production in select strains of mice as well as lymphocyte proliferation measured by a popliteal lymph node (PLN) assay. However, the proliferation and antibody production was dependent on the presence of T cells. Probably, in a similar manner, T cells from Hg-treated rats can adoptively transfer enhancing activity to syngeneic recipients that have increased autoantibody production (Pelletier et al., 1988b). Likewise, the polyclonal antibody effect of $HgCl_2$ in Brown–Norway rats was not obtained after depletion of T cells (Hirsch et al., 1982). The ability of Hg to induce the production of numerous types of autoantibodies is one of the best developed models of metal-induced autoimmunity (Pelletier et al., 1988a; Hultman et al., 1989; Reuter et al., 1989). The ability of Hg to induce autoantibodies is regulated by genes in the I region of the MHC (Goter-Robinson et al., 1986; Mirtcheva et al., 1989). Hg also stimulates IgE production, which is known to be under tight control by T cells (Prouvost-Danon et al., 1981; Pietsch et al., 1989).

In addition to assessment of the number of B cells and the serum Ig concentration, direct B cell effects can be determined by responsiveness to T cell-independent stimulators such as LPS in mice. Pb acetate (0.24–4.8 mM drinking water for 3 wk) was reported to suppress the T cell-independent antibody response to DNP–Ficoll, a macrophage-dependent antigen, but not to LPS, a macrophage-independent antigen (Blakley and Archer, 1981). A similar result was obtained with Cd (Blakley and Tomar, 1986). Exposure of rats to TBT produced an enhanced response to a T cell-dependent antigen, but no modulation of the response to a T cell-independent antigen (Smialowicz et al., 1990). LPS-induced B cell proliferation also was not inhibited by Pb (Koller et al., 1979). Assessment of the LPS-induced B cell proliferation in mice exposed to $NiCl_2$ in utero indicated suppression (Smialowicz et al., 1986); however, exposure of adult mice or rats to $NiCl_2$ did not cause any B cell inhibition (Smialowicz et al., 1984,1987). These data suggest that Ni may suppress B cell development, but not mature B cells. In general, mature B cells appear to be more resistant to the toxic effects of metals than T cells. An in vitro analysis of mouse mitogen-induced lymphoproliferation indicates that T cells are more sensitive than B cells to Cd; however, similar sensitivities were obtained with Hg, Pb, Ni, Co, As, and molybdenum (Mo) (Otsuka and Ohsawa, 1991). A similar study reported that mouse B cells were more sensitive to Cu (Yamauchi and Yamamoto, 1990). An in vitro deficiency of Cu, Mn, and Zn did not affect mouse B cell proliferation, but T cell responsiveness was inhibited (Flynn, 1984). An in vitro analysis of human B cell and T cell proliferation indicated that B cells have a greater requirement for Ca and Mg than T cells (Carpentieri et al., 1988). Reports of in vitro metal effects on lymphocytes prior to the availability of fetal bovine serum with low LPS (endotoxin) suggested that some metals can directly induce B cell activation and proliferation (Shenker et al., 1977; Gallagher et al., 1979; Lawrence, 1981a). However, these results would not likely occur in the absence of LPS or some other bacterial antigens. Most work now suggests that heavy metals that induce lymphocyte proliferation do so on T cells, not B cells. However, some metals are still thought to stimulate B cell proliferation. Beryllium can induce lymphocyte proliferation in nude mice (T cell deficient) and is a polyclonal B cell activator (Newman and Campbell, 1987).

The basis for the apparent higher degree of resistance of mature B cells to most metals is presently unknown. A resistance to metals does not appear to correlate with other sensitivities, because B cells are more sensitive to radiation (Lawrence, 1981b) and oxidative stressors (Duncan and Lawrence, 1988) than T cells. Signal transduction events are not likely to be substantially different between T cells and B cells; in fact, Zn and Au also can induce translocation of PKC in B cells (Forbes et al., 1991), as discussed earlier for T cells. The subcellular mechanisms involved in cell resistance to metals usually are limited to induction of MT. B cells and T cells can be induced to produce MT; thus, the mechanisms of metal resistance remain to be elucidated. Likewise, the influence of metals on B cell development remain to be determined. Clearly, numerous metals have positive and negative influences on T and B cell development, as well as on the functions of the immunologically mature lymphoid subsets.

References

Agarwal, K., Sharma, A., and Talukder, G. (1990). Clastogenic effects of copper sulfate on the bone marrow chromosomes of mice in vivo. *Mutation Res.* **243**, 1–6.

Amigorena, S., Choquet, D., Teillaud, J. L., Korn, H., and Fridman, W. H. (1990). Ion channels and B cell mitogenesis. *Mol. Immunol.* **27**, 1259–1268.

Aw, T. Y., Nicotera, P., Manzo, L., and Orrenius, S. (1990). Tributyltin stimulates apoptosis in rat thymocytes. *Arch. Biochem. Biophys.* **283**, 46–50.

Bala, S., Failla, M. L., and Lunney, J. K. (1991). Alterations in splenic lymphoid cell subsets and activation antigens in copper-deficient rats. *J. Nutr.* **121**, 745–753.

Baldwin, A. S., LeClair, K. P., Singh, H., and Sharp, P. A. (1990). A large protein containing zinc finger domains binds to related sequence elements in the enhancers of the class I major histocompatibility complex and kappa immunoglobulin genes. *Mol. Cell. Biol.* **10**, 1406–1414.

Bencko, V., Wagner, V., Wagnerova, M., and Ondrejcak, V. (1990). Immunological profiles in workers occupationally exposed to inorganic mercury. *J. Hyg. Epidemiol. Microbiol. Immunol.* **34**, 9–15.

Benson, J. M., Carpenter, R. C., Hahn, F. F., Haley, P. J., Hanson, R. C., Hobbs, C. H., Pickrell, J. A., and Dunnick, J. K. (1987). Comparative inhalation toxicity of nickel subsulfide to F344/N rats and B6C3F1 mice exposed for 12 days. *Fund. Appl. Toxicol.* **9**, 251–265.

Berg, J. M. (1990). Zinc finger domains: Hypothesis and current knowledge. *Annu. Rev. Biophys. Biophys. Chem.* **19**, 405–421.

Blakley, B. R., and Archer, D. L. (1981). The effect of lead acetate on the immune response in mice. *Toxicol. Appl. Pharmacol.* **61**, 18–26.

Blakley, B. R., and Tomar, R. S. (1986). The effect of cadmium on antibody responses to antigens with different cellular requirements. *Int. J. Immunopharmacol.* **8**, 1009–1015.

Blazka, M. E., and Shaikh, Z. A. (1991). Differences in cadmium and mercury uptake by hepatocytes: role of calcium channels. *Toxicol. Appl. Pharmacol.* **110**, 355–363.

Blunden, S. J., and Chapman, A. (1986). Organotin compounds in the environment. *In* "Organometallic Compounds in the Environment" (P. J. Craig, ed.), pp. 112–159. Longman Group, Essex, England.

Boyer, I. J. (1989). Toxicity of dibutyltin, tributyltin and other organotin compounds to humans and to experimental humans. *Toxicology* **55**, 253–298.

Bozelka, B. E., Burkholder, P. M., and Chang, L. W. (1978). Cadmium, a metallic inhibitor of antibody-mediated immunity in mice. *Environ. Res.* **17**, 390–402.

Bravo, I., Carvalho, G. S., Barbosa, M. A., and DeSousa, M. (1990). Differential effects of eight metal ions on lymphocyte differentiation antigens in *in vitro*. *J. Biomed. Mat. Res.* **24**, 1059–1068.

Brummerstedt, E. (1977). Animal model of human disease. Acrodermatitis enteropathica, zinc malabsorption. *Am. J. Pathol.* **87**, 725–728.

Burchiel, S. W., Hadley, W. M., Cameron, C. L., Fincher, R. H., Lim, T., Elias, L., and Stewart, C. C. (1987). Analysis of heavy metal immunotoxicity by multi-parameter flow cytometry: Correlation of flow cytometry and immune function data in B6CF1 mice. *Int. J. Immunopharmacol.* **9**, 597–610.

Carpentieri, U., Myers, J., Daeschner, C. W., and Haggard, M. E. (1988). Effects of iron, copper, zinc, calcium, and magnesium on human lymphocytes in culture. *Biol. Trace Elem. Res.* **16**, 165–176.

Chopikashvili, L. V., Vasil'eva, I. M., L'vova, G. N., Zasukhina, G. D., and Babyleva, L. A. (1989). Decrease in repair processes in lymphocytes of workers exposed to heavy metals. *Genetika* **25**, 2247–2250.

Chow, S. C., Kass, G. E. N., McCabe, M. J., and Orrenius, S. (1992). Tributytin increases cytosolic free Ca^{2+} concentration in thymocytes by mobilizing intracellular Ca^{2+}, activating a Ca^{2+} entry pathway, and inhibiting Ca^{2+} efflux. *Arch. Biochem. Biophys.* **298**, 143–149.

Chowdhury, B. A., Friel, J. K., and Chandra, R. K. (1987). Cadmium-induced immunopathology is prevented by zinc administration in mice. *J. Nutr.* **117**, 1788–1794.

Cifone, M. G., Alesse, E., Di Eugenio, R., Napolitano, T., Morrone, S., Paolini, R., Santoni, G., and Santoni, A. (1989). *In vivo* cadmium treatment alters natural killer cell activity and large granular lymphocyte number in the rat. *Immunopharmacol.* **18**, 149–156.

Coghlan, A. (1990). Lethal paint makes for the open sea. *New Scientist* **8**, 16–18.

Cohen, J. J., and Duke, R. C. (1984). Glucocorticoid activation of a calcium-dependent endonuclease in thymocyte nuclei leads to cell death. *J. Immunol.* **132**, 38–42.

Cossarizza, A., Monti, D., Montagnani, G., Ortolani, C., Masi, M., Zannotti, M., and Franceschi, C. (1990). Precocious aging of the immune system in Down Syndrome: Alteration of B lymphocytes, T lymphocyte subsets and cells with NK markers. *Am. J. Med. Genet. Suppl.* **7**, 213–218.

Csermely, P., Gueth, S., and Somogyi, J. (1987). The tumor promoter tetradecanoyl-phorbol-acetate (TPA) elicits the redistribution of zinc in subcellular fractions of rabbit thymocytes measured by x-ray fluorescence. *Biochem. Biophys. Res. Commun.* **144**, 863–868.

Csermely, P., Szamel, M., Resch, K., and Somogy, J. (1988a). Zinc can increase the activity of protein kinase C and contributes to its binding to plasma membranes in T lymphocytes. *J. Biol. Chem.* **263**, 6487–6490.

Csermely, P., Szamel, M., Resch, K., and Somogyi, J. (1988b). Zinc increases the affinity of phorbol ester receptor in T lymphocytes. *Biochem. Biophys. Res. Commun.* **154**, 578–583.

Deknudt, G., and Gerber, G. B. (1979). Chromosomal aberrations in bone marrow cells of mice given a normal or a calcium deficient diet supplemented with various heavy metals. *Mutation Res.* **68**, 163–168.

DePasquale-Jardieu, P., and Fraker, P. J. (1979). The role of corticosterone in the loss in immune function in the zinc-deficient A/J mouse. *J. Nutr.* **109**, 1847–1855.

Duncan, D. D., and Lawrence, D. A. (1988). Four sulfhydryl-modifying compounds cause different structural damage but similar functional damage in murine lymphocytes. *Chem. Biol. Interact.* **68**, 137–152.

Ewers, U., Stiller-Winkler, R., and Idel, H. (1982). Serum immunoglobulins, C3 and salivary IgA levels in lead workers. *Environ. Res.* **29,** 351–357.

Finkel, T. H., Kubo, R. T., and Cambier, J. C. (1991). T-cell development and transmembrane signaling: Changing biological responses through an unchanging receptor. *Immunol. Today* **12,** 79–85.

Fisher, M., MacNeil, I., Suda, T., Cupp, J. E., Shortman, K., and Zlotnik, A. (1991). Cytokine production by mature and immature thymocytes. *J. Immunol.* **146,** 3452–3456.

Flynn, A. (1984). Control of *in vitro* lymphocyte proliferation by copper, magnesium and zinc deficiency. *J. Nutr.* **114,** 2034–2042.

Forbes, I. J., Zalewski, P. D., Giannakis, C., and Betts, W. H. (1990a). Zinc induces specific association of PKC with membrane cytoskeleton. *Biochem. Int.* **22,** 741–748.

Forbes, I. J., Zalewski, P. D., Giannakis, C., Petkoff, H. S., and Cowled, P. A. (1990b). Interaction between protein kinase C and regulatory ligand is enhanced by a chelatable pool of intracellular zinc. *Biochim. Biophys. Acta* **1053,** 113–117.

Forbes, I. J., Zalewski, P. D., and Giannakis, C. (1991). Role for zinc in a cellular response mediated by protein kinase C in human B lymphocytes. *Exp. Cell Res.* **195,** 224–229.

Freedman, L. P., Luisi, B. F., Korszun, Z. R., Basavappa, R., Sigler, P. B., and Yamamoto, K. R. (1988). The function and structure of the metal coordination sites within the glucocorticoid receptor DNA binding domain. *Nature (London)* **334,** 543–546.

Friedman, R. L., Manly, S. P., McMahon, M., Kerr, I. M., and Stark, G. R. (1984). Transcriptional and posttranscriptional regulation of interferon-induced gene expression in human cells. *Cell* **38,** 745–755.

Gallagher, K., Matarazzo, W. J., and Gray, I. (1979). Trace metal modification of immunocompetence. II. Effect of Pb, Cd, and Cr on RNA turnover, hexokinase activity, and blastogenesis during B-lymphocyte transformation in vitro. *Clin. Immunol. Immunopathol.* **13,** 369–377.

Goldman, M., Druet, P., and Gleichmann, E. (1991). Th2 cells in systemic autoimmunity: Insights from allogenic diseases and chemically-induced autoimmunity. *Immunol. Today* **12,** 223–227.

Goter-Robinson, C. J., Balazs, T., and Egorov, I. K. (1986). Mercuric chloride, gold sodium thiomalate and D-penicillamine-induced antinuclear antibodies in mice. *Toxicol. Appl. Pharmacol.* **86,** 159–169.

Guillemin, F., Bene, M. C., Aussedat, R., Bannwarth, B., and Pourel, J. (1987). Hypogammaglobulinemia associated with gold therapy: evidence for a partial maturation blockade of B cells. *J. Rheumatol.* **14,** 1034–1035.

Haley, P. J., Shopp, G. M., Benson, J. M., Cheng, Y. S., Bice, D. E., Luster, M. I., Dunnick, J. K., and Hobbs, C. H. (1990). The immunotoxicity of three nickel compounds following 13-week inhalation exposure in the mouse. *Fund. Appl. Toxicol.* **15,** 476–487.

Hayakawa, K., and Hardy, R. R. (1988). Normal, autoimmune and malignant CD5 B cells: The Ly-1 B lineage. *Annu. Rev. Immunol.* **6,** 196–218.

Haynes, D. C., Gershwin, M. E., Golub, M. S., Cheung, A. T., Hurley, L. S., and Hendricks, A. G. (1985). Studies of marginal zinc deprivation in rhesus monkeys. VI. Influence on the immunochemistry of infants in the first year. *Am. J. Clin. Nutr.* **42,** 252–262.

Hays, E. F., and Margaretten, N. (1985). Long-term oral cadmium produces bone marrow hypoplasia in mice. *Exp. Hematol.* **13,** 229–234.

Herkovits, J., and Perez-Coll, C. S. (1990). Zinc protection against delayed development produced by cadmium. *Biol. Trace Elem. Res.* **24,** 217–221.

Hirsch, F., Couderc, J., Sapin, C., Fournie, G., and Druet, P. (1982). Polyclonal effect of HgCl$_2$ in the rat, its possible role in an experimental autoimmune disease. *Eur. J. Immunol.* **12,** 620–625.

Ho, I-C., Vorhees, P., Marin, N., Oakley, B. K., Tsai, S-F., Orkin, S. H., and Leiden, J. M. (1991). Human GATA-3: A lineage-restricted transcription factor that regulates the expression of the T cell receptor α gene. *Embo J.* **10,** 1187–1192.

Ho, Y., Kurita, H., Yoshida, T., Shima, S., Niiya, Y., Toriumi, H., and Nakayasu, T. (1982). Studies on serum specific protein levels in lead-exposed workers. *Jap. J. Ind. Health* **24**, 390–391.

Huebner, K., Druck, T., Croce, C. M., and Thiesen, H-J. (1991). Twenty-seven nonoverlappingmzinc finger cDNAs from human T cells map to nine different chromosomes with apparent clustering. *Am. J. Hum. Genet.* **48**, 726–740.

Huerta, P., Galan, P., Alcala, A. J., Ribas, B., and Teijon, J. M. (1988). Effects of the administration of cadmium and zinc on the concentration of zinc in the thymus of rats. *Biol. Trace Elem. Res.* **18**, 95–103.

Hultman, P., Enestrom, S., Pollard, K. M., and Tan, E. M. (1989). Anti-fibrillarin in mercury-treated mice. *Clin. Exp. Immunol.* **78**, 470–472.

Hutchens, T. W., Li, C. M., Yoshiaki, S., and Yip, T. (1989). Multiple DNA-binding estrogen receptor forms resolved by interaction with immobilized metal ions. *J. Biol. Chem.* **264**, 17206–17212.

Imbra, R. J., and Karin, M. (1987). Metallothionein gene expression is regulated by serum and activators of protein kinase C. *Mol. Cell. Biol.* **7**, 1358–1363.

Itoh, N., Yonehara, S., Ishii, A., Yonehara, M., Mizushima, S., Sameshima, M., Hase, A., Seto, Y., and Nagata, S. (1991). The polypeptide encoded by the cDNA for human cell surface antigen Fas can mediate apoptosis. *Cell* **66**, 233–243.

June, C. H., Fletcher, M. C., Ledbetter, J. A., and Samelson, L. E. (1990). Increases in tyrosine phosphorylation are detectable before phospholipase C activation after T cell receptor stimulation. *J. Immunol.* **144**, 1591–1599.

Kantor, A. (1991). A new nomenclature for B cells. *Immunol. Today* **12**, 388.

Karin, M., Haslinger, A., Holtgreve, H., Cathala, G., Slater, E., and Baxter, J. D. (1984a). Activation of heterologous promoter in response to dexamethasone and cadmium by metallothionein gene 5'-flanking DNA. *Cell* **36**, 371–379.

Karin, M., Haslinger, A., Holtgreve, H., Richards, R. I., Krauter, P., Westphal, H. M., and Besto, M. (1984b). Characterization of DNA sequences through which cadmium and glucocorticoid hormones induce human metallothionein-IIA gene. *Nature (London)* **308**, 513–519.

Karin, M., Imbra, R. J., Hegy, A., and Wong, G. (1985). Interleukin-1 regulates human metallothionein gene expression. *Mol. Cell. Biol.* **5**, 2866–2869.

Kass, G. E. N., Nicotera, P., and Orrenius, S. (1990). Effects of xenobiotics on signal transduction and Ca^{2+}-mediated processes in mammalian cells. *Int. Symp. Princess Takamatsu Cancer Res. Fund.* **21**, 213–226.

Kimber, I., Stonard, M. D., Gidlow, D. A., and Niewola, Z. (1986). Influence of chronic low level exposure to lead on plasma immunoglobulin concentration and cellular imune function in man. *Int. Arch. Occup. Environ. Health* **57**, 117–125.

Kipps, T. J. (1989). The CD5 B cell. *Adv. Immunol.* **47**, 117–185.

Kizaki, H., Tadakuma, T., Odaka, C., Muramatsu, J., and Ishimura, Y. (1989). Activation of a suicide process of thymocytes through DNA fragmentation by calcium ionophores and phorbol esters. *J. Immunol.* **143**, 1790–1794.

Knight, J. A., Rezwke, W. N., Wong, S. H. Y., Hopper, S. M., Zahoria, O., and Sunderman, F. W., Jr. (1987). Acute thymic involution and increased lipoperoxide in thymus of nickel chloride-treated rats. *Res. Commun. Chem. Pathol. Pharmacol.* **55**, 291–302.

Koller, L. D., Roan, J. G., and Exon, J. H. (1976). Humoral antibody response in mice after single dose exposure to lead or cadmium. *Proc. Soc. Exp. Biol. Med.* **151**, 339–342.

Koller, L. D., Roan, J. G., and Kerkvliet, N. I. (1979). Mitogen stimulation of lymphocytes in CBA mice exposed to lead and cadmium. *Environ. Res.* **19**, 177–188.

Kosuda, L. L., Wayne, A., Nahounou, M., Greiner, D. L., and Bigazzi, P. E. (1991). Reduction of the RT6.2 suset of T lymphocytes in Brown Norway rats with mercury-induced renal autoimmunity. *Cell. Immunol.* **135**, 154–167.

Kowolenko, M., Tracy, L., and Lawrence, D. (1991). Early effects of lead on bone marrow cell responsiveness in mice challenged with *Listeria monocytogenes*. *Fund. Appl. Toxicol.* **17,** 75–82.

Kowolenko, M., McCabe, M. J., and Lawrence, D. A. (1992). Metal-induced alterations of immunity. In "Clinical Immunotoxicology" (D. S. Newcombe, N. R. Rose, and J. C. Bloom, eds.), pp. 401–419. Raven Press, New York.

Krajnc, E. L., Wester, P. W., Loeber, J. G., van Leeuwen, F. X. R., Vos, J. G., Vaessen, H. A. M. G., and van Der Heijden, C. A. (1984). Toxicity of bis(tri-*n*-butyltin)oxide in the rat. I. Short-term effects on general parameters and on the endocrine and lymphoid systems. *Toxicol. Appl. Pharmacol.* **75,** 363–386.

Lawrence, D. A. (1981a). Heavy metal modulation of lymphocyte activities. II. Lead, an *in vitro* mediator of B-cell activation. *Int. J. Immunopharmacol.* **3,** 153–161.

Lawrence, D. A. (1981b). Antigen activation of T cells. *Hdbk Cancer Immunol.* **8,** 257–320.

Luecke, R. W., and Fraker, P. J. (1979). The effect of varying dietary zinc levels on growth and antibody-mediated response in two strains of mice. *J. Nutr.* **109,** 1373–1376.

Lukasewycz, O. A., Prohaska, J. R., Meyer, S. G., Schmidtke, J. R., Hatfield, S. M., and Marder, P. (1985). Alterations in lymphocyte subpopulations in copper-deficient mice. *Infect. Immun.* **48,** 644–647.

Luster, M. I., Faith, R. E., and Kimmel, C. A. (1978). Depression of humoral immunity in rats following chronic development lead exposure. *J. Environ. Pathol. Toxicol.* **1,** 397–402.

Lutton, J. D., Ibraham, N. G., Friedland, M., and Levere, R. D. (1984). The toxic effects of heavy metals on rat bone marrow in vitro erythropoiesis: Protective role of hemin and zinc. *Environ. Res.* **35,** 97–103.

Lynes, M. A., Garvey, J. S., and Lawrence, D. A. (1990). Extracellular metallothionein effects on lymphocyte activities. *Mol. Immunol.* **27,** 211–219.

Markovac, J., and Goldstein, G. W. (1988). Picomolar concentrations of lead stimulate brain protein kinase C. *Nature (London)* **334,** 71–73.

Marine, J., and Winoto, A. (1991). The human enhancer binding protein GATA-3 binds to several T cell receptor regulatory elements. *Proc. Natl. Acad. Sci. USA* **88,** 7284–7288.

Marinovich, M., Sanghvi, A., Colli, S., Tremoli, E., and Galli, C. L. (1990). Cytoskeletal modifications induced by organotin compounds in human neutrophils. *Toxicol. In Vitro* **4,** 109–116.

Mathieson, B. J., and Fowlkes, B. J. (1984). Cell surface antigen expression on thymocytes: Development and phenotypic differentiation of intrathymic subsets. *Immunol. Rev.* **82,** 141–173.

Maytin, E. V., and Young, D. A. (1983). Separate glucocorticoid, heavy metal, and heat shock domains in thymic lymphocytes. *J. Biol. Chem.* **258,** 12718–12722.

McCabe, M. J., Jr., and Lawrence, D. A. (1991). Lead, a major environmental pollutant, is immunomodulatory by its differential effects on CD4$^+$ T cell subsets. *Toxicol. Appl. Pharmacol.* **111,** 13–23.

McCabe, M. J., Jr., Nicotera, P., and Orrenius, S. (1992). Calcium-dependent cell death: Role of the endonuclease, protein kinase C, and chromatin structure. *Ann. N.Y. Acad. Sci.* **663,** 269–278.

McConkey, D. J., Hartzell, P., Jondal, M., and Orrenius, S. (1989). Inhibition of DNA fragmentation in thymocytes and isolated thymocyte nuclei by agents that stimulate protein kinase C. *J. Biol. Chem.* **264,** 13399–13402.

Milicevic, N. M., and Milicevic, Z. (1989). Histochemistry of the acutely involved thymus in nickel chloride-treated rats. *J. Comp. Pathol.* **101,** 143–150.

Miller, K., Scott, M. P., and Foster, J. R. (1984). Thymic involution in rats given diets containing dioctyltin dichloride. *Clin. Immunol. Immunopathol.* **30,** 62–70.

Mirtcheva, J., Pfeiffer, C., De Bruijn, J. A., Jacquesmart, F., and Gleichmann, E. (1989). Immunological alterations inducible by mercury compounds. III. H-2A acts as an immune response and H-2E as an immune suppression locus for $HgCl_2$-induced antinucleolar autoantibodies. *Eur. J. Immunol.* **19,** 2257–2261.

Miszta, H. (1990). *In vitro* effect of copper on the stromal cells of bone marrow in rats. *Toxicol Ind. Health* **6,** 33–39.

Mudzinski, S. P., Rudofsky, U. H., Mitchell, D. G., and Lawrence, D. A. (1986). Analysis of lead effects on *in vivo* antibody mediated immunity in several mouse strains. *Toxicol. Appl. Pharmacol.* **83,** 321–330.

Murakami, K., Whiteley, M. K., and Routtenberg, A. (1987). Regulation of protein kinase activity by cooperative interaction of Zn^{2+} and Ca^{2+}. *J. Biol. Chem.* **262,** 13902–13906.

Murray, M. J., Wilson, F. D., Fisher, G. L., and Erickson, K. L. (1983). Modulation of murine lymphocyte and macrophage proliferation by parenteral zinc. *Clin. Exp. Immunol.* **53,** 744–749.

Mustelin, T., and Altman, A. (1990). Dephosphorylation and activation of the T cell tyrosine kinase pp56^{lck} by the leukocyte common antigen CD45. *Oncogene* **5,** 809–813.

Mustelin, T., Coggeshall, K. M., and Altman, A. (1989). Rapid activation of the T cell tyrosine protein kinase pp56^{lck} by the CD45 phospho-tyrosine phosphatase. *Proc. Natl. Acad. Sci. USA* **86,** 6302–6307.

Mustelin, T., Coggeshall, K. M., Isakov, N., and Altman, A. (1990). Tyrosine phosphorylation is required for T cell antigen receptor-mediated activation of phospholipase C. *Science* **247,** 1584–1587.

Newmann, L. S., and Campbell, P. A. (1987). Mitogenic effect of beryllium sulfate on mouse B lymphocytes but not T lymphocytes *in vitro*. *Int. Arch. Allergy Appl. Immunol.* **84,** 223–227.

Nikolic-Zugic, J. (1991). Phenotypic and functional stages in the intrathymic development of $\alpha\beta$ T cells. *Immunol. Today* **12,** 65–70.

Ohsawa, M., Sato, K., Takahashi, K., and Ochi, T. (1983). Modified distribution of lymphocyte subpopulations in blood and spleen from mice exposed to cadmium. *Toxicol. Lett.* **19,** 29–35.

Otsuka, F., and Ohsawa, M. (1991). Differential susceptibility of T- and B-lymphocyte proliferation to cadmium: relevance to zinc requirement in T-lymphocyte proliferation. *Chem. Biol. Interact.* **78,** 193–205.

Parker, P. J., Coussens, L., Totty, N., Rhee, L., Young, S., Chen, E., Stabel, S., Waterfield, M. D., and Ullrich, A. (1986). The complete primary structure of protein kinase C—the major phorbol ester receptor. *Science* **233,** 853–859.

Pietsch, P., Vohr, H., Degitz, K., and Gleichmann, E. (1989). Immunological alterations inducible by mercury compounds. II. $HgCl_2$ and gold sodium thiomalate enhance serum IgE and IgG concentrations in susceptible mouse strains. *Int. Arch. Allergy Appl. Immunol.* **90,** 47–53.

Pelletier, L., Pasquier, R., Guettier, C., Vial, M., Mandet, C., Nochy, D., Bazin, H., and Druet, P. (1988a). $HgCl_2$ induces T and B cells to proliferate and differentiate in BN rats. *Clin. Exp. Immunol.* **71,** 336–342.

Pelletier, L., Pasquier, R., Rossert, J., Vial, M., Mandet, and Druet, P. (1988b). Autoreactive T cells in mercury-induced autoimmunity. *J. Immunol.* **140,** 750–754.

Penninks, A., Kuper, F., Spit, B. J., and Seinen, W. (1985). On the mechanism of dialkyltin-induced thymus involution. *Immunopharmacol.* **10,** 1–10.

Pernelle, J., Creuzet, C., Loeb, J., and Gacon, G. (1991). Phosphorylation of the lymphoid kinase p56^{lck} is stimulated by micromolar concentrations of Zn^{2+}. *FEBS Lett.* **281,** 278–282.

Pounds, J. G. (1984). Effect of lead intoxication on calcium homeostasis and calcium-mediated cell function: A review. *Neurotoxicol.* **5,** 295–332.

Powers, M. F., and Beavis, A. D. (1991). Triorganotins inhibit the mitochondrial inner membrane anion channel. *J. Biol. Chem.* **266,** 17250–17256.

Prasad, A. S. (1984). Discovery and importance of zinc in human nutrition. *Fed. Proc.* **43,** 2829–2834.

Prasad, A. S., Meftah, S., Abdallah, J., Kaplan, J., Brewer, G. J., Bach, J. F., and Dardenne, M. (1988). Serum thymulin in human zinc deficiency. *J. Clin. Invest.* **82**, 1202–1210.

Prouvost-Danon, A., Abadie, A., Sapin, C., Bazin, H, and Druet, P. (1981). Induction of IgE synthesis and potentiation of anti-ovalbumin IgE antibody response by HgCl$_2$ in the rat. *J. Immunol.* **126**, 699–702.

Raffray, M., and Cohen, G. M. (1991). Bis(tri-*n*-butyltin)oxide induces programmed cell death (apoptosis) in immature rat thymocytes. *Arch. Toxicol.* **65**, 135–139.

Ramakrishnan, L., Wu, Q., Yue, A., Cooper, M. D., and Rosenberg, N. (1990). BP-1/6C3 expression defines a differentiation stage of transformed pre-B cells and is not related to malignant potential. *J. Immunol.* **145**, 1603–1608.

Reigart, J. R., and Graber, C. D. (1976). Evaluation of the humoral immune response of children with low level lead exposure. *Contam. Toxicol.* **16**, 112–117.

Reuter, R., Tessars, G., Vohr, H., Gleichmann, E., and Luhrmann, R. (1989). Mercuric chloride induces autoantibodies against U3 small nuclear ribonucleoprotein in susceptible mice. *Proc. Natl. Acad. Sci. USA* **86**, 237–241.

Ringenberg, Q. S., Doll, D. C., Patterson, W. P., Perry, M. C., and Yarbro, J. W. (1988). Hematologic effects of heavy metal poisoning. *Southern Med. J.* **81**, 1132–1139.

Rossi, A., Manzo, L., Orrenius, O., Vahter, M., and Nicotera, P. (1991). Modifications of cell signalling in the cytotoxicity of metals. *Pharmacol. Toxicol.* **68**, 424–429.

Schlick, E., and Friedberg, K. D. (1982). Bone marrow cells of mice under the influence of low lead dose. *Arch. Toxicol.* **49**, 227–236.

Schuhmann, D., Kubicka-Muranyi, M., Mirtschewa, J., Gunther, J., Kind, P., and Gleichmann, E. (1990). Adverse immune reactions to gold. I. Chronic treatment with an Au(I) drug sensitizes mouse T cells not to Au(I) but to Au(III) and induces autoantibody formation. *J. Immunol.* **145**, 2132–2139.

Screpanti, I., Morrone, S., Meco, D., Santoni, A., Gulino, A., Paolini, R., Crisnati, A., Mathieson, B. J., and Frati, L. (1989). Steroid sensitivity of thymocyte subpopulations during intrathymic differentiation. Effects of 17β-estradiol and dexamethasone on subsets expressing T cell antigen receptor or IL-2 receptor. *J. Immunol.* **142**, 3378–3383.

Seinen, W., and Penninks, A. H. (1979). Immune suppression as a consequence of a selective cytotoxic activity of certain organometallic compounds on thymus and thymus-dependent lymphocytes. *Ann. N.Y. Acad. Sci.* **320**, 499–517.

Seinen, W., Vos, J. G., Brands, R, and Hooykaas, H. (1979). Lymphocytotoxicity and immunosuppression by organotin compounds: Suppression of GVH activity, blast transformation and E-rosette formation by di-*n*-butyltin dichloride and di-*n*-octyltin dichloride. *Immunopharmacol.* **1**, 343–354.

Sellins, K. S., and Cohen, J. J. (1987). Gene induction by γ-irradiation leads to DNA fragmentation in lymphocytes. *J. Immunol.* **139**, 3199–3206.

Shenker, B. J., Matarazzo, W. J., Hirsch, R. L., and Gray, I. (1977). Trace metal modification of immunocompetence. I. Effect of trace metals in the cultures on in vitro transformation of B lymphocytes. *Cell. Immunol.* **34**, 19–24.

Shimizu, T., Kubota, S. M., Tanizawa, A., Sano, H., Kasai, Y., Hashimoto, H., Akiyama, Y., and Mikawa, H. (1990). Inhibition of both etoposide-induced DNA fragmentation and activation of poly(ADP)-ribose) synthesis by zinc ion. *Biochem. Biophys. Res. Commun.* **169**, 1172–1177.

Shipp, M. A., Stefano, G. B., D'Adamio, L., Switzer, S. N., Howard, F. D., Sinisterra, J., Scharrer, B., and Reinherz, E. L. (1990). Downregulation of enkephalin-mediated inflammatory responses by CD10/neutral endopeptidase 24.11. *Nature (London)* **347**, 394–396.

Shiraishi, N., Yamamoto, H., Takeda, Y., Kondoh, S., Hagashi, H., Hashimoto, K., and Aono, K. (1986). Increased metallothionein content in rat liver and kidney following X-irradiation. *Toxicol. Appl. Pharmacol.* **85**, 128–134.

Shiraishi, N., Hayashi, H., Hiraki, Y., Aono, K., Itano, Y., Kosaka, F., Noji, S., and Taniguchi,

S. (1989). Elevation in metallothionein messenger RNA in rat tissues after exposure to X-irradiation. *Toxicol. Appl. Pharmacol.* **98,** 501–506.

Smialowicz, R. J., Rogers, R. R., Riddle, and Stott, G. A. (1984). Immunological effects of nickel. I. Suppression of cellular and humoral immunity. *Environ. Res.* **33,** 413–427.

Smialowicz, R. J, Rogers, R. R., Riddle, M. M., Rowe, D. G., and Luebke, R. W. (1986). Immunological studies in mice following *in utero* exposure to NiCl$_2$. *Toxicology* **38,** 293–303.

Smialowicz, R. J., Rogers, R. R., Rowe, D. G., Riddle, M. M., and Luebke, R. W. (1987). The effects of nickel on immune function in the rat. *Toxicology* **44,** 271–281.

Smialowicz, R. J., Riddle, M. M., Rogers, R. R., Luebke, R. W., Copeland, C. B., and Ernst, G. G. (1990). Immune alterations in rats following subacute exposure to tributyltin oxide. *Toxicology* **64,** 169–178.

Smith, J. B., Dwyer, S. D., and Smith, L. (1989). Cadmium evokes inositol polyphosphate formation and calcium mobilization. Evidence for a cell surface receptor that cadmium stimulates and zinc antagonizes. *J. Biol. Chem.* **264,** 7115–7118.

Snoeij, N. J., Van Iersel, A. A. J., Penninks, A. H., and Seinen, W. (1985). Toxicity of triorganotin compounds: Comparative *in vivo* studies with a series of trialkyltin compounds and triphenyltin chloride in male rats. *Toxicol. Appl. Pharmacol.* **81,** 274–286.

Snoeij, N. J., Punt, P. M., Penninks, A. H., and Seinen, W. (1986). Effects of tri-*n*-butyltin chloride on energy metabolism, macromolecular synthesis, precursor uptake and cyclic AMP production in isolated rat thymocytes. *Biochim. Biophys. Acta* **852,** 234–243.

Stelzer, K. J., and Pazdernik, T. L. (1983). Cadmium-induced immunotoxicity. *Int. J. Immunopharmacol.* **5,** 541–548.

Subramanian, R. V. (1985). Biologically active organotin polymers. *Ann. N.Y. Acad. Sci.* **446,** 134–148.

Suzuki, K., Tadakuma, T., and Kizaki, H. (1991). Modulation of thymocyte apoptosis by isoproterenol and prostaglandin E$_2$. *Cell. Immunol.* **134,** 235–240.

Tinwell, H., and Ashby, J. (1990). Inactivity of copper sulphate in a mouse bone-marrow micronucleus assay. *Mutation Res.* **245,** 223–226.

Tonks, N. K., Diltz, C. D., and Fisher, F. D. (1990). CD45, an integral membrane protein tyrosine phosphatase. *J. Biol. Chem.* **265,** 10674–10680.

Turner, J. M., Brodsky, M. H., Irving, B. A., Levin, S. D., Perlmutter, R. M., and Littman, D. R. (1990). Interaction of the unique N-terminal region of tyrosine kinase p56[lck] with cytoplasmic domains of CD4 and CD8 is mediated by cysteine motifs. *Cell* **60,** 755–765.

Valle, B. L., and Auld, D. S. (1990). Zinc coordination, function, and structure of zinc enzymes and other proteins. *Biochemistry* **29,** 5647–5659.

Vos, J. G., De Klerk, A., Krajnc, E. I., Kruizinga, W., van Ommen, B., and Rozing, J. (1984). Toxicity of bis(tri-*n*-butyltin) oxide in the rat. II. Suppression of thymus-dependent immune responses and of parameters of non-specific resistance after short term exposure. *Toxicol. Appl. Pharmacol.* **75,** 387–408.

Warner, G. L., and Lawrence, D. A. (1986). Stimulation of murine lymphocyte responses by cations. *Cell. Immunol.* **101,** 425–439.

Watanabe-Fukunaga, R., Brannan, C. I., Copeland, N. G., Jenkins, N. A., and Nagata, S. (1992). Lymphoproliferation disorder in mice explained by defects in Fas antigen that mediates apoptosis. *Nature (London)* **356,** 314–317.

Welch, P. A., Burrows, P. D., Namen, A., Gillis, S., and Cooper, M. D. (1990). Bone marrow stromal cells and interleukin 7 induce coordinate expression of the BP-1/6C3 antigen and pre-B cell growth. *Int. Immunol.* **2,** 697–705.

Williams, W. R., Kagamimori, S., Watanabe, M., Shinmura, T., and Hagino, N. (1983). An immunological study on patients with chronic cadmium disease. *Clin. Exp. Immunol.* **53,** 651–658.

Winchurch, R. A. (1988). Activation of thymocyte responses to interleukin-1 by zinc, *Clin. Immunol. Immunopathol.* **47,** 174–180.

Winchurch, R. A., Thomas, D. J., Adler, W. H., and Lindsay, T. J. (1984). Supplemental zinc restores antibody formation in cultures of aged spleen cells. *J. Immunol.* **133**, 569–571.

Winchurch, R. A., Togo, J., and Adler, W. H. (1987). Supplemental zinc restores antibody formation in cutures of aged spleen cells. II. Effects on mediator production. *Eur. J. Immunol.* **17**, 127–132.

Wirth, J. J., Fraker, P. J., and Kierszenbaum, F. (1984). Changes in the levels of marker expression by mononuclear phagocytes in zinc deficient mice. *J. Nutr.* **114**, 1826–1833.

Wu, Q., Li, L., Cooper, M. D., Pierres, M., and Gorvei, J. P. (1991). Aminopeptidase A activity of the murine B lymphocyte differentiation antigen BP-1/6C3. *Proc. Natl. Acad. Sci. USA* **88**, 676–680.

Wyllie, A. H. (1980). Glucocorticoid-induced thymocyte apoptosis is associated with endogenous endonuclease activation. *Nature (London)* **284**, 555–556.

Xu, P. Y., Xiao, B. L., and Wang, Z. Q. (1989). Changes in histopathology and enzyme histochemistry of thymus in cadmium exposure mice. *Hua-Hsi-I-Ko-Ta-Hsueh-Hsueh-Pao* **20**, 429–432.

Yagminas, A. P., Franklin, C. A., Villeneuve, D. C., Gilman, A. P., Little, P. B., and Valli, V. E. O. (1990). Subchronic oral toxicity of triethyl lead in the male weanling rat. Clinical, biochemical, hematological and histopathological effects. *Fund. Appl. Toxicol.* **15**, 580–596.

Yamada, H., and Koizumi S. (1991). Metallothionein induction in human peripheral blood lymphocytes by heavy metals. *Chem. Biol. Interact.* **78**, 347–354.

Yamada, Y. K., Shimizu, F., Kawamura, R., and Kubota, K. (1981). Thymic atrophy in mice induced by cadmium administration. *Toxicol. Lett.* **8**, 49–55.

Yamada, Y. K., Murakami, N., Shimizu, F., and Kubota, K. (1982). The role of corticosterone in cadmium-induced thymic atrophy in mice. *Toxicol. Lett.* **12**, 225–229.

Yamauchi, T., and Yamamoto, I. (1990). CuSO4 as an inhibitor of B cell proliferation. *Jpn. J. Pharmacol.* **54**, 455–460.

Yan, A., and Davis, P. (1990). Gold induced marrow suppression: a review of 10 cases. *J. Rheumatol.* **17**, 47–51.

Yoshida, K., Sakurai, H., and Toyama, T. (1980). Immunological parameters in lead workers. *Jap. J. Ind. Health* **22**, 488–493.

Zalewski, P. D., Forbes, I. J., Giannakis, C., Cowled, P. A., and Betts, W. H. (1990). Synergy between zinc and phorbol ester in translocation of protein kinase C to cytoskeleton. *FEBS Lett.* **273**, 131–134.

Zalewski, P. D., Forbes, I. J., Giannakis, C., and Betts, W. H. (1991). Regulation of protein kinase C by Zn^{2+}-dependent interaction with actin. *Biochem. Int.* **24**, 1103–1110.

Zareba, G., and Chmielnicka, J. (1989). Effects of tin and lead on organ levels of essential minerals in rabbits. *Biol. Trace Elem. Res.* **20**, 233–242.

9

Xenobiotic-Induced Skin Toxicity

Jeffrey D. Laskin and Diane E. Heck

I. Introduction

The most common route of exposure to xenobiotics is through the skin. As the largest organ in the body, this tissue protects an individual from the external environment. Many xenobiotics with which humans are in contact are capable of inducing skin toxicity, ranging from ultraviolet (uv) light to detergents, metals, and organic chemicals (Emmett, 1986). After dermal xenobiotic exposure, many different factors that are dependent on the host as well as on the material are important in determining whether or not toxic reactions will develop in the skin. For example, the ability of a xenobiotic to penetrate the tissue and/or disrupt its structure may limit toxicity. This ability in turn depends on the dose of the xenobiotic, the duration of exposure, and the chemical and/or physical characteristics of the xenobiotic (Dugard, 1987; Adams, 1993; Fitzpatrick et al., 1993). The ability of the host to metabolize and eliminate the xenobiotic may also limit toxicity (Noonan and Webster, 1987). Determinants of skin toxicity of uv light, depend on wavelength and the physical characteristics of the skin (Everett et al., 1969; Gallo et al., 1989; Moan and Berg, 1992; Harber, 1993; Norris et al., 1993) Additional host factors that may act as determinants of toxicity are genetic and/or underlying disease states (Mathias, 1987). Note that skin toxicity may also arise after other routes of exposure to xenobiotics (Emmett, 1979; Blacker et al., 1993). For example, many commonly used drugs, either alone or in combination with sunlight, elicit skin inflammatory reactions after oral administration (Table I).

The ability of xenobiotics to penetrate the outermost layer of skin and interact with its various cellular components is critical in initiating skin toxicity. Target cells may be localized in the dermal and/or epidermal compartments of the tissue and consist not only of immune cells, but also of

Table I   Examples of Drugs Inducing Skin Toxicity

Drug	Reference
Psoralens + UV A light	Pathak and Fitzpatrick (1992)
Penicillins	Weiss and Adkinson (1988)
Phenytoin	Wilson et al. (1978)
Ampicillin	Hodak (1983)
Sulfonamides	Park et al. (1987)
Vitamin K	Barnes and Sarkany (1976)

cells thought to act simply as structural elements of the skin, such as fibroblasts and keratinocytes (Rongone, 1987; Barker et al., 1991). Xenobiotics may directly induce structural damage to the tissue or, more commonly, induce dermal inflammatory reactions. Many of these reactions are initiated by highly specific mechanisms in skin cells. For example, two potent dermatotoxins—2,3,7,8-tetrachlorodibenzo-p-dioxin (TCDD) and the potent tumor promoter 12-O-tetradecanoyl-phorbol-13-acetate (TPA) initiate their biological activity by binding to highly specific cellular receptors in epidermal cells (Molloy et al., 1987; Marks and Furstenburger, 1990; Pohjanvirta and Tuomisto, 1990; Puhvel and Conner, 1991; Burbach et al., 1992). Other xenobiotics may induce damage by nonspecific mechanisms. For example, strong acids or bases denature proteins and lipids and alter the structural integrity of the tissue (Adams, 1993).

II. Barriers to Xenobiotic Toxicity

The major barrier to xenobiotics in the skin is the epidermis, which consists of a relatively thin layer of cells overlying the dermis. The tissue is a stratified squamous epithelium composed predominantly of specialized cells known as keratinocytes. These cells differentiate to form a tough cornified cell layer that serves as the principle barrier to the external environment. Cornified cells are continuously shed and replaced by differentiating stem cells in a well-regulated process of cell replenishment (Holbrook and Wolff, 1993). The major structural proteins produced by the keratinocytes are a group of proteins known as keratins, which have important structural and functional roles in the maintenance of tissue integrity. Keratins comprise a diverse group of water-insoluble proteins that are found in all mammalian epithelial cells (Fuchs and Green, 1978,1980; Molloy and Laskin, 1987,1988,1992; Molloy et al., 1987; Fuchs, 1990,1992; Fuchs and Coulombe, 1992; Steinert, 1993). Consisting of 20 or more polypeptides in the molecular weight range of 40,000–70,000, these proteins are translated from distinct mRNAs that are derived from a large multigene family. Keratinocytes express both acidic and basic keratin subunits that associate to form the intermediate filaments, a major network of the cytoskeletal architecture. Keratins play a major role in cytoskeletal organization and in the overall structural integrity of the epidermis.

The highly keratinized cornified cells of the stratum corneum are generally considered to be primarily responsible for limiting permeability of chemical toxins (Elias et al., 1981; Dugard, 1987; Adams, 1993; Fitzpatrick et al., 1993). Temperature, stratum corneum hydration, direct damage induced by the chemical, binding of the chemical to the stratum corneum, and broken or diseased skin are among several important factors that control penetration of a chemical into the skin. Also important are the characteristics of the toxicant. Thus, in addition to such physical properties such as lipid solubility, molecular size, and charge, chemical reactivity may also contribute to penetration (Behl et al., 1980; Dugard, 1987; Adams, 1993; Fitzpatrick et al., 1993). For example, an alkylating agent may disrupt cell membranes and/or denature proteins. As indicated earlier, this action may compromise the integrity of the stratum corneum (Frei, 1991).

III. Responses of Skin to Xenobiotics

The reactions of the skin to xenobiotics range from subtle alterations in tissue architecture, such as epidermal thickening and altered keratinization, to gross inflammatory reactions characterized by edema and erythema and, in some instances, tissue destruction and necrosis (Adams, 1993). Both physical and chemical insult to the skin can dramatically alter growth and differentiation processes in the tissue. For example, topical application of the irritant TPA induces rapid alterations in tissue structure. Within 24 hr, increased basal cell proliferation is observed, in addition to alterations in the normal process of keratinocyte maturation. These changes are associated with an increase in thickness of the epidermis as well as in the number of nucleated cell layers (Raick et al., 1972; Raick, 1973; Argyris, 1980; Astrup and Iverson, 1983). Marked edema and erythema in the tissue, as well as leukocyte infiltration, are also apparent. Among the biochemical changes that occur in the skin following treatment with these irritants are alterations in epidermal DNA, RNA, and protein biosynthesis, phospholipid metabolism, sulfated proteoglycan biosynthesis, and keratinization. Although inflammation is necessary for tissue repair and healing, chronic inflammation has been associated with carcinogenesis (Rohrschneider et al., 1972; Balmain et al., 1977; Laskin et al., 1981,1991; Trush and Kensler, 1991).

Over the last several years, active investigation into the complex interplay which occurs between the different cell types comprising the skin, has led to the discovery of an array of inflammatory molecules that mediate the toxic effects of xenobiotics (Taylor, 1991; Bos and Kapenberg, 1993). Initially, skin inflammatory reactions were thought to be regulated to a large extent by immune cells, including resident immune cells (i.e., Langerhans cells) and infiltrating leukocytes (i.e., lymphocytes, macrophages, and polymorphonuclear leukocytes, Kupper, 1990; Clark, 1991). During xenobiotic-induced inflammation, each of these cell types can become functionally active and release a variety of soluble immune mediators (Kilgus et al., 1993; Friedman et al., 1993). It has now become evident that keratinocytes and melanocytes participate directly in controlling inflammatory reactions in the skin (Lugar and Schwarz, 1990; McKenzie and Sauder, 1990; Knighton and Fiegel, 1991; McKay and Leigh, 1991). The contribution of each of the different cell types to skin toxicity is characteristic of the host as well as of the xenobiotic.

Leukocyte infiltration is one of the hallmarks of the inflammatory response. In early stages of chemical-induced inflammation, granulocyte infiltration predominates. This event is followed by infiltration of lymphocytes and macrophages (Keshav et al., 1990; Stein and Keshav, 1992; Oberg et al., 1993). Macrophages and granulocytes are phagocytic cells that release a variety of highly toxic reactive intermediates (see subsequent discussion) as well as an array of soluble immune mediators (Kupper, 1990; Van Deurem et al., 1992; Aderem, 1993; Duff, 1993; Ogawa, 1993). The ability of these cells to engulf foreign substances is critical not only for tissue repair, but also for localized antimicrobial activity (Stein and Keshav, 1992). Macrophages also process and present antigens to lymphocytes, an important event for both humoral and cell-mediated immune responses as well as for contact-mediated hypersensitivity reactions (Kapp and Zeck-Kapp, 1990). During xenobiotic-induced skin inflammation, lymphocytes as well as macrophages also release a number of soluble factors that amplify the inflammatory process. In particular, these cells produce a variety of intercellular messenger proteins referred to as cytokines. These small proteins include interleukins, growth factors, and chemoattractants that regulate immune responses to other cell types as well as the growth, differentiation, and immunological activity of resident skin cells including keratinocytes and melanocytes (Barker et al., 1991; Dudley and Wiedmeier, 1991; Rees, 1992).

Migration of phagocytic cells as well as lymphocytes into the skin during inflammation and tissue repair is regulated by the localized release of leukocyte chemoattractants as well as by expression of leukocyte adhesion/recognition molecules (Dustin et al., 1988; Nickoloff and Griffiths, 1990; Norris, 1990; Singer et al., 1990; Katz et al., 1991; Barker and McDonald, 1992; Caughman et al., 1992; Schroder, 1992a). Many different leukocyte chemoattractants can be generated in the skin including lipid mediators such as leukotriene B_4, 12-hydroxyeicosatetraenoic acid (12-HETE), platelet activating factor, and diacylglycerol as well as chemotactic proteins such as NAP-

1/IL-8 (neutrophil attractant protein 1/interleukin 8), macrophage inflammatory proteins (MIP-1α and -1β) and monocyte chemotactic protein 1 (MCP-1); Hammarstrom *et al.*, 1975; Brain *et al.*, 1983; Mallet *et al.*, 1984; Larsen *et al.*, 1989; Schroder, 1992a,b). Localization and immobilization of immune cells in different compartments of the skin after injury or during chronic inflammation is dependent on appropriate temporal and spatial expression of a variety of intercellular adhesion molecules or integrins such as ICAM-1 and HLA-DR. Changes in the expression of these intercellular adhesion molecules following xenobiotic-induced toxicity is an important determinant of the type of leukocytes that accumulate in the skin (Dustin *et al.*, 1988; Norris, 1990; Griffiths *et al.*, 1991; Boehncke *et al.*, 1992). Leukocyte binding can lead to cellular activation and the additional release of cytotoxic effector molecules as well as additional cytokines (Keshav *et al.*, 1990; Fiers, 1991).

Studies have demonstrated that keratinocytes can also actively take part in xenobiotic-induced skin inflammatory reactions. Once exposed to inflammatory cytokines, these cells acquire functional characteristics of activated immune cells. For example, in response to interferon (γ-IFN) released by infiltrating lymphocytes, keratinocytes are induced to express HLA-DR as well as ICAM-1 (Griffiths *et al.*, 1989; Larjava, 1991; Tamaki *et al.*, 1992). Keratinocytes can also be induced to process and present antigens to lymphocytes, to release highly toxic free radicals, and to express and respond to a variety of inflammatory cytokines. These cytokines—which include granulocyte–macrophage colony stimulating factor (GM-CSF), tumor necrosis factor α (TNFα), transforming growth factors (TGF) α and β, IL-1α, IL-1β, IL-3, IL-6, and IL-8—affect a large array of metabolic processes in the skin (Camp *et al.*, 1990; Schall, 1991; Colditz and Watson, 1992; Enk and Katz, 1992; Breathnach, 1993; Friedman *et al.*, 1993). Some of these processes are important in the regulation of keratinocyte growth and differentiation. Keratinocytes also constitutively produce and store cytokines such as IL-1 that are thought to function in initiating inflammatory responses induced after direct cellular damage induced by xenobiotics (Sauder *et al.*, 1982; Gahring *et al.*, 1985; Granstein *et al.*, 1986; Bell *et al.*, 1987). IL-1 causes the release of additional cytokines and chemotactic factors and stimulates the expression of cell adhesion molecules at the site of xenobiotic-induced toxicity, which may initiate an inflammatory reaction in the skin (Dinarello and Wolff, 1993). The progression and resolution of xenobiotic-induced toxicity is regulated by the complex interplay between anti-inflammatory cytokines and inflammatory mediators released by keratinocytes and leukocytes (Dinarello *et al.*, 1993). For example, both keratinocytes and macrophages release growth factors that suppress the production of inflammatory mediators by macrophages and keratinocytes (Kingsworth and Slavin, 1991; Heck *et al.*, 1992).

IV. Consequences of Xenobiotic Toxicity

The release of free radicals by both immune cells and immunologically activated keratinocytes is thought to be an important mechanism by which xenobiotic-induced irritation and inflammation leads to skin tissue damage. Although these free radicals function in host defense, excessive production may damage the tissue and compromise normal functioning (Flohe et al., 1985; Sinclair et al., 1990; Bulkley, 1993). At least two major classes of free radical species are produced in the skin: reactive oxygen intermediates and reactive nitrogen intermediates (Table II). Lipid peroxidation reactions generated by reactive oxygen intermediates, which include superoxide anion, hydrogen peroxide, and superoxide anion, are known lead to cell membrane damage (Willson, 1985). Reactive oxygen intermediates also cause oxidation of proteins as well as of DNA bases, which may lead to mutations and cancer (Kensler and Taffe, 1986; Ribilloud et al., 1990; Barnes, 1992; Cheng et al., 1992; Frenkel, 1992). Elevated levels of reactive oxygen intermediates are typically found in epidermal cells following irritant exposure (Kensler and Taffe, 1986; Trush and Kensler, 1991).

For many years, researchers thought that nitric oxide was simply a combustion product of fossil fuels that contributed to the formation of acid rain and photochemical smog. This reactive nitrogen intermediate is now known to be produced in mammals and is an important regulatory and cytotoxic molecule (Snyder and Bredt, 1992). Nitric oxide is produced endogenously by a number of different tissues and cells for the control of a variety of physiological functions including the regulation of blood pressure, gastric motility, respiration, neurotransmission, memory, and bone marrow cell growth and development (Feng and Hedner, 1990; Culotta and Koshland, 1992; Marletta, 1992; Punjabi et al., 1992). In the skin nitric oxide production is likely to be important in tissue homeostasis as well as in nonspecific host defense (Heck et al., 1992). Thus, following injury or inflammation, leukocytes infiltrating into the skin produce nitric oxide to kill various

Table II   Reactive Mediators in Skin Toxicity

Compound	References
Reactive oxygen intermediates	
hydrogen peroxide	Chance et al. (1978)
hydroperoxides	Willson (1985)
hydroxyl radicals	Flohe et al. (1985)
superoxide anion	Bandy et al. (1990)
Reactive nitrogen intermediates	
nitric oxide	Mulligan et al. (1991), Marletta (1992)
peroxynitrite	Ischiropoulous et al. (1992)

pathogens (Nathan, 1992). However, recent work has revealed that activated keratinocytes are a major source of nitric oxide (Heck *et al.*, 1992). Nitric oxide is produced in cells from the amino acid L-arginine by the enzyme nitric oxide synthase (Nathan, 1992). In the presence of NADPH and several other cofactors, nitric oxide synthase oxidizes the terminal guanido nitrogen of L-arginine into nitric oxide, leaving citrulline as a by-product. A constitutive isoform of nitric oxide synthase is present in brain and endothelial cells and requires calcium and calmodulin for activity, whereas an inducible isoform is present in macrophages that does not require these cofactors (Marletta, 1992; Nathan, 1992). Keratinocytes appear to express a constitutive type of nitric oxide synthase which requires calcium and calmodulin as well as glutathione for activity. They may also express an inducible type isoform. Nitric oxide production by keratinocytes is dependent on L-arginine and is blocked by competitive inhibitors of nitric oxide synthase, including the substrate analog N^G-monomethy-L-arginine. Of interest is the fact that nitric oxide causes a suppression of keratinocyte growth, suggesting that nitric oxide production in the skin may play a role in the regulation of keratinocyte proliferation during the wound healing process. Nitric oxide production by keratinocytes is also inhibited by growth factors such as epidermal growth factor and insulin-like growth factor 1, two potent keratinocyte growth promoting agents. These cytokines also reverse nitric oxide-induced growth inhibition. The ability of epidermal growth factor to suppress nitric oxide production by keratinocytes may be important in the resolution of inflammation during wound healing (Heck *et al.*, 1992).

V. Cellular Defenses against Xenobiotic-Induced Tissue Damage

Skin tissue also possesses a variety of defense mechanisms that have the capacity to protect against xenobiotic-induced tissue damage, in particular, that caused by free radicals (Table III). For example, epidermal keratinocytes are a rich source of cytochrome P450 and toxic chemicals penetrating the stratum corneum may be metabolized (Noonan and Webster, 1987; Miles and Wolf, 1991; Guengerich, 1992). Keratinocytes also possess high levels of glutathione, which can bind xenobiotics as well as detoxify reactive oxygen intermediates (Meister, 1992; Rushmore and Pickett, 1993; Vessey and Lee, 1993). Note, however, that a number of toxins deplete cells of glutathione; this process may indirectly lead to tissue injury (Best *et al.*, 1991). Various enzymes are present in the skin that also have the capacity of detoxify reactive oxygen intermediates including catalase, superoxide dismutase, and glutathione peroxidase (Rushmore and Pickett, 1993; Vessey and Lee, 1993; Table III). In contrast, nitric oxide binds to both heme and nonheme iron-containing proteins as well as to protein thiols and

Table III   Detoxification Mechanisms for Free Radicals in the Skin

Mechanism	References
Reactive oxygen intermediates	
catalase, superoxide dismutase	Chance et al. (1978), Boveris and Cadenas (1982)
glutathione peroxidase, glutathione	Kensler and Taffe (1986), Shindo et al. (1993)
Reactive nitrogen intermediates	
heme proteins (soluble guanylyl cyclase; hemoglobin)	Marletta (1992), Nathan (1992), Stamler et al. (1992), Girard and Potier (1993)
iron–sulfur proteins (NADPH:ubiquinone oxidoreductase; NADPH:succinate oxidoreductase; cis-aconitase)	
nonheme iron proteins (ferritin; ribonucleotide reductase)	
protein thiols (tissue type plasminogen activator, dehydrogenase)	
superoxide anion	Radi et al. (1991)
nitration of phenolics	Smith and Beckman (1992)

superoxide anion (Nathan, 1992). Although this binding may serve to lower intracellular concentrations of nitric oxide, it may also result in inhibition of target proteins (Table III). The reaction of nitric oxide with superoxide anion may also lead to the formation of peroxynitrite. This highly toxic radical is produced during xenobiotic-induced inflammation and, although it detoxifies superoxide anion, may actually potentiate cellular injury and tissue damage (Ischiropoulous et al., 1992; Zhu et al., 1992).

VI. Summary

In summary, xenobiotic-induced skin toxicity is mediated by a complex network of cells and regulatory molecules that interact within the tissue. This process is dependent on the ability of the xenobiotic to penetrate into the skin and react with its various cellular components. Cells that are important in initiating inflammatory responses include not only immune cells localized throughout the skin, but also the epidermal keratinocytes. Each of these cell types contributes to toxicity by the ability to release soluble immune mediators and regulatory factors as well as toxic free radical species. The skin protects itself against toxicity by a variety of mechanisms. In fact, many xenobiotics may function by interfering with these processes. A number of important issues remain unresolved about the mechanisms of skin toxicity, including (1) the identification of the precise sequence of steps by which diverse groups of xenobiotics trigger toxic responses, (2) the role of each skin cell type and of various soluble mediators such as prostaglandins, cytokines, and growth factors in toxicity; (3) the factors that control alterations in keratinocyte growth and differentiation; and (4) the precise mechanisms controlling wound healing and the resolution of inflammation. Any model proposed on the mechanism of action xenobiotics in the skin must take into account the multifactorial basis not only of cutaneous inflammatory reactions but also of processes that regulate growth and development of the skin tissue.

References

Adams, R. A. (1993). Disorders due to drugs and chemical agents. In "Dermatology in General Medicine" (T. B. Fitzpatrick, A. Z. Eisen, K. Wolff, I. M. Freedberg, and K. F. Austen, eds.), pp. 1767–1783. McGraw-Hill, New York.

Aderem, A. A. (1993). How cytokines signal messages within cells. *J. Infect. Dis.* **167**, s2–s7.

Argyris, T. S. (1980). Epidermal growth following a single application of 12-O-tetradecanoyl-phorbol-13-acetate. *Am. J. Pathol.* **98**, 639–646.

Astrup, E. G., and Iverson, O. H. (1983). Cell population kinetics in hairless mouse epidermis following a single topical application of 12-O-tetradecanoyl-phorbol-13-acetate II. *Virchow's Arch. Cell Pathol.* **42**, 1–8.

Balmain, A., Alonso, A., and Fisher, J. (1977). Histone phosphorylation, DNA and RNA synthesis during phases of proliferation and differentiation induced in mouse epidermis by the tumor promoter 12-O-tetradecanoyl-phorbol-13-acetate. *Cancer Res.* **37**, 1548–1555.

Bandy, B., Moon, J., and Davidson, A. J. (1990). Multiple actions of superoxide dismutase: Why can it both inhibit and stimulate reduction of oxygen by hydroquinones? *Adv. Free Rad. Biol. Med.* **9**, 143–148.

Barker, J. N., and McDonald, D. M. (1992). Cutaneous lymphocyte trafficking in the inflammatory dermatoses. *Br. J. Dermatol.* **126**, 211–215.

Barker, J. N. W. N., Mitra, R. S., Griffiths, C. E. M., Dixit, V. M., and Nickoloff, B. J. (1991). Keratinocytes as initiators of inflammation. *Lancet* **337**, 211–214.

Barnes, D. A. (1992). Damage-limiting exercises. *Nature (London)* **359**, 12–13.

Barnes, H. M., and Sarkany, I. (1976). Adverse skin reactions from vitamin K_1. *Br. J. Dermatol.* **95**, 653–658.

Behl, C. R., Flynn, G. L., Kurihara, T., Harper, N., Smith, W., Higuchi, W. I., Ho., N. F. H., and Pierson, C. L. (1980). Hydration and percutaneous absorption. I. Influence of hydration on alkanol permeation through hairless mouse skin. *J. Invest. Dermatol.* **75**, 346–352.

Bell, T. V., Harley, C. B., Stetso, D., and Sauder, D. N. (1987). Expression of mRNA homologous to interleukin-1 in human epidermal cells. *J. Invest. Dermatol.* **88**, 375–379.

Best, A., Haenen, G. R., and Lunec, J. (1991). Oxidants and antioxidants: State of the art. *Am. J. Med.* **91**, 2s–13s.

Blacker, K. L., Stern, R. S., and Wintroub, B. U. (1993). Cutaneous reactions to drugs. In "Dermatology in General Medicine" (T. B. Fitzpatrick, A. Z. Eisen, K. Wolff, I. M. Freedberg, and K. F. Austen, eds.), pp. 1783–1794. McGraw-Hill, New York.

Boehncke, W. H., Kellner, I., Konter, U., and Sterry, W. (1992). Differential expression of adhesion molecules on infiltrating cells in inflammatory dermatosis. *J. Am. Acad. Dermatol.* **26**, 907–913.

Bos, J. D., and Kapenberg, J. (1993). The skin immune system: Progress in cutaneous biology. *Immunol. Today* **14**, 75–78.

Boveris, A., and Cadenas, E. (1982). Production of superoxide radicals and hydrogen peroxide in mitochondria. *In* "Superoxide Dismutase" (L. W. Oberley, eds.), Vol. 2, pp. 15–30. CRC Press, Boca Raton, Florida.

Brain, S. D., Camp, R. D. R., and Dowd, P. M. (1983). Leukotriene B_4 and monohydroxy eicosatetraenoic acid-like material are released in biologically active amounts from the lesional skin of patients with psoriasis. *Br. J. Dermatol.* **83**, 313–317.

Breathnach, S. M. (1993). The skin immune system and psoriasis. *Clin. Exp. Immunol.* **91**, 343–345.

Bulkley, G. B. (1993). Free radicals and other reactive oxygen metabolites: Clinical relevance and the therapeutic efficacy of antioxidant therapy. *Surgery* **113**, 479–483.

Burbach, K. M., and Poland, A., and Bradfield, C. A. (1992). Cloning of the Ah-receptor cDNA reveals a distinctive ligand-activated transcription factor. *Proc. Natl. Acad. Sci. USA* **89**, 8185–8189.

Camp, R. D. R., Fincham, N. J., Ross, J. S., Bacon, K. B., and Gearing, A. J. H. (1990). Leukocyte chemoattractant cytokines of the epidermis. *J. Invest. Dermatol.* **95**, 108S–110S.

Caughman, S. W., Li, L. J., and Degitz, K. (1992). Human intercellular adhesion molecule-1 gene and its expression in the skin. *J. Invest. Dermatol.* **98**, 61s–65s.

Chance, B., Sies, H., and Boveris, A. (1978). Hydroperoxide metabolism in mammalian organs. *Physiol. Rev.* **59**, 527–605.

Cheng, K. C., Cahill, D. S., Kasai, H., Nishimura, S., and Loeb, L. A. (1992). 8-Hydroxydeoxyguanosine, an abundant form of oxidative DNA damage causes G-T and A-T substitutions. *J. Biol. Chem.* **267**, 166–172.

Clark, R. A. (1991). The commonality of cutaneous wound repair and lung injury. *Chest* **99**, 575–605.

Colditz, I. G., and Watson, D. L. (1992). The effect of cytokines and chemotactic agonists on the migration of T-lymphocytes into skin. *Immunology* **76**, 272–278.

Culotta, E., and Koshland, D. E. (1992). NO news is good news. *Science* **258**, 1862–1865.

Dinarello, C. A., and Wolff, S. M. (1993). The role of IL-1 in disease. *N. Engl. J. Med.* **328**, 106–113.

Dinarello, C. A., Gelfand, J. A., and Wolff, S. M. (1993). Anticytokine strategies in the treatment of the systemic inflammatory response syndrome. *J. Am. Med. Assoc.* **18**, 29–35.

Dudley, D. J., and Wiedmeier, S. (1991). The ontogeny of the immune response: Perinatal perspectives. *Sem. Perinatol.* **15**, 184–195.

Duff, G. W. (1993). Cytokines and anticytokines. *Br. J. Rheumatol.* **32**, 15–20.

Dugard, P. H. (1987). Skin permeability theory in relation to measurements of percutaneous adsorption in toxicology. In "Dermatotoxicology" (F. N. Marzulli, and H. I. Maibach, eds.), pp. 95–134. Hemisphere, New York.

Dustin, M. L., Singer, K. H., Tuck, D. T., and Springer, T. A. (1988). Adhesion of T lymphoblasts to epidermal keratinocytes is regulated by interferon-gamma and is mediated by intercellular adhesion molecule-1 (ICAM-1). *J. Exp. Med.* **167**, 1323–1340.

Elias, P. M., Cooper, E. R., Korc, A., and Brown, B. E. (1981). Percutaneous transport in relation to stratum corneum structure and lipid composition. *J. Invest. Dermatol.* **76**, 297–301.

Emmett, E. A. (1979). Phototoxicity from exogenous agents. *Photochem. Photobiol.* **30**, 429–436.

Emmett, E. A. (1986). Toxic responses of the skin. *In* "Casarett and Doull's Toxicology. The Basic Science of Poisons" (C. D. Klassen, M. O. Amdur, and J. Doull eds.), pp. 412–431. Macmillan, New York.

Enk, A. H., and Katz, S. I. (1992). Early molecular events in the induction phase of contact sensitivity. *Proc. Natl. Acad. Sci. USA* **89**, 1398–1402.

Everett, M. A., Sayre, R. M., and Olson, R. L. (1969). Physiologic responses of human skin to ultraviolet light. *In* "The Biologic Effects of Ultraviolet Radiation" (F. Urbach, ed.), pp. 181–186. Pergamon Press, New York.

Feng, Q., and Hedner, T. (1990). Endothelium derived relaxing factor (EDRF) and nitric oxide

(NO). I. Physiology, pharmacology and pathophysiological implications. *Clin. Physiol.* **10,** 407–426.

Fiers, W. (1991). Tumor necrosis factor. Characterization at the molecular, cellular and *in vivo* level. *FEBS Lett.* **285,** 199–212.

Fitzpatrick, T. B., Eisen, A. Z., Wolff, K., Freedberg, I. M., and Austen, K. F. (1993). Dermatology in the perspective of general medicine. *In* "Dermatology in General Medicine," (T. B. Fitzpatrick, A. Z. Eisen, K. Wolff, I. M. Freedberg, and K. F. Austen, eds.), pp. 1–6. McGraw-Hill, New York.

Flohe, L., Beckman, R., Giertz, H., and Loschen, G. (1985). Oxygen centered free radicals as mediators of inflammation. *In* "Oxidative Stress," (H. Sies, ed.), pp. 403–428. Academic Press, Orlando, Florida.

Frei, E. (1991). The modulation of alkylating agents. *Sem. Hematol.* **28,** 22–24.

Frenkel, K. (1992). Carcinogen-mediated formation and oxidative DNA damage. *Pharmacol. Therapeut.* **53,** 127–166.

Friedmann, P. S., Strickland, I., Memomoa, A. A., and Johnson, P. M. (1993). Early time course of recruitment of immune surveillance in human skin after chemical provocation. *Clin. Exp. Immunol.* **91,** 351–356.

Fuchs, E. (1990). Epidermal differentiation: The bare essentials. *J. Cell Biol.* **111,** 2807–2814.

Fuchs, E. (1992). Genetic skin disorders of keratin. *J. Invest. Dermatol.* **99,** 671–674.

Fuchs, E., and Coulombe, P. A. (1992). Of mice and men: Genetic skin diseases of keratin. *Cell* **69,** 899–902.

Fuchs, E., and Green, H. (1978). The expression of keratin genes in epidermis and cultured epidermal cells. *Cell* **15,** 887–897.

Fuchs, E., and Green, H. (1980). Changes in keratin gene expression during terminal differentiation of the keratinocyte. *Cell* **19,** 1033–1042.

Gahring, L. C., Buckley, A., and Daynes, R. A. (1985). Presence of epidermal derived thymocyte-activating factor/IL-1 in normal human stratum corneum. *J. Clin. Invest.* **76,** 1585–1589.

Gallo, R. L., Staszewski, R., and Granstein, R. D. (1989). Physiology and pathology of skin photoimmunology. *In* "Skin and the Immune System," (J. D. Bos, ed.), pp 381–402. CRC Press, Boca Raton, Florida.

Girard, P., and Potier, P. (1993). NO, thiols and disulfides. *FEBS Lett.* **320,** 7–8.

Granstein, R. D., Margolis, R., Mizel, S. B., and Sauder, D. N. (1986). *In vivo* inflammatory activity of epidermal cell-derived thymocyte activating factor (ETAF) and recombinant IL-1 in the mouse. *J. Clin. Invest.* **77,** 1020–1027.

Griffiths, C. E., Voorhees, J. J., and Nickoloff, B. J. (1989). Gamma-interferon induces different keratinocyte cellular patterns of expression of HLA-DR and intercellular adhesion molecule-1 (ICAM-1) antigens. *Br. J. Dermatol.* **120,** 1–8.

Griffiths, C. E. M., Barker, J. N. W. N., Kunkel, S., and Nickoloff, B. J. (1991). Modulation of leukocyte adhesion molecules, a T cell chemotaxin (IL-8) and a regulatory cytokine (TNF-α) in allergic contact dermatitis (rhus dermatitis). *Br. J. Dermatol.* **124,** 519–526.

Guengerich, F. P. (1992). Human cytochrome P-450 enzymes. *Life Sci.* **50,** 1471–1478.

Hammarstrom, S., Hamberg, M., Samuelsson, B., Duell, E. A., Stawiski, M., and Voorhees, J. J. (1975). Increased concentrations of nonesterified arachidonic acid, 12-L-hydroxy-5,8,10,14-eicosatetraenoic acid, prostaglandin E2 and prostaglandin F2 in epidermis of psoriasis. *Proc. Natl. Acad. Sci. USA* **72,** 5130–5134.

Harber, L. C. (1993). Abnormal responses to ultraviolet radiation: Drug-induced photosensitivity. *In* "Dermatology in General Medicine" (T. B. Fitzpatrick, A. Z. Eisen, K. Wolff, I. M. Freedberg, and K. F. Austen, eds.), pp 1677–1689. McGraw-Hill, New York.

Heck, D. E., Laskin, D. L., Gardner, C. R., and Laskin, J. D. (1992). Epidermal growth factor suppresses nitric oxide and hydrogen peroxide production by keratinocytes. *J. Biol. Chem.* **267,** 21277–21280.

Hodak, E. (1983). Bullous pemphigoid: An adverse effect of ampillicin. *Clin. Exp. Dermatol.* **15**, 50–55.

Holbrook, K. A., and Wolff, K. (1993). *In* "The Structural and Development of Skin" "Dermatology in General Medicine," (T. B. Fitzpatrick, A. Z. Eisen, K. Wolff, I. M. Freedberg, and K. F. Austen, eds.), pp. 97–145. McGraw-Hill, New York.

Ischiropoulous, H., Zhu, L., and Beckman, J. S. (1992). Peroxynitrite formation from macrophage derived nitric oxide. *Arch. Biochem. Biophys.* **289**, 446–451.

Kapp, A., and Zeck-Kapp, G. (1990). Activation of the oxidative metabolism in human polymorphonuclear neutrophilic granulocytes: The role of immunomodulating cytokines. *J. Invest. Dermatol.* **95**, 94s–99s.

Katz, A. M., Rosenthal, D., and Sauder, D. N. (1991). Cell adhesion molecules. Structure, function and implication in a variety of cutaneous and other pathologic conditions. *Int. J. Dermatol.* **30**, 153–160.

Kensler, T. W., and Taffe, B. G. (1986). Free radicals in tumor promotion. *Adv. Free Rad. Biol. Med.* **2**, 347–387.

Keshav, S., Chung, L. P., and Gordon, S. (1990). Macrophage products and inflammation. *Diagn. Microbiol. Infect. Dis.* **13**, 439–447.

Kilgus, O., Payer, E., Schreiber, S., Elbe, A., Strohal, R., and Stingl, G. (1993). In vivo cytokine expression in normal and perturbed murine skin. *J. Invest. Dermatol.* **100**, 674–680.

Kingsworth, A. N., and Slavin, J. (1991). Peptide growth factors and wound healing. *Br. J. Surg.* **78**, 1286–1290.

Knighton, D. R., and Fiegel, V. D. (1991). Regulation of cutaneous wound healing by growth factors and the microenvironment. *Invest. Radiol.* **26**, 604–611.

Kupper, T. S. (1990). Immune and inflammatory processes in cutaneous tissues. Mechanisms and speculations. *J. Clin. Invest.* **86**, 1783–1789.

Larjava, H. (1991). Expression of beta 1 integrins in normal human keratinocytes. *Am. J. Med. Sci.* **301**, 63–681.

Larsen, C. G., Anderson, A. O., Oppenheim, J. J., and Matsushima, K. (1989). Production of interleukin-8 by human dermal fibroblasts and keratinocytes in response to interleukin 1 or tumor necrosis factor. *Immunology* **69**, 31–38.

Laskin, J. D., Mufson, R. A., Piccinini, L., Engelhardt, D. L., and Weinstein, I. B. (1981). Effects of the tumor promoter 12-O-tetradecanoyl-phorbol-13-acetate on newly synthesized proteins in mouse epidermis. *Cell* **25**, 441–449.

Laskin, J. D., Dokidis, A., and Laskin, D. L. (1991). Alterations in epidermal sulfated proteoglycan production following topical application of the tumor promoter 12-O-tetradecanoyl-phorbol-13-acetate. *Cancer Biochem. Biophys.* **12**, 69–79.

Luger, T. A., and Schwarz, T. (1990). Evidence for an epidermal cytokine network. *J. Invest. Dermatol.* **95**, 100s–104s.

Mallet, A. I., Cunningham, F. M., and Daniel, R. (1984). Rapid isocratic high performance liquid chromatographic purification of platelet activating factor (PAF) and lyso-PAF from human skin. *J. Chromatog.* **309**, 160–164.

Marks, F., and Furstenburger, G. (1990). The conversion stage of skin carcinogenesis. *Carcinogenesis* **11**, 2085–2092.

Marletta, M. A. (1992). Mammalian synthesis of nitrite, nitric oxide and N-nitrosylating agents. *Chem. Res. Toxicol.* **1**, 249–257.

Mathias, T. C. (1987). Clinical and experimental aspects of cutaneous irritation. *In* "Dermatotoxicology" (F. N. Marzulli, and H. I. Maibach, eds.), pp. 173–185. Hemisphere, New York.

McKay, I. A., and Leigh, I. M. (1991). Epidermal cytokines and their roles in cutaneous wound healing. *Br. J. Dermatol.* **124**, 513–518.

McKenzie, R. C., and Sauder, D. N. (1990). The role of keratinocyte cytokines in inflammation and immunity. *J. Invest. Dermatol.* **95**, 105s–107s.

Meister, A. (1992). On the antioxidant effects of ascorbic acid and glutathione. *Biochem. Pharmacol.* **44,** 1905–1915.

Miles, J. S., and Wolf, C. R. (1991). Developments and perspectives on the role of cytochrome P-450s in chemical carcinogenesis. *Carcinogenesis* **12,** 2195–2199.

Moan, J., and Berg, K. (1992). Photochemotherapy of cancer: Experimental research. *Photochem. Photobiol.* **55,** 931–948.

Molloy, C. J., and Laskin, J. D. (1987). Specific alterations in keratin biosynthesis in mouse epidermis in vivo and in explant culture following a single exposure to the tumor promoter 12-O-tetradecanoyl-phorbol-13-acetate. *Cancer Res.* **47,** 4674–4680.

Molloy, C. J., and Laskin, J. D. (1988). Keratin polypeptide expression in mouse epidermis and cultured epidermal cells. *Differentiation* **37,** 86–97.

Molloy, C. J., and Laskin, J. D. (1992). Altered expression of a mouse epidermal cytoskeletal protein is a sensitive marker for proliferation induced by tumor promoters. *Carcinogenesis* **13,** 963–968.

Molloy, C. J., Gallo, M. A., and Laskin, J. D. (1987). Alterations in the expression of specific epidermal keratin markers in the hairless mouse by the topical application of the tumor promoters 2,3,7,8-tetrachlorodibenzo-*p*-dioxin and the phorbol ester 12-O-tetradecanoyl-phorbol-13-acetate. *Carcinogenesis* **9,** 1193–1199.

Mulligan, M. S., Hevel, J. M., Marletta, M. A., and Ward, P. A. (1991). Tissue injury caused by immune complexes is L-arginine dependent. *Proc. Natl. Acad. Sci. USA* **88,** 6338–6342.

Nathan, C. (1992). Nitric oxide as a secretory product of mammalian cells. *FASEB J.* **6,** 3051–3064.

Nickoloff, B. J., and Griffiths, E. M. (1990). Abnormal cutaneous topobiology: The molecular basis for dermatopathologic mononuclear cell patterns in inflammatory skin disease. *J. Invest. Dermatol.* **95,** 128s–131s.

Noonan, P. K., and Wester, R. C. (1987). Cutaneous biotransformations and some pharmacological and toxicological implications. *In* "Dermatotoxicology" (F. N. Marzulli, and H. I. Maibach, eds.), pp. 71–90. Hemisphere, New York.

Norris, D. A. (1990). Cytokine modulation of adhesion molecules in the regulation of immunological cytotoxicity of epidermal targets. *J. Invest. Dermatol.* **95,** 111S–120S.

Norris, P. G., Gange, R. W., and Hawk, J. L. M. (1993). Acute effects of ultraviolet radiation on the skin. *In* "Dermatology in General Medicine," (T. B. Fitzpatrick, A. Z. Eisen, K. Wolff, I. M. Freedberg, and K. F. Austen, eds.), pp. 1651–1658. McGraw-Hill, New York.

Oberg, F., Botling, J., and Nilsson, K. (1993). Macrophages and the cytokine network. *Transplant Proc.* **25,** 2044–2047.

Ogawa, M. (1993). Differentiation and proliferation of hematopoietic stem cells. *Blood* **81,** 2844–2853.

Park, B. K., Coleman, J. W., and Kitteringham, N. R. (1987). Drug disposition and drug hypersensitivity, *Biochem. Pharmacol.* **36,** 581–590.

Pathak, M. A., and Fitzpatrick, T. B. (1992). The evolution of photochemotherapy with psoralens and UVA (PUVA): 2000 BC to 1992 AD. *Photochem. Photobiol.* **14,** 3–22.

Pohjanvirta, R., and Tuomisto, J. (1990). Mechanism of action of 2,3,7,8-tetrachlorodibenzo-*p*-dioxin (TCDD). *Toxicol. Appl. Pharmacol.* **105,** 508–509.

Puhvel, S. M., and Connor, M. J. (1991). Vitamin A deficiency and the induction of cutaneous toxicity in murine skin by TCDD. *Toxicol. Appl. Pharmacol.* **107,** 106–116.

Punjabi, C. J., Laskin, D. L., Heck, D. E., and Laskin, J. D. (1992). Production of nitric oxide by murine bone marrow cells. *J. Immunol.* **149,** 2179–2184.

Radi, R., Beckman, J. S., Bush, K. M., and Freeman, B. A. (1991). Peroxynitrite and oxidation of sulfhydryls. The cytotoxic potential of superoxide and nitric oxide. *J. Biol. Chem.* **266,** 4244–4250.

Raick, A. N. (1973). Ultrastructural, histological and biochemical alterations produced by

12-O-tetradecanoyl-phorbol-13-acetate on mouse epidermis and their relevance to tumor promotion. *Cancer Res.* **33**, 269–286.

Raick, A. N., Thumm, K., and Chivers, B. R. (1972). Early effects of 12-O-tetradecanoyl-phorbol-13-acetate on the incorporation of tritiated precursors into DNA, and the thickness of the interfollicular epidermis, and their relation to tumor promotion in mouse skin. *Cancer Res.* **32**, 1562–1568.

Rees, R. C. (1992). Cytokines as biological response modifiers. *J. Clin. Pathol.* **45**, 93–98.

Ribilloud, T., Asselineau, D., Miquel, C., Calvayrac, R., Darmon, M., and Vuillaume, M. (1990). Deficiency in catalase activity correlates with the appearance of tumor phenotype in human keratinocytes. *Int. J. Cancer* **45**, 952–956.

Rohrschneider, L. R., O'Brien, T. H., and Boutwell, R. K. (1972). The stimulation of phospholipid metabolism in mouse skin following phorbol ester treatment. *Biochim. Biophys. Acta* **280**, 57–63.

Rongone, R. L. (1987). Skin structure, function, and biochemistry. *In* "Dermatotoxicology," (F. N. Marzulli, and H. I. Maibach, eds.), pp. 1–46. Hemisphere, New York.

Rushmore, T. H., and Pickett, C. B. (1993). Glutathione-S-transferases. structure, regulation, and therapeutic implications. *J. Biol. Chem.* **268**, 11475–11478.

Sauder, D. N., Carter, C., Katz, S. I., and Oppenheim, J. J. (1982). Epidermal cell production of thymocyte activating factor (ETAF). *J. Invest. Dermatol.* **79**, 34–39.

Schall, T. J. (1991). Biology of the RANTES/sis cytokine family. *Cytokine* **3**, 165–183.

Schroder, J.-M. (1992a). Chemotactic cytokines in the epidermis. *Exp. Dermatol.* **1**, 12–19.

Schroder, J.-M. (1992b). Generation of NAP-1 and related peptides in psoriasis and other inflammatory skin diseases. *Cytokines* **4**, 54–76.

Shindo, Y., Witt, E., and Packer, L. (1993). Antioxidant defense mechanisms in murine epidermis and dermis and their response to ultraviolet light. *J. Invest. Dermatol.* **100**, 260–265.

Sinclair, A. J., Barnett, A. H., and Lunec, J. (1990). Free radicals and antioxidant systems in health and disease. *Br. J. Hosp. Med.* **43**, 334–344.

Singer, K. H., Le, P. T., Denning, S. M., Whichard, L. P., and Haynes, B. F. (1990). The role of adhesion molecules in epithelial-T cell interactions in thymus and skin. *J. Invest. Dermatol.* **94**, 85s–90s.

Smith, C. D., and Beckman, J. S. (1992). Peroxynitrite-mediated tyrosine nitration catalyzed by superoxide dismutase. *Arch. Biochem. Biophys.* **298**, 431–437.

Snyder, S. H., and Bredt, D. S. (1992). Biological roles of nitric oxide. *Sci. Am.* **266**(5) 68–71, 74–77.

Stamler, J. S., Simon, D. I., Osborn, J. A., Mullins, M. E., Jaraki, O., Michel, T., Singel, D. J., and Loscalzo, J. (1992). S-Nitrosylation of proteins with nitric oxide: Synthesis and characterization of biologically active compounds. *Proc. Natl. Acad. Sci. USA* **89**, 444–448.

Stein, M., and Keshav, S. (1992). The versatility of macrophages. *Clin. Exp. Allergy* **22**, 19–27.

Steinert, P. M. (1993). Structure, function and dynamics of keratin intermediate filamets. *J. Invest. Dermatol.* **100**, 729–734.

Tamaki, K., Saitoh, A., and Yasaka, N. (1992). Differential effect of griseofulvin on gamma-interferon-induced HLA-DR and intercellular adhesion molecule-1 expression of human keratinocytes. *Br. J. Dermatol.* **126**, 450–455.

Taylor, R. T. (1991). Cytokine networks: Immunobiology surfaces. *J. NIH Res.* **3**, 71–74.

Trush, M. A., and Kensler, T. W. (1991). An overview of the relationship between oxidative stress and chemical carcinogenesis. *Adv. Free Rad. Biol. Med.* **10**, 201–209.

Van Deurem, M., Dofferhoff, A. S., and Van Der Meer, J. W. (1992). Cytokines and the response to infection. *J. Pathol.* **168**, 349–356.

Vessey, D. A., and Lee, K. H. (1993). Inactivation of enzymes of the glutathione antioxidant system by treatment of cultured human keratinocytes with peroxides. *J. Invest. Dermatol.* **100**, 829–833.

Weiss, M. E., and Adkinson, N. F. (1988). Immediate hypersensitivity reactions to penicillin and related antibiotics. *Clin. Allergy* **18,** 515–540.

Willson, R. L. (1985). Organic free radicals as ultimate agents in oxygen toxicity. *In* "Oxidative Stress" (H. Sies, ed.), pp. 44–71. Academic Press, Orlando, Florida.

Wilson, J. T., Hojer, B., Tomson, G., Rane, A., and Sjoqvist, F. (1978). High incidence of a concentration dependent skin reaction in children treated with phenytoin. *Br. Med. J.* **1,** 1583–1586.

Zhu, L., Gunn, C., and Beckman, J. S. (1992). Bactericidal activity of peroxynitrite. *Arch. Biochem. Biophys.* **2,** 452–457.

10

Pathogenesis of Atherosclerosis: A Cytokine Hypothesis

George Ku and Richard L. Jackson

I. Introduction

The development of atherosclerosis involves a complicated series of cellular events requiring years to exhibit its final clinical sequelae; coronary heart disease and myocardial ischemia (for review, see Nilsson, 1986; Munro and Cotran, 1988; Halliwell, 1989; Hansson et al., 1989; Haudenschild, 1990; Ip et al., 1990; Steinberg and Witztum, 1990; Takano and Mineo, 1990; Woolf, 1990; Fisher, 1991). The advanced atherosclerotic lesion is a fibrous plaque made up of various cell types and extracellular matrix components including proteoglycans, collagen, and elastin. Beneath the fibrous cap are smooth muscle cells (SMC), macrophages, T lymphocytes, and, in some cases, a necrotic core of cellular debris. The earliest detectable atherosclerotic lesion in humans is the fatty streak that is composed of cholesteryl ester-loaded macrophages. During the last 140 years (Table I), scientific understanding of the pathogenesis of atherosclerosis has advanced from a histological description of lesions to definition of the disease in terms of the interactions of vascular cells, that is, endothelial cells (EC) and SMC, with blood-borne monocytes/macrophages and T lymphocytes. Breakthroughs in cell and molecular biology have provided evidence that cell adhesion molecules, growth factors, and cytokines modulate cellular function in the arterial wall. In this chapter, the evidence that these protein factors play a role in the pathogenesis of atherosclerosis is reviewed.

II. "Response-to-Injury" Hypothesis

The first cellular hypothesis to explain the initiation of atherosclerosis was the "response-to-injury" hypothesis (Ross and Glomset, 1976). This

Xenobiotics and Inflammation

Table I   Atherosclerosis Hypotheses

Hypothesis	Reference
Encrustation Theory	Rokitansky (1852)
Imbibition Theory	Virchow (1856)
Modified Encrustation Theory	Beneke (1890)
Thrombosis Hypothesis	Duguid (1949)
Response-to-Injury Hypothesis	Ross and Glomset (1976)
Modified Response-to-Injury Hypothesis	Ross (1986)
Oxidized Lipoproteins Theory	Steinberg *et al.* (1989)

hypothesis proposed that endothelial injury and subsequent loss of EC is a critical event in the disease process. As a result of EC loss, platelet-derived growth factor (PDGF) induces SMC proliferation. Formulation of this hypothesis was based primarily on the observations that (1) fibrous plaques are characterized by intimal SMC proliferation, (2) PDGF is a potent mitogen for SMC *in vitro*, and (3) injured endothelial surfaces facilitate platelet attachment, leading to platelet aggregation, degranulation, and release of PDGF.

Although the "response-to-injury" hypothesis is consistent with angioplasty-induced arterial SMC proliferation response (Liu *et al.*, 1989), researchers now accept that SMC proliferation resulting from hypercholesterolemia can proceed without endothelial injury (Walker *et al.*, 1986). One limitation of this hypothesis is that little or no significance was assigned to the influx of circulating low density lipoproteins (LDL) and chemotaxis of monocytes into the arterial intima, both of which are hallmarks of atherosclerosis. In a modified version of the "response-to-injury" hypothesis (Ross, 1986), endothelial injury includes subtle changes in EC function such as the expression of cell surface adhesion molecules for monocytes and lymphocytes, thus acknowledging an atherogenic role of pro-inflammatory and immunoregulatory cell types and conceptually expanding the hypothesis from a monomial one, that is, PDGF alone, to one that has a multifactorial mechanism.

III. Infiltration and Modification of Low Density Lipoproteins Hypothesis

Reseachers have well established that lipid accumulation is a hallmark of atherosclerosis and that hypercholesterolemia is a major risk factor for the disease (National Cholesterol Education Program Expert Panel, 1988). In humans, plasma LDL levels are positively correlated with the risk of atherosclerotic heart disease. LDL carry the bulk of cholesteryl esters in the circulation and are considered the major atherogenic lipoproteins. A defect in the clearance of plasma LDL because of the absence of LDL receptors or because of a mutated LDL apolipoprotein B (apo B), so the lipoprotein does not bind to the LDL receptor, is associated with accelerated atherosclerosis (Kita *et al.*, 1981; Rapacz *et al.*, 1986; Buja *et al.*, 1990). The mechanism by which LDL penetrate the arterial wall is based in part on studies performed with co-culture systems of EC and SMC (Merrilees and Scott, 1981; Davies *et al.*, 1985; Weinberg and Bell, 1986; Hajjar *et al.*, 1987; Hough *et al.*, 1990). These co-culture systems show that EC LDL receptors are not significantly involved in the transendothelial transport of LDL, a finding consistent with whole animal studies in New Zealand white rabbits and in Watanabe heritable hyperlipidemic (WHHL) rabbits (Wiklund *et al.*, 1985; Navab *et al.*, 1986). In crossing the endothelial barrier by an LDL receptor-independent mechanism, about half the particles require energy. The remaining half probably move through junctions between and/or through the EC. The co-culture system also reveals that LDL passage through the EC monolayer is saturable.

During the influx of LDL into the subendothelial compartment, LDL are assumed to be modified by EC and, perhaps to a lesser extent, by monocytes. The mechanism of cellular modification of LDL has been the subject of intensive investigation (Henriksen *et al.*, 1983; Parthasarathy *et al.*, 1986a). Researchers know that LDL modification can be prevented by antioxidants such as butylated hydroxytoluene (Morel *et al.*, 1984), α-tocopherol (Steinbrecher *et al.*, 1984), or probucol (Parthasarathy *et al.*, 1986b), suggesting that cell modification involves an oxidative process. In terms of the mechanism of oxidative modification, oxidation may be mediated by a lipoxygenase and/or free radical process. A role for lipoxygenase is supported by the findings that soybean lipoxygenase causes most of the changes induced by EC on LDL (Sparrow *et al.*, 1988; Rankin *et al.*, 1991) and that lipoxygenase inhibitors are effective in blocking the cell-induced oxidative modification of LDL *in vitro* (Parthasarathy *et al.*, 1989). However, analysis of lipids from human atherogenic lesions shows a racemic mixture of hydroxy fatty acids (see subsequent discussion), arguing against an enzymatic mechanism for LDL modification (Sparrow and Olszewski, 1992) but consistent with a free radical-mediated process (Morel *et al.*, 1984; Heinecke *et al.*, 1986; Hiramatsu *et al.*, 1987; Cathcart *et al.*, 1989; Panasenko *et al.*, 1991).

Oxidation of LDLs results in the formation of various lipid hydroperoxy and hydroxy acids such as the linoleate-derived 9- and 13-hydroperoxyocta-decadienoic acid (HPODE) and hydroxyoctadecadienoic acid (HODE; Lenz *et al.*, 1990; Ku *et al.*, 1991). Depending on the extent of oxidation, hydroperoxy fatty acids can be further oxidized to a complex mixture of saturated and unsaturated aldehydes (Carpenter *et al.*, 1990). These aldehydes then can form Schiff base adducts with lysine residues on apo B (Steinbrecher, 1987; Steinbrecher *et al.*, 1987). These modified LDL (MLDL) bind to the scavenger receptor on monocytes/macrophages (Parthasarathy *et al.*, 1986a; Steinbrecher *et al.*, 1989). However, with minimal oxidation, limited amounts of lipid aldehydes are produced. Minimally modified LDL (MMLDL) have intact apo B; thus the lipoproteins retains affinity for the LDL receptor.

IV. Minimally Modified Low Density Lipoprotein-Induced Expression of Endothelial Cell Adhesion Molecules and Release of Chemotactic Factors

MMLDL prepared by prolonged storage at 4°C have been shown to be pathologically relevant in the early stage of atherogenesis, since MMLDL produced by this method induce EC to express granulocyte (G), macrophage (M) and granulocyte–macrophage (GM) colony stimulating factor (CSF) *in vitro* (Rajavashisth *et al.*, 1990). These growth factors affect the differentiation, proliferation, migration, and metabolism of macrophages/granulocytes and the migration and proliferation of EC (Wang *et al.*, 1988; Bussolino *et al.*, 1989). Further, injection of MMLDL into mice induces a 7- to 26-fold increase of M-CSF, supporting a biological role for MMLDL (Liao *et al.*, 1991).

MMLDL is not chemotactic. However, MMLDL stimulate EC and SMC to release monocyte chemotactic peptide 1 (MCP-1), which attracts monocytes but not neutrophils into the subendothelial space (Cushing *et al.*, 1990; Leonard and Yoshimura, 1990). The mechanism of monocyte chemoattraction by MCP-1 is poorly understood, although this process seems likely to be different from that of formyl methionine peptide attractants since MCP-1 does not induce the release of superoxide anion. Using a coculture system of EC and SMC, anti-MCP-1 completely inhibits monocyte chemotaxis before and after exposure to MMLDL, suggesting that MCP-1 could account for all the chemotactic activity, at least in the early stage of atherogenesis (Cushing *et al.*, 1990). In addition to MMLDL, interleukin 4 (IL-4) also induces the synthesis and secretion of MCP-1 by human EC (Rollins and Pober, 1991), supporting a role for T lymphocytes in the pathogenesis of atherosclerosis.

V. Monocyte Infiltration and Fatty Streak Formation

Researchers generally accept that monocyte invasion into the subendothelial space is an important event in the pathogenesis of atherosclerosis (Gerrity, 1981a,b; Faggiotto *et al.*, 1984; Gerrity *et al.*, 1985; Rosenfeld *et al.*, 1987). Interestingly, the sites of monocyte invasion are identical to those previously enriched with LDL (Schwenke and Carew, 1989), consistent with a chemotactic role for entrapped LDL. Further, oxidized LDL (OLDL) have been shown to be chemotactic for monocytes (Quinn *et al.*, 1987).

The events that follow the influx of LDL and monocyte/macrophages into the arterial wall are still undefined, although most investigators agree that these processes play a crucial role in the formation of the fatty streak. At the cellular level, fatty streaks are predominantly made up of cholesteryl ester-loaded macrophages resulting from scavenger receptor-mediated uptake of MLDL (Brown *et al.*, 1980; Parthasarathy *et al.*, 1986a). The presence of MLDL in atherosclerotic lesions has been supported by *in vivo* evidence. For example, (1) antibodies prepared against OLDL recognize proteins in atherosclerotic lesions of LDL receptor-deficient rabbits (Boyd *et al.*, 1989; Palinski *et al.*, 1989), (2) LDL isolated from atherosclerotic lesions share biological properties with OLDL (Ylä-Herttuala *et al.*, 1989), and (3) malondialdehyde-altered proteins that colocalize with apo B are present in atheroma of WHHL rabbits (Haberland *et al.*, 1988; Mao *et al.*, 1991). In terms of the pathological significance of the fatty streak, formation of the initial fatty lesion could be the unfortunate consequence of the clearance of MLDL from the body, that is, this formation could be a protective mechanism to down-regulate the atherogenic signals of MLDL, such as cytokine induction.

VI. Induction of Cytokine Release by Modified Low Density Lipoproteins

Structural identification of the complex mixture of oxygenated fatty acid derivatives in human atherosclerotic plaques reveals that more than 95% of the oxygenated fatty acids is derived from linoleic acid; 9- and 13-HODE are present in a ratio of about 1:1 (H. Kühn, personal communication). Since 9-HODE is a strong pro-inflammatory mediator *in vivo* (Moch *et al.*, 1990) and can be released by EC (Kaduce *et al.*, 1989), macrophages in the lesion could be stimulated by 9-HODE during the scavenger receptor-mediated uptake of OLDL. This notion is supported by the finding that both 9-HODE and cholesteryl-9-HODE induce human macrophage interleukin 1β (IL-1β) mRNA expression and secretion (Ku *et al.*, 1991). Consistent with the presence of 9-HODE in OLDL but not in acetylated LDL (ALDL), metal ion-oxidized and cell-modified LDL, that is, OLDL, induce IL-1β release whereas ALDL are ineffective, indicating that scavenger receptor binding is itself insufficient for the induction of IL-1β.

VII. Interleukin 1β-Induced Smooth Muscle Cell Proliferation

Northern blot analyses of aortic lesions obtained from cholesterol-fed nonhuman primates show a significant increase of IL-1β mRNA levels relative to aorta from control animals (Ross *et al.*, 1990). In addition, a 640-

fold increase of IL-1β mRNA levels has been reported in human atherosclerotic lesions (Wang et al., 1989). These data suggest a strong relationship between IL-1β levels and the pathogenesis of atherosclerosis. As a regulatory protein with a broad spectrum of biological effects (Dinarello, 1991), IL-1β released in the subendothelial space could enhance the expression of adhesion molecules on EC (Bochner et al., 1991), stimulate the release of EC-derived chemotactic factors such as G-CSF and M-CSF (Bagby et al., 1986; Zsebo et al., 1988), further potentiate IL-1β secretion by an autocrine mechanism (Dinarello et al., 1987; Warner et al., 1987a,b), and up-regulate the expression of PDGF and its receptor (Libby et al., 1988; Raines et al., 1989; Ikeda et al., 1990). Therefore, IL-1β release could bring additional damage to the arterial wall as a result of an inflammatory response.

VIII. Activation of T Lymphocytes during Atherogenesis

Histological examination of atherosclerotic lesions using monoclonal antibodies against T lymphocyte surface markers has shown the presence of both helper and cytotoxic T cells in fibrous plaques (Grown et al., 1986; Jonasson et al., 1986; Emeson and Robertson, 1988; van der Wal, 1989). Direct participation of T cells in the pathogenesis of atherosclerosis is supported by findings that these cells express interleukin 2 (IL-2) receptors and that interferon γ (IFNγ) is detected in lesions. Both of these findings are associated with a state of T cell activation (Hansson et al., 1989). With respect to the activating signal for T lymphocytes, the putative candidates are (1) modified apo B in OLDL, (2) cell debris in the necrotic area of lesion, (3) atherosclerotic plaque-associated heat shock proteins (Berberian et al., 1990), and (4) viral antigens, particularly of the herpes-type virus (Benditt et al., 1983; Yamashiroya et al., 1988; Hendrix et al., 1990). In terms of a viral etiology of atherosclerosis, circumstantial evidence suggests circulating antiviral antibodies in atherosclerotic patients. Except for the virus-induced neo-antigens, all other possible candidate antigens for T cell activation are shielded from circulating T cells by an intact endothelium. Therefore, T lymphocyte involvement in atherogenesis probably occurs in the advanced phase of atherosclerosis that is characterized by endothelial injury and necrosis of the fibrous plaque.

IX. Antioxidants as Antiatherosclerosis Agents

Several years ago (Mizel and Farrar, 1979), before the term IL-1 was adopted, immunological research was characterized by an intense interest in the role of extracellular factors in lymphocyte activation (for review, see Silverstein, 1991). Investigators reported that the mitogenic effect of phytohemagglutinin (PHA) on murine thymocytes could be enhanced 100-fold by the addition of supernatant fractions from sodium periodate (NaIO$_4$)-treated macrophage cultures (Novogrodsky and Gery, 1972). Researchers suggested that a NaIO$_4$-induced Schiff base might be involved in the initiation of blastogenesis. Periodate-induced mitogenesis could also be explained by postulating that NaIO$_4$ induces the release of IL-1, which stimulates IL-2 secretion leading to T lymphocyte proliferation. This hypothesis is supported by a report that periodic acid (H$_5$IO$_6$), a strong oxidizing agent, stimulates the production of IL-1β by human peripheral blood mononuclear cells (Malinin et al., 1989). A putative role for oxidative events in IL-1 induction is also suggested by the findings that the antioxidant probucol inhibits ex vivo lipopolysaccharide (LPS)-induced IL-1 release by murine peritoneal macrophages, and phorbol myristate acetate (PMA) induces IL-1β release by THP-1 cells in vitro (Ku et al., 1988,1990; Akeson et al., 1991). An atherogenic role for IL-1, and inhibition of IL-1 expression and secretion, may explain the antiatherosclerotic properties of probucol in animal models (Table II). Since probucol prevents LDL oxidation and the formation of cytotoxic metabolites, OLDL-induced oxidative injury to EC should be prevented by this antioxidant and is consistent with results of in vitro studies (Kuzuya et al., 1991).

X. Summary

Figure 1 summarizes the "cytokine hypothesis." By referring to the IL-1 induction effect of 9-HODE and cholesteryl-9-HODE, which are released by EC and contained in MLDL, respectively, this hypothesis unifies two hallmarks of atherosclerosis, namely, oxidative modification of lipoproteins and vascular SMC proliferation. According to this hypothesis, hypercholesterolemia promotes LDL infiltration across a presumably intact endothelium. EC induce minimal modification of LDL. The subsequent MMLDL facilitate monocyte infiltration via stimulation of adhesion molecules (Cybulsky and Gimbrone, 1991) and chemotactic factors. In the subendothelial space, monocytes differentiate into macrophages that modify LDL and MMLDL to MLDL or OLDL. In the processes of oxidative modification and uptake of oxidatively modified LDL, macrophages are stimulated by 9-HODE and cholesteryl-9-HODE to release IL-1β. Therefore, the significance of foam cell formation resides in the process and less on the product, that is, foam cells might even be a protective mechanism to down-regulate the IL-1 induction signal in MLDL. The cytokine hypothesis also accommodates a role for PDGF in the absence of endothelial injury and platelet degranulation, since IL-1β up-regulates PDGF release (Wilcox et al., 1988; Wilcox, 1991) and PDGF receptor expression by vascular SMC. However, in the event of endothelial injury, the IL-1-mediated inflammatory response

Table II Probucol and Atherosclerosis

Reference	In vivo model				Probucol		Antiatherogenic effect
	Animal	n/Group	Atherogenic regimen	Weeks	Dosage (%)	Route	(% lesion of control)[a]
Kita (1987)	WHHL rabbit	4	Standard chow	26	1	Diet	13, $p < 0.01$
Carew et al (1987)	WHHL rabbit	10	Standard chow	33	1	Diet	35, $p < 0.001$
Finckh et al. (1991)	WHHL rabbit	3	Standard chow	52	1	Diet	53, ND[b]
Mao et al. (1991)	Hybrid WHHL rabbit[c]	9	Standard chow	10	1	Diet	31, $p < 0.05$
Kritchevsky (1971)	Dutch belted rabbit	9	2% cholesterol chow	3	1	Diet	67, $p < 0.01$
Daugherty et al. (1989)	New Zealand albino rabbit	8	2% cholesterol chow	8	1	Diet	21, $p < 0.01$
Stein et al. (1989)	New Zealand albino rabbit	12	1% cholesterol chow	14	1	Diet	100
Towara et al. (1986)	Japanese albino rabbit	7	0.5% cholesterol chow	9	0.5	Diet	54, $p < 0.01$
Shankar et al. (1989)	Wistar rat	20	4% cholesterol chow	3	0.5	Diet	50, $p < 0.005$
Wissler and Vesselinovitch (1983)	Rhesus monkey	5	2% cholesterol chow	52	60[d]	Oral	72, ND

[a] Normalized to 100%.
[b] ND, Not determined.
[c] F$_1$ hybrid of Japanese WHHL and British Half-Lop rabbits; 50% atherosclerotic lesion will develop in 10–12 wk.
[d] Dosage in mg/kg.

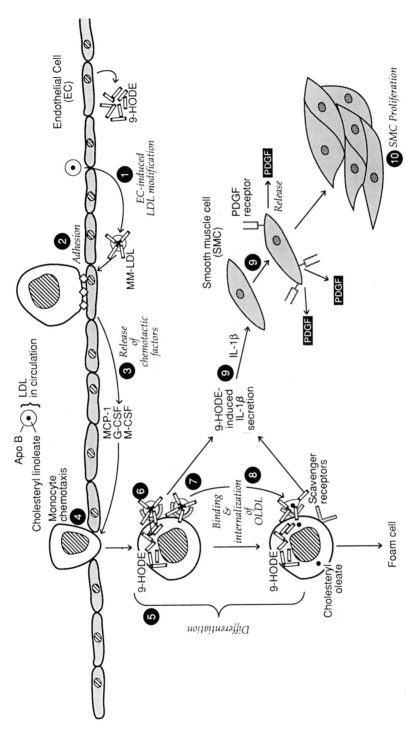

Fig. 1 Essential events in atherosclerosis. (1) LDL infiltration, MM-LDL formation. (2) MM-LDL-induced expression of endothelial cell adhesion molecules. (3) Release of endothelial cell MCP-1 and G- and M-CSF. (4) Monocyte chemotaxis. (5) Monocyte differentiation. (6) Binding of MM-LDL to LDL receptor, delivery of 9-HODE. (7) Oxidative modification of MM-LDL. (8) Binding of OLDL to scavenger receptor. (9) Release of IL-1β, stimulation of PDGF release. (10) Smooth muscle cell (SMC) proliferation. See text for abbreviations.

241

brings platelets and T lymphocytes into play, resulting in SMC proliferation and T lymphocyte-mediated autoimmune attack, leading to further fibrous plaque formation.

XI. Future Direction in the Prevention of Atherosclerosis

In this chapter, the evidence that oxidative modification of LDL plays a central role in the initiation of a cascade of events leading to the formation of atherosclerosis has been reviewed. LDL particles rich in polyunsaturated fatty acids could be speculated to be more accessible to oxidative attack and, theoretically, to be more atherogenic than LDL particles enriched in monounsaturated fatty acids such as oleic acid. The notion of dietary modification to prevent oxidative modification of LDLs is supported by findings that LDLs isolated from the plasma of rabbits fed an oleic acid-enriched diet are more resistant to oxidation than rabbits fed a linoleic acid-enriched diet (Parthasarathy et al., 1990). Another possible approach to protect LDLs from oxidation is supplementing the diet with antioxidants such as α-tocopherol, ascorbic acid, and β-carotene. Obtaining high α-tocopherol levels in LDLs with a α-tocopherol-enriched diet is difficult. This approach only marginally enhances resistance of LDLs to oxidation (Esterbauer et al., 1990). Alternatively, a better absorbed hydrophobic anti-oxidant and/or a regenerable α-tocopherol analog would be useful to protect LDLs from oxidation. The third approach in the prevention of atherosclerosis is that of blocking macrophage infiltration of the endothelium by down-regulating the expression of endothelial cell surface adhesion molecules. In this regard, more research is needed to elucidate the mechanisms of induction of adhesion molecules and of the monocyte chemotactic process. Finally, a tangible approach to disrupting the atherogenic cascade involves blocking the synthesis, the secretion, and/or the action of IL-1 by antioxidants or IL-1 receptor antagonists, thus down-regulating the injury to the endothelium and the signal for SMC proliferation.

Acknowledgments

The authors are grateful to Rosanne Dennin and Sara Gaskey for preparation of the manuscript. We are thankful to Andrew Stein for excellent graphical assistance.

References

Akeson, A. L., Woods, C. W., Mosher, L. B., Thomas, C. E., and Jackson, R. L. (1991). Inhibition of IL-1β expression in THP-1 cells by probucol and tocopherol. *Atherosclerosis* **86**, 261–270.

Bagby, G. C., Jr., Dinarello, C. A., Wallace, P., Wagner, C., Hefeneider, S., and McCall, E. (1986). Interleukin 1 stimulates granulocyte macrophage colony-stimulating activity release by vascular endothelial cells. *J. Clin. Invest.* **78**, 1316–1323.

Benditt, E. P., Barrett, T., and McDougall, J. K. (1983). Viruses in the etiology of atherosclerosis. *Proc. Natl. Acad. Sci. USA* **80**, 6386–6390.

Beneke, R. (1890). Die Ursachen der Thrombusorganisation. *Beitr. Pathol. Anat.* **7**, 27–159.

Berberian, P. A., Myers, W., Tytell, M., Challa, V., and Bond, M. G. (1990). Immunohisto-chemical localization of heat shock protein-70 in normal-appearing and atherosclerotic specimens of human arteries. *Am. J. Pathol.* **136**, 71–80.

Bochner, B. S., Luscinskas, F. W., Gimbrone, M. A., Jr., Newman, W., Sterbinsky, S. A., Derse-Anthony, C. P., Klunk, D., and Schleimer, R. P. (1991). Adhesion of human baso-phils, eosinophils, and neutrophils to interleukin 1-activated human vascular endothe-lial cells: Contributions of endothelial cell adhesion molecules. *J. Exp. Med.* **173**, 1553–1556.

Boyd, H. C., Gown, A. M., Wolfbauer, G., and Chait, A. (1989). Direct evidence for a pro-tein recognized by a monoclonal antibody against oxidatively modified LDL in athero-sclerotic lesions from a Watanabe heritable hyperlipidemic rabbit. *Am. J. Pathol.* **135**, 815–825.

Brown, M. S., Basu, S. K., Falck, J. R., Ho, Y. K., and Goldstein, J. L. (1980). The scavenger cell pathway for lipoprotein degradation: Specificity of the binding site that mediates the uptake of negatively-charged LDL by macrophages. *J. Supermol. Struct.* **13**, 67–81.

Buja, L. M., Clubb, F. J., Bilheimer, D. W., and Willerson, J. T. (1990). Pathobiology of human familial hypercholesterolaemia and a related animal model, the Watanabe heritable hyperlipidaemic rabbit. *Eur. Heart J. (Suppl. E)* **11**, 41–52.

Bussolino, F., Wang, J. M., Defilippi, P., Turrini, F., Sanavio, F., Edgell, C.-J. S., Aglietta, M., Arese, P., and Mantovani, A. (1989). Granulocyte- and granulocyte-macrophage-colony stimulating factors induce human endothelial cells to migrate and proliferate. *Nature (London)* **337**, 471–473.

Carew, T. E., Schwenke, D. C., and Steinberg, D. (1987). Antiatherogenic effect of probucol unrelated to its hypocholesterolemic effect: Evidence that antioxidants *in vivo* can selectively inhibit low density lipoprotein degradation in macrophage-rich fatty streaks and slow the progression of atherosclerosis in the Watanabe heritable hyperlipidemic rabbit. *Proc. Natl. Acad. Sci. USA* **84**, 7725–7729.

Carpenter, K. L. H., Ballantine, J. A., Fussell, B., Enright, J. H., and Mitchinson, M. J. (1990). Oxidation of cholesteryl linoleate by human monocyte-macrophages *in vitro*. *Atherosclerosis* **83**, 217–229.

Cathcart, M. K., McNally, A. K., Morel, D. W., and Chisolm, G. M., III (1989). Superoxide anion participation in human monocyte-mediated oxidation of low-density lipoprotein and conversion of low-density lipoprotein to a cytotoxin. *J. Immunol.* **89**, 1963–1969.

Cushing, S. D., Berliner, J. A., Valente, A. J., Territo, M. C., Navab, M., Parhami, F., Gerrity, R., Schwartz, C. J., and Fogelman, A. M. (1990). Minimally modified low density lipoprotein induces monocyte chemotactic protein 1 in human endothelial cells and smooth muscle cells. *Proc. Natl. Acad. Sci. USA* **87**, 5134–5138.

Cybulsky, M. I., and Gimbrone, M. A., Jr. (1991). Endothelial expression of a mononuclear leukocyte adhesion molecule during atherogenesis. *Science* **251**, 788–791.

Daugherty, A., Zweifel, B. S., and Schonfeld, G. (1989). Probucol attenuates the development of aortic atherosclerosis in cholesterol-fed rabbits. *Br. J. Pharmacol.* **98**, 612–618.

Davies, P. F., Truskey, G. A., Warren, H. B., O'Connor, S. E., and Eisenhaure, B. H. (1985). Metabolic cooperation between vascular endothelial cells and smooth muscle cells in co-culture: Changes in low density lipoprotein metabolism. *J. Cell Biol.* **101**, 871–879.

Dinarello, C. A. (1991). Interleukin-1 and interleukin-1 antagonism. *Blood* **8**, 1627–1652.

Dinarello, C. A., Ikejima, T., Warner, S. J. C., Orencole, S. F., Lonnemann, G., Cannon, J. G., and Libby, P. (1987). Interleukin 1 induces interleukin 1. I. Induction of circulating interleukin 1 in rabbits *in vivo* and in human mononuclear cells in vitro. *J. Immunol.* **87,** 1902–1910.

Duguid, J. B. (1949). Pathogenesis of atherosclerosis. *Lancet* **2,** 925–927.

Emeson, E. E., and Robertson, A. L., Jr. (1988). T lymphocytes in aortic and coronary intimas. *Am. J. Pathol.* **130,** 369–374.

Esterbauer, H., Dieber-Rotheneder, M., Waeg, G., Puhl, H., and Tatzber, F. (1990). Endogenous antioxidants and lipoprotein oxidation. *Biochem. Soc. Trans.* **18,** 1059–1061.

Faggiotto, A., Ross, R., and Harker, L. (1984). Studies of hypercholesterolemia in the nonhuman primate. I. Changes that lead to fatty streak formation. *Arteriosclerosis* **4,** 323–340.

Finckh, B., Niendorf, A., Rath, M., and Beisiegel, U. (1991). Antiatherosclerotic effect of probucol in WHHL rabbits: Are there plasma parameters to evaluate this effect? *Eur. J. Clin. Pharmacol.* **49** (*Suppl.* 1), 577–580.

Fisher, R. (1991). Atherosclerosis: Cellular aspects and potential intervention. *Cerebrovasc. Brain Metab. Rev.* **3,** 114–133.

Gerrity, R. G. (1981a). The role of the monocyte in atherogenesis. I. Transition of blood-borne monocytes into foam cells in fatty lesions. *Am. J. Pathol.* **81,** 181–190.

Gerrity, R. G. (1981b). The role of the monocyte in atherogenesis. II. Migration of foam cells from atherosclerotic lesions. *Am. J. Pathol.* **81,** 191–200.

Gerrity, R. G., Goss, J. A., and Soby, L. (1985). Control of monocyte recruitment by chemotactic factor(s) in lesion-prone areas of swine aorta. *Arteriosclerosis* **5,** 55–66.

Grown, A. M., Tsukata, T., and Ross, R. (1986). Human atherosclerosis. II. Immunocytochemical analysis of the cellular composition of human atherosclerotic lesions. *Am. J. Pathol.* **125,** 191–196.

Haberland, M. E., Fong, D., and Cheng, L. (1988). Malondialdehyde-altered protein occurs in atheroma of Watanabe heritable hyperlipidemic rabbits. *Science* **241,** 215–218.

Hajjar, D. P., Marcus, A. J., and Hajjar, K. A. (1987). Interactions of arterial cells: Studies on the mechanisms of endothelial cell modulation of cholesterol metabolism in co-cultured smooth muscle cells. *J. Biol. Chem.* **262,** 6976–6981.

Halliwell, B. (1989). Current status review: From radicals, reactive oxygen species and human disease: A critical evaluation with special reference to atherosclerosis. *Br. J. Exp. Pathol.* **70,** 737–757.

Hansson, G. K., Jonasson, L., Seifert, P. S., and Stemme, S. (1989). Immune mechanism in atherosclerosis. *Arteriosclerosis* **9,** 567–578.

Haudenschild, C. C. (1990). Pathogenesis of atherosclerosis: State of the art. *Cardiovasc. Drugs Ther.* **4,** 993–1004.

Heinecke, J. W., Baker, L., Rosen, H., and Chait, A. (1986). Superoxide-mediated modification of low density lipoprotein by arterial smooth muscle cells. *J. Clin. Invest.* **77,** 757–761.

Hendrix, M. G., Salimans, M. M., van B. C. P., and Bruggeman, C. A. (1990). High prevalence of latently present cytomegalovirus in arterial walls of patients suffering from grade III atherosclerosis. *Am. J. Pathol.* **136,** 23–27.

Henriksen, T., Mahoney, E. M., and Steinberg, D. (1983). Enhanced macrophage degradation of biologically modified low density lipoprotein. *Arteriosclerosis* **3,** 149–159.

Hiramatsu, K., Rosen, H., Heinecke, J. W., Wolfbauer, G., and Chait, A. (1987). Superoxide initiates oxidation of low density lipoprotein by human monocytes. *Arteriosclerosis* **7,** 55–60.

Hough, G. P., Ross, L. A., Navab, M., and Fogelman, A. M. (1990). Transport of low density lipoproteins across endothelial monolayers. *Eur. Heart J.* (*Suppl.* E) **11,** 62–71.

Ikeda, U., Ikeda, M., Ooohara, T., Kano, S., and Yaginuma, T. (1990). Mitogenic action of interleukin-1α on vascular smooth muscle cells mediated by PDGF. *Atherosclerosis* **84,** 183–188.

Ip, J. H., Fuster, V., and Chesebro, J. H. (1990). Exploration of the atherosclerotic plaque. *Biomed. Pharmacother.* **44,** 343–352.

Jonasson, L., Holm, J., Skalli, O., Bonders, G., and Hansson, G. K. (1986). Regional accumulation of T cells, macrophages, and smooth muscle cells in the human atherosclerotic plaque. *Arteriosclerosis* **6**, 131–137.

Kaduce, T. L., Figard, P. H., Leifur, R., and Spector, A. A. (1989). Formation of 9-hydroxyoctadecadienoic acid from linoleic acid in endothelial cells. *J. Biol. Chem.* **264**, 6823–6830.

Kita, T., Brown, M. S., Watanabe, Y., and Goldstein, J. L. (1981). Deficiency of low density lipoprotein receptors in liver and adrenal gland of the WHHL rabbit, an animal model of familial hypercholeaterolemia. *Proc. Natl. Acad. Sci. USA* **78**, 2268–2272.

Kita, T., Nagano, Y., Yokode, M., Ishii, K., Kume, N., Ooshima, A., Yoshida, H., and Kawai, C. (1987). Probucol prevents the progression of atherosclerosis in Watanabe heritable hyperlipidemic rabbit, an animal model for familial hypercholesterolemia. *Proc. Natl. Acad. Sci. USA* **84**, 5928–5931.

Kritchevsky, D., Kim, H. K., and Tepper, S. A. (1971). Influence of 4,4'-(isopropylidenedithio)bis(2,6-di-*t*-butylphenol) (Dh-581) on experimental atherosclerosis in rabbits. *Proc. Soc. Exp. Biol. Med.* **136**, 1216–1221.

Ku, G., Doherty, N. S., Schmidt, L. F., Jackson, R. L., and Dinerstein, R. J. (1990). Ex vivo lipopolysaccharide-induced interleukin-1 secretion from murine peritoneal macrophages inhibited by probucol, a hypocholesterolemic agent with anti-oxidant properties. *FASEB J.* **4**, 1645–1649.

Ku, G., Akeson, A. L., Mano, M., Thomas, C. E., and Jackson, R. L. (1991). Products of oxidized linoleate mediate the release of interleukin-1 beta from human macrophages. *Trans. Assoc. Am. Phys.* **CIV**, 107.

Ku, G., Thomas, C. E., Akeson, A. L., and Jackson, R. L. (1992). Induction of interleukin-1 beta expression from human peripheral blood monocyte-derived macrophages by 9-hydroxyoctadecadienoic acid. *J. Biol. Chem.* **267**, 14183–14187.

Lenz, M. L., Huges, H., Mitchell, J. R., Via, D. P., Guyton, J. R., Taylor, A. A., Gotto, A. M., Jr., and Smith, C. V. (1990). Lipid hydroperoxy and hydroxy derivatives in copper-catalyzed oxidation of low density lipoprotein. *J. Lipid Res.* **31**, 1043–1050.

Leonard, E. J., and Yoshimura, T. (1990). Human monocyte chemoattractant protein-1 (MCP-1). *Immunol. Today* **11**, 97–101.

Liao, F., Berliner, J. A., Mehrabian, M., Navab, M., Demer, L. L., and Lusis, A. J., and Fogelman, A. M. (1991). Minimally modified low density lipoprotein is biologically active in vivo in mice. *J. Clin. Invest.* **87**, 2253–2257.

Libby, P., Warner, S. J. C., and Friedman, G. B. (1988). Interleukin 1: A mitogen for human vascular smooth muscle cells that induces the release of growth-inhibitory prostanoids. *J. Clin. Invest.* **81**, 487–498.

Liu, M. W., Roubin, G. S., and King, S. B., III. (1989). Restenosis after coronary angioplasty: Potential biologic determinants and role of intimal hyperplasia. *Circulation* **79**, 1374–1387.

Malinin, G. I., Hornicek, F. J., and Malinin, T. I. (1990). Production of interleukin-1β by periodic acid-oxidized human peripheral blood mononuclear cells. *Mol. Cell. Biochem.* **95**, 177–182.

Mao, S. J. T., Yates, M. T., Rechtin, A. E., Jackson, R. L., and van Sickle, W. A. (1991). Antioxidant activity of probucol and its analogs in hypercholesterolemic Watanabe rabbits. *J. Med. Chem.* **34**, 298–302.

Merrilees, M. J., and Scott, L. (1981). Interaction of aortic endothelial and smooth muscle cells in culture. Effect on glycoaminoglycan levels. *Atherosclerosis* **39**, 147–161.

Mizel, S. B., and Farrar, J. J. (1979). Revised nomenclature for antigen-nonspecific T-cell proliferation and helper factors. *Cell. Immunol.* **48**, 433–436.

Moch, D., Schewe, T., Kuhn, H., Schmidt, D., and Buntrock, P. (1990). The linoleic acid metabolite $9D_s$-hydroxy-10,12(E,Z)-octadecadienoic acid is a strong proinflammatory mediator in an experimental wound healing model of the rat. *Biomed. Biochim. Acta* **49**, 201–207.

Morel, D. W., DiCorleto, P. E., and Chisolm, G. M. (1984). Endothelial and smooth muscle cells alter low density lipoprotein *in vitro* by free radical oxidation. *Arteriosclerosis* **4**, 357–364.

Munro, J. M., and Cotran, R. S. (1988). Biology of disease: The pathogenesis of atherosclerosis, atherogenesis and inflammation. *Lab. Invest.* **58**, 249–261.

National Cholesterol Education Program Expert Panel (1988). Report of the National Cholesterol Education Program Expert Panel on detection, evaluation, and treatment of high blood cholesterol in adults. *Arch. Intern. Med.* **148**, 36–69.

Navab, M., Hough, G. P., Berliner, J. A., Frank, J. A., Fogelman, A. M., Haberland, M. E., and Edwards, P. A. (1986). Rabbit beta-migrating very low density lipoprotein increases endothelial macromolecular transport without altering electrical resistance. *J. Clin. Invest.* **78**, 389–397.

Nilsson, J. (1986). Growth factors and the pathogenesis of atherosclerosis. *Atherosclerosis* **62**, 185–199.

Novogrodsky, A., and Gery, I. (1972). Enhancement of mouse thymus cells response to periodate treatment by a soluble factor. *J. Immunol.* **109**, 1278–1281.

Palinski, W., Rosenfeld, M. E., Ylä-Herttuala, S., Gurtner, G. C., Socher, S. S., Butler, S. W., Parthasarathy, S., Carew, T. E., Steinberg, D., and Witztum, J. L. (1989). Low density lipoprotein undergoes oxidative modification in vivo. *Proc. Natl. Acad. Sci. USA* **86**, 1372–1376.

Panasenko, O. M., Vol'nova, T. V., Azizova, O. A., and Vladimirov, Y. A. (1991). Free radical modification of lipoproteins and cholesterol accumulation in cells upon atherosclerosis. *Adv. Free Rad. Biol. Med.* **10**, 137–148.

Parthasarathy, S., Printz, D. J., Boyd, D., Joy, L., and Steinberg, D. (1986a). Macrophage oxidation of low density lipoprotein generates a modified form recognized by the scavenger receptor. *Arteriosclerosis* **6**, 505–510.

Parthasarathy, S., Yound, S. G., Witztum, J. L., Pittman, R. C., and Steinberg, D. (1986b). Probucol inhibits oxidative modification of low density lipoprotein. *J. Clin Invest.* **77**, 641–644.

Parthasarathy, S., Wieland, E., and Steinberg, D. (1989). A role for endothelial cell lipoxygenase in the oxidative modification of low density lipoprotein. *Proc. Natl. Acad. Sci. USA* **86**, 1046–1050.

Parthasarathy, S., Khoo, J. C., Miller, E., Barnett, J., Witztum, J. L., and Steinberg, D. (1990). Low density lipoprotein rich in oleic acid is protected against oxidative modification: Implications for dietary prevention of atherosclerosis. *Proc. Natl. Acad. Sci. USA* **87**, 3894–3898.

Quinn, M. T., Parthasarathy, S., Fong, L. G., and Steinberg, D. (1987). Oxidatively modified low density lipoproteins: A potential role in recruitment and retention of monocyte/macrophages during atherogenesis. *Proc. Natl. Acad. Sci. USA* **84**, 2995–2998.

Raines, E. W., Dower, S. K., and Ross, R. (1989). Interleukin-1 mitogenic activity for fibroblasts and smooth muscle cells is due to PDGF-AA. *Science* **243**, 393–396.

Rajavashisth, T. B., Andalibi, A., Territo, M. C., Berliner, J. A., Navab, M., Fogelman, A. M., and Lusis, A. J. (1990). Induction of endothelial cell expression of granulocyte and macrophage colony-stimulating factors by modified low-density lipoproteins. *Nature* (*London*) **344**, 254–257.

Rankin, S. M., Parthasarathy, S., and Steinberg, D. (1991). Evidence for a dominant role of lipoxygenase(s) in the oxidation of LDL by mouse peritoneal macrophages. *J. Lipid Res.* **32**, 449–456.

Rapacz, J., Hasler-Rapacz, J., Taylor, K. M., Checovich, W. J., and Attie, A. D. (1986). Lipoprotein mutations in pigs are associated with elevated plasma cholesterol and atherosclerosis. *Science* **234**, 1573–1577.

Rokitanoky, C. V. (1852). "A Manual of Pathological Anatomy," Vol. 3. Sydenbam Society, London.

Rollins, B. J., and Pober, J. S. (1991). Interleukin-4 induces the synthesis and secretion of MCP-1/JE by human endothelial cells. *Am. J. Pathol.* **138,** 1315–1319.

Rosenfeld, M. E., Tsukada, T., Gown, A. M., and Ross, R. (1987). Fatty streak initiation in Watanabe heritable hyperlipemic and comparably hypercholesterolemic fat-fed rabbits. *Arteriosclerosis* **7,** 9–23.

Ross, R. (1986). The pathogenesis of atherosclerosis—An update. *N. Engl. J. Med.* **314,** 488–500.

Ross, R., and Glomset, J. A. (1976). The pathogenesis of atherosclerosis. *N. Engl. J. Med.* **295,** 369–377, 420–425.

Ross, R., Masuda, J., Raines, E. W., Gown, A. M., Katsuda, S., Sasahara, M., Malden, L. T., Masuko, H., and Sato, H. (1990). Localization of PDGF-B protein in macrophages in all phases of atherogenesis. *Science* **248,** 1009–1012.

Schwenke, D. C., and Carew, T. E. (1989). Initiation of atherosclerotic lesions in cholesterol-fed rabbits. *Arteriosclerosis* **9,** 895–907.

Shankar, R., Sallis, J. D., Stanton, H., and Thomson, R. (1989). Influence of probucol on early experimental atherogenesis in hypercholesterolemic rats. *Atherosclerosis* **78,** 91–97.

Silverstein, A. M. (1991). History of immunology. The dynamics of conceptual change in twentieth century immunology. *Cell. Immunol.* **132,** 515–531.

Sparrow, C. P., and Olszewski, J. (1992). Cellular oxidative modification of low density lipoprotein does not require lipoxygenase. *Proc. Natl. Adac. Sci. USA* **89,** 128–131.

Sparrow, C. P., Parthasarathy, S., and Steinberg, D. (1988). Enzymatic modification of low density lipoprotein by purified lipoxygenase plus phospholipase A$_2$ mimics cell-mediated oxidative modification. *J. Lipid Res.* **29,** 745–753.

Stein, Y., Stein, O., Delplangue, B., Fesmire, J. D., Lee, D. M., and Alaupovic, P. (1989). Lack of effect of probucol on atheroma formation in cholesterol-fed rabbits kept at comparable cholesterol levels. *Atherosclerosis* **75,** 145–155.

Steinberg, D., and Witztum, J. L. (1990). Lipoproteins and atherogenesis. Current concepts. *J. Am. Med. Assoc.* **264,** 3047–3052.

Steinberg, D., Parthasarathy, S., Carew, T. E., Khoo, J. C., and Witztum, J. L. (1989). Beyond cholesterol. Modifications of low-density lipoprotein that increase its atherogenicity. *N. Engl. J. Med.* **320,** 915–924.

Steinbrecher, U. P. (1987). Oxidation of human low density lipoprotein results in derivatization of lysine residues of apolipoprotein B by lipid peroxide decomposition products. *J. Biol. Chem.* **262,** 3603–3608.

Steinbrecher, U. P., Parthasarathy, S., Leake, D. S., Witztum, J. L., and Steinberg, D. (1984). Modification of low density lipoprotein by endothelial cells involves lipid peroxidation and degradation of low density lipoprotein phospholipids. *Proc. Natl. Acad. Sci. USA* **81,** 3883–3887.

Steinbrecher, U. P., Witztum, J. L., Parthasarathy, S., and Steinberg, D. (1987). Decrease in reactive amino groups during oxidation or endothelial cell modification of LDL. *Arteriosclerosis* **7,** 135–143.

Steinbrecher, U. P., Lougheed, M., Kwan, W-C., and Dirks, M. (1989). Recognition of oxidized low density lipoprotein by the scavenger receptor of macrophages results from derivatization of apolipoprotein B by products of fatty acid peroxidation. *J. Biol. Chem.* **264,** 15216–15223.

Takano, T., and Mineo, C. (1990). Atherosclerosis and molecular pathology: Mechanisms of cholesteryl ester accumulation in foam cells and extracellular space of atherosclerotic lesions. *J. Pharmacobiol.-Dyn.* **13,** 385–413.

Towara, K., Ishihara, M., Ogawa, H., and Tomikawa, M. (1986). Effect of probucol, pantetheine and their combinations on serum lipoprotein metabolism and on the incidence of atheromatous lesions in the rabbits. *Jpn. J. Pharmacol.* **41,** 211–222.

van der Wal, A. C. (1989). Atherosclerotic lesions in human. *In situ* immunophenotypic analysis suggesting an immune mediated response. *Lab. Invest.* **61,** 166–171.

Virchow, R. (1856). Ueber die Verstopfung der Lungenarterie. In "Gesammelte Abhandlungen zur Wissenschaftlichen Medicin." Meidinger Sohn, Frankfurt.

Walker, L. N., Reidy, M. A., and Bowyer, D. E. (1986). Morphology and cell kinetics of fatty streak lesion formation in the hypercholesterolemic rabbit. Am. J. Pathol. 125, 450–459.

Wang, A. M., Doyle, M. V., and Mark, D. F. (1989). Quantitation of mRNA by the polymerase chain reaction. Proc. Natl. Acad. Sci. USA 86, 9717–9721.

Wang, J. M., Griffin, J. D., Rambaldi, A., Chen, Z. G., and Mantovani, A. (1988). Induction of monocyte migration by recombinant macrophage colony-stimulating factor. J. Immunol. 141, 575–579.

Warner, S. J. C., Auger, K. R., and Libby, P. (1987a). Human interleukin 1 induces interleukin 1 gene expression in human vascular smooth muscle cells. J. Exp. Med. 165, 1316–1331.

Warner, S. J. C., Auger, K. R., and Libby, P. (1987b). Interleukin 1 induces interleukin 1. Recombinant human interleukin 1 induces interleukin 1 production by adult human vascular endothelial cells. J. Immunol. 139, 1911–1917.

Weinberg, C. B., and Bell, E. (1986). A blood vessel model constructed from collagen and cultured vascular cells. Science 231, 397–400.

Wiklund, O., Carew, T. E., and Steinberg, D. (1985). Role of the low density lipoprotein receptor in penetration of low density lipoprotein into rabbit aortic wall. Arteriosclerosis 5, 135–141.

Wilcox, J. N. (1992). Analysis of local gene expression in human atherosclerotic plaques by in situ hybridization. J. Vasc. Surg. 15, 913–916.

Wilcox, J. N., Smith, K. M., Williams, L. T., Schwartz, S. M., and Gordon, D. (1988). Platelet-derived growth factor mRNA detection in human atherosclerotic plaques by in situ hybridization. J. Clin. Invest. 82, 1134–1143.

Wissler, R. W., and Vesselinovitch, D. (1983). Combined effects of cholestyramine and probucol on regression of atherosclerosis in Rhesus monkey aortas. Appl. Pathol. 1, 89–96.

Woolf, N. (1990). Pathology of atherosclerosis. Br. Med. Bull. 46, 960–985.

Yamashiroya, H. M., Ghosh, L., Yang, R., and Robertson, A. L. J. (1988). Herpesviridae in the coronary arteries and aorta of young trauma victims. Am. J. Pathol. 130, 71–77.

Ylä-Herttuala, S., Palinski, W., Rosenfeld, M. E., Parthasarathy, S., Carew, T. E., Butler, S., Witztum, J. L., and Steinberg, D. (1989). Evidence for the presence of oxidatively modified low density lipoprotein in atherosclerotic lesions of rabbit and man. J. Clin. Invest. 84, 1086–1095.

Zsebo, K. M., Yuschenkoff, V. N., Schiffer, S., Chang, D., McCall, E., Dinarello, C. A., Brown, M. A., Altrock, B., and Bagby, G. C., Jr. (1988). Vascular endothelial cells and granulopoiesis: Interleukin-1 stimulates release of G-CSF and GM-CSF. Blood 71, 99–103.

11

Ozone-Induced Inflammatory Response in Pulmonary Cells

Hillel S. Koren, Robert B. Devlin, and Susanne Becker

I. Introduction

Ozone is a major component of photochemical smog and is often found at ambient concentrations as high as 0.20 part per million (ppm) in many urban areas and occasionally as high as 0.40 ppm in the Los Angeles area [United States Environmental Protection Agency (U.S. EPA), 1986]. The current National Ambient Air Quality Standards (NAAQS) for ozone allow, on average, one exceedance per year of 0.12 ppm averaged over the hour of highest concentration. Examination of air quality data for 1983 for the 38 United States Standardized Metropolitan Statistical Areas (SMSA) that have populations greater than one million reveals that the second highest 1-hr average value for ozone exceeded 0.12 ppm for 35 of the 38 SMSAs (U.S. EPA, 1986). These values ranged from 0.10 in Philadelphia, Fort Lauderdale, and Seattle to 0.25 in Newark, 0.28 in Houston, and 0.37 ppm in Los Angeles. Clearly, millions of Americans are being exposed recurrently to levels of ozone that have been judged to be harmful by the U.S. EPA.

Researchers widely accept that humans exposed to known concentrations of ozone under controlled conditions exhibit reversible changes that affect the large and small airways, as well as the alveolar region of the lung. These changes include reduction in respiratory function performance, narrowing of large airways, increased nonspecific airway reactivity, alveolar inflammation, damage to pulmonary epithelial cells, and increased leakage of vascular components into the lung. However, whether recurrent exposure to ozone results in induction of chronic disease is not known.

Disclaimer: This document has been reviewed in accordance with U.S. Environmental Protection Agency policy and has been approved for publication. Mention of trade names or commercial products does not constitute endorsement or recommendation for use.

The advent of fiberoptic bronchoscopy has allowed sampling of fluids lining the respiratory tract for analysis of many markers (for review, see Reynolds, 1987) by a technique termed bronchoalveolar lavage (BAL). The use of markers in the lining fluids allows measurement of the degree of inflammation, which is useful in determining the progress of an inflammatory response and in ranking inhaled compounds in animal and human studies. Inflammatory responses in the nose and in the upper respiratory tract can be detected by site-specific sampling of the lining fluids. The biochemical and cellular content of the epithelial lining fluid can also provide information about the type of inflammatory response and the stage of a disease process.

Some of the most characteristic findings in BAL in response to exposure to ozone include an influx of neutrophils, increased permeability, and decreased macrophage phagocytic activity. Production of eicosanoids, some cytokines, fibronectin, lactic dehydrogenase (LDH), coagulation factors, elastase, and plasminogen activator is increased (Seltzer *et al.*, 1986; Koren *et al.*, 1989). Changes in those markers have been reported in humans exposed to levels of ozone as low as 0.08 ppm (Devlin *et al.*, 1991). The involvement of neutrophils and macrophages in the inflammatory response has been known for some time. Since the earliest descriptions of inflammation, injury to epithelial cells has been implicated. However, examples of surface epithelial cells as active effectors in inflammation and host defense are rare (Hunter *et al.*, 1985; Henke *et al.*, 1988; Churchill *et al.*, 1989; Duniec *et al.*, 1989; Hansbrough *et al.*, 1989). Nevertheless, data provide evidence that epithelial cells may play an active role in the inflammatory response to ozone and that they can cause initiation of mediator release by other cells (R. B. Devlin, unpublished observation).

In addition to the *in vivo* studies conducted in environmentally controlled exposure chambers, *in vitro* exposure studies performed with isolated cells can be useful in understanding cellular and molecular mechanisms, and also may be helpful in trying to extrapolate responses among species. The *in vitro* studies described in this chapter focus on the effects of ozone exposure on three cell types: the alveolar macrophage, which is the principal cell type found in normal human BAL fluid (85–90%) and plays a key role in host defenses and inflammation; the alveolar lymphocyte, which is not typically found in large numbers (approximately 10%) in BAL fluid; and the epithelial cell, which is the predominant cell lining the respiratory tract. Epithelial cells are capable of secreting various mediators and cytokines and, therefore, are thought to be important in initiating and perpetuating the inflammatory response in the lung in response to ozone exposure.

The two groups of markers that have drawn much attention in recent years relative to the ozone-induced inflammatory response are the various products of the arachidonic acid metabolites (eicosanoids; for review, see

Henderson, 1987; Holtzman, 1991) and the cytokines (for review, see Kelley, 1990). Products of the arachidonic acid pathway, particularly the prostaglandins, have been shown to be potent mediators of inflammation (for review, see Slauson, 1982; Fantone and Ward, 1984). Products of the lipoxygenase pathway, such as leukotriene B_4 (LTB$_4$), are also known to have strong chemotactic activity for neutrophils (Garcia et al., 1987).

Cytokines are extracellular signaling proteins secreted by effector cells. These molecules have as their primary function the ability to modify the behavior of other closely adjacent cells. Many of the cytokines exhibit potent activity as chemotaxins for specific cell types (Deuel et al., 1982; Hunninghake, 1984; Wahl et al., 1987). Tumor necrosis factor α (TNFα), for example, is a pro-inflammatory cytokine produced primarily by cells of the mononuclear phagocyte series in response to endotoxin exposure (for review, see Beutler and Cerami, 1986; Le and Vilcek, 1987). TNFα has also been implicated as a critical component in silica-induced pulmonary fibrosis (Piguet et al., 1990). Therefore, the in vitro work described in this chapter concentrates on cytokines and eicosanoids.

The body of literature already mentioned clearly demonstrates that the biological response to such an active molecule as ozone is complex and only partly understood. In an attempt to provide a framework for this review, some of the key elements (both cellular and soluble) that may be involved in the acute and chronic inflammatory response to ozone have been illustrated (Figure 1). This figure represents the response of the various cell types to a single exposure (acute) and multiple or continuous exposures (chronic) to this oxidant. The illustration also indicates the general categories of substances (e.g., cytokines, oxygen species) that are produced by the various cell types and their possible effects on other cell types. In addition, the figure shows potential relationships between the various biological responses to pathological situations such as fibrosis. Although this scheme is based on data obtained from animal studies (especially in terms of chronic exposures) and human studies, it also indicates certain relationships such as cell–cell communications that are less well established and are, therefore, more speculative.

The general topic of ozone-induced health effects has been reviewed (Lippmann, 1989; Wright et al., 1990). The focus of this review, however, differs from those mentioned. In this chapter, issues that specifically pertain to the inflammatory response of lung cells following exposure to ozone will be addressed. The chapter highlights the roles of AMs, polymorphonuclear neutrophils (PMN), and epithelial cells and their products (primarily eicosanoids and cytokines) in the inflammatory cascade, comparing animal and human data and in vivo and in vitro data. The relationship of the inflammatory response induced by ozone to that induced by other inhaled environmental materials will be discussed as well.

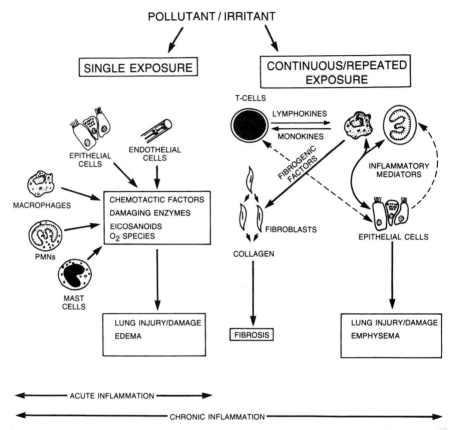

Fig. 1 Schematic representation of possible relationships between various pulmonary cell types and how they can lead to acute or chronic effects in the lung. Dotted lines symbolize hypothetical interactions between cell types.

II. Inflammatory Effects of Ozone on Humans and Animals Exposed *in Vivo*

A. Human Studies

1. *Inflammation as Assessed by Bronchoalveolar Lavage*

Seltzer *et al.* (1986) were the first to demonstrate that exposure of humans to ozone resulted in inflammation in the lung. In this study, 10 volunteers were exposed to 0.4 ppm or 0.6 ppm ozone for 2 hr while undergoing exercise; BAL was performed 3 hr later. BAL fluid from subjects exposed to ozone contained 7.8-fold more neutrophils than BAL fluid from the same subjects exposed to filtered air. Additionally, BAL fluid from ozone-exposed subjects contained increased levels of prostaglandin E_2 (PGE$_2$), $F_{2\alpha}$ (PGF$_{2\alpha}$), and thromboxane B_2 (TxB_2). A report by Koren *et al.* (1989) also described inflammatory changes in the lungs of humans exposed to ozone. In this study, 11 subjects were exposed to 0.4 ppm ozone for 2 hr while undergoing intermittent exercise at 70 L/min designed to simulate heavy outdoor exercise by adults. In this study, BAL was performed 18 hr after ozone exposure. Subjects exposed to ozone had an 8-fold increase in neutrophils in the BAL fluid, confirming the observations of Seltzer *et al.* (1986). In addition, Koren *et al.* (1989) reported a 2-fold increase in BAL fluid protein, albumin, and IgG levels, indicative of increased epithelial cell permeability as a result of ozone exposure. Also, a 12-fold increase in interleukin 6 (IL-6) levels was seen in the BAL fluid. Although IL-1 and TNFα, two potent inflammatory proteins, were not detected in the BAL fluid of any subject, a 2-fold increase in the pro-inflammatory eicosanoid PGE_2 and in the complement component C3a was detected. This study also provided evidence for stimulation of fibrogenic processes in the lung by demonstrating significant increases in two components of the coagulation pathway, tissue factor and factor VII (McGee *et al.*, 1990), as well as increased levels of urokinase plasminogen activator and fibronectin (Koren *et al.*, 1989). Collectively, these two studies demonstrate that exposure of humans to moderate levels of ozone results in an extensive inflammatory reaction in the lung, involving substantial increases in neutrophils and pro-inflammatory compounds such as IL-6 and PGE_2. Further, these studies demonstrate that cells and soluble mediators capable of damaging pulmonary tissue are increased after ozone exposure, as are compounds that play a role in fibrotic and fibrinolytic processes.

2. Inflammation Induced by Ambient Levels of Ozone

In a subsequent study, Devlin *et al.* (1991) reported an inflammatory response in humans exposed for multihour periods to ozone concentrations at or below the current NAAQS concentration of 0.12 ppm. In this study, 10 volunteers were exposed to filtered air and 0.10 and 0.08 ppm ozone for 6.6 hr while undergoing moderate exercise (40 L/min), and underwent BAL 18 hr later. An additional 8 subjects were exposed to filtered air and 0.08 ppm ozone. Increased levels of neutrophils and IL-6 were found in BAL fluid of subjects exposed to 0.10 and 0.08 ppm ozone. Increases also occurred in most of the other compounds reported by Koren *et al.* (1989), including fibronectin and PGE_2. In this study, alveolar macrophage phagocytic capability was also monitored. Researchers reported that macrophages removed from humans exposed to both ozone concentrations had decreased ability to phagocytose *Candida albicans* opsonized with complement. Comparison of the magnitude of inflammatory changes observed in this study and in the study by Koren *et al.* (1989) when normalized for differences in concentration, duration of exposure, and ventilation suggest that lung inflammation from ozone may have no threshold to background levels. Although the mean changes in IL-6 and neutrophils reported by Devlin *et al.* (1991) were low, a considerable range of response was seen among the individuals participating in the study. Although some of the subjects showed little or no response to ozone, others had increases in IL-6 or PMNs that were as large as or larger than those reported by Koren *et al.* (1989) for subjects who were exposed to 0.4 ppm ozone. These data suggest that, although the population as a whole may have a small inflammatory response to low levels of ozone, a significant subpopulation may be very sensitive to these low levels.

3. Time Course of Inflammatory Response

The time course of the inflammatory response to ozone in humans has not been fully explored. Studies in which BAL was performed 1 hr (Devlin *et al.*, 1990; Koren *et al.*, 1992) or 3 hr (Seltzer *et al.*, 1986) after exposure to 0.4 ppm ozone demonstrate that the inflammatory response is quickly initiated; the data reported by Koren *et al.* (1989) indicate that, even 18 hr after exposure, inflammatory mediators such as IL-6 and PMNs are still substantially elevated. Schelegle *et al.* (1991) exposed 5 subjects to filtered air or 0.3 ppm ozone for 1 hr with a ventilation of 60 L/min. Each subject was exposed to ozone on three separate occasions and BAL was performed either 1, 6, or 24 hr after exposure. In addition, BAL fluid was separated into two fractions: the first 60-ml wash was designated the "proximal airways" fraction (PA) and the remaining 360-ml (6 × 60 ml) washes were pooled and designated the "distal airways and alveolar surface" fraction (DAAS). The percentage of PMNs in the PA sample was statistically elevated at 1, 6, and 24 hr after ozone exposure, with a peak response at 6 hr. The percentage PMNs in the DAAS sample was elevated at only the 6- and 24-hr time points, with equivalent elevations at each time. However, more extensive studies are needed better to define the kinetics of appearance and disappearance of the various inflammatory mediators observed in the lungs of humans exposed to ozone.

4. Effect of Anti-inflammatory Agents on Ozone-Induced Inflammation

Previous studies (Schelegle *et al.*, 1987; Eschenbacher *et al.*, 1989) have shown that indomethacin, an anti-inflammatory agent that inhibits cyclooxygenase products of arachidonic acid metabolism, is capable of blunting the well-documented decrements in pulmonary function observed in humans exposed to ozone. In one study, human volunteers were given ibuprofen, another anti-inflammatory agent that blocks cyclooxygenase metabolism, or a placebo 90 min prior to and in the middle of a 2-hr exposure to 0.4 ppm ozone. BAL was performed 1 hr after the exposure. As expected, subjects given ibuprofen had blunted decrements in lung function after ozone exposure compared with the same subjects given a placebo (Hazucha *et al.*, 1991). BAL fluid from subjects given ibuprofen also had reduced levels of the cyclooxygenase product PGE_2, TxB_2, and IL-6, but no decreases were observed in PMNs, fibronectin, permeability, LDH, or macrophage phagocytic function (Madden *et al.*, 1991b). Additional studies are needed to determine the role, if any, played by PGE_2 and IL-6 in pulmonary function decrements and in increases in PMNs, fibronectin, and other components in the BAL fluid of humans after ozone exposure.

5. *Use of Nasal Lavage to Assess Ozone-Induced Inflammation in the Upper Respiratory Tract*

BAL has proven to be a powerful research tool with which to analyze changes in the lung after exposure of humans to xenobiotics. However, because BAL is expensive, is somewhat invasive, and requires specialized personnel and facilities, it is usually done only with small numbers of subjects and in selected medical centers. Therefore, interest is increasing in the use of nasal lavage (NAL) as a tool in assessing xenobiotic-induced inflammation in the upper respiratory tract, which is the primary portal for inspired air and, therefore, the first region of the respiratory tract to come in contact with airborne xenobiotics. NAL is simple and rapid, is noninvasive, and allows collection of multiple sequential samples from the same person. Graham *et al.* (1988) reported increased levels of PMNs in the NAL fluid of 41 humans exposed to 0.5 ppm ozone for 4 hr on 2 consecutive days, with NAL performed immediately before and immediately after each exposure as well as 22 hr after the second exposure. NAL fluid contained elevated PMN levels after all ozone exposures, with peak values occurring immediately after the second day of exposure. Bascom *et al.* (1990) exposed 12 subjects to filtered air or 0.5 ppm ozone for 4 hr, followed immediately by NAL. These investigators reported a 7-fold increase in PMNs, a 20-fold increase in eosinophils, and a 10-fold increase in mononuclear cells following ozone exposure, as well as a 2.5-fold increase in albumin. Graham and Koren (1990) compared inflammatory mediators present in the NAL and BAL fluids of humans exposed to ozone. The same 11 subjects who were exposed to 0.4 ppm ozone for 2 hr with BAL performed 18 hr later, as described earlier (Koren *et al.*, 1989), also underwent NAL immediately before, immediately after, and 18 hr after each exposure (Graham and Koren, 1990). Significant increases in PMNs were detected in the NAL fluid taken both immediately after exposure as well as on the next day. Increases in NAL and BAL PMNs were similar (6.6- and 8-fold, respectively), demonstrating a qualitative correlation between changes in the lower airways as assessed by BAL and in the upper respiratory tract as assessed by NAL. Further, all individuals who had increased PMNs in BAL fluid also had increased PMNs in NAL fluid, although the NAL PMN increase could not quantitatively predict the BAL PMN increase. Albumin, a marker of epithelial cell permeability, was increased 18 hr later, but not immediately after exposure. No changes in PGE_2, plasminogen activator, or leukotrienes $C_4/D_4/E_4$ were detected (Graham and Koren, 1990). However, tryptase, a constituent of mast cells contained in the same granules as histamine, was found in elevated levels immediately after ozone exposure, but not 18 hr later (Koren *et al.*, 1990). These studies suggest that NAL may be a sensitive and reliable tool with which to detect inflammation in the upper airways of humans exposed to xenobiotics.

In addition to measuring NAL fluid for the presence of inflammatory cells and soluble mediators, nasal brush scrapings can be performed in which several thousand cells are removed. These cells can then be analyzed by techniques such as RNA *in situ* hybridization or polymerase chain reaction (PCR), which are capable of analyzing mRNAs present in only a few thousand cells. mRNAs encoding cytokines and other relevant mediators have been quantified in human upper airway cells that were removed by brush scraping (Becker *et al.*, 1993). This approach may extend both the sensitivity and the range of end points that can be assayed in humans.

B. Animal Studies

Although considerable information is available about the inflammatory effects of ozone on humans, controlled exposure of laboratory animals to ozone is useful to study mechanisms of ozone toxicity as well as to explore more fully the pattern of response to ozone. Studies of animals exposed to ozone for long periods of time (months or years) may also yield information about whether repeated but reversible inflammatory responses to ozone over a period of time can result in chronic lung damage indicative of fibrosis. Differences in response among various animal species and humans can also be ascertained. Responses that require highly invasive procedures or sacrifice can only be measured in animals.

1. Inflammatory Response to Acute Ozone Exposure

Researchers have documented well that animals exposed acutely to ozone develop a rapid inflammatory response, as well as derangements in epithelial cells lining the airways and alveoli. Early morphological studies demonstrated that a 2-hr exposure of rats to 0.5 ppm ozone resulted in significant alveolar type I cell damage (Stephens *et al.*, 1974a), and that exposure for 6 hr resulted in inflammation as assessed by increased levels of mononuclear cells in the airways (Stephens *et al.*, 1974b). Other studies showed that acute exposure of dogs to ozone results in a rapid and reversible influx of PMNs into the airway mucosa (Holtzman *et al.*, 1983a) and BAL fluid (Fabbri *et al.*, 1984). BAL fluid protein, an index of lung injury and alteration in epithelial cell permeability, was shown to increase in rats exposed to 0.4 ppm ozone for 6 hr (Guth *et al.*, 1986). Since then, many additional studies have confirmed and extended these findings.

Animals exposed to ozone also have been shown to have increased BAL fluid levels of prostaglandins. Kleeberger *et al.* (1988) reported that ozone delivered to lobar segments of dogs resulted in increased PGD_2 and perhaps

LTB_4 in BAL fluid obtained from those segments. Schlesinger *et al.* (1990) reported that rabbits exposed to 1 ppm ozone for 2 hr had increased levels of PGE_2 and $PGF_{2\alpha}$ in the BAL fluid recovered immediately after exposure. However, increases in arachidonic acid metabolites may depend on the age of the animal. Gunnison *et al.* (1990) exposed rats and rabbits, ranging in age from neonates to young adults, to 1 ppm ozone for 2 hr. In both species, younger animals had large increases in PGE_2 and $PGF_{2\alpha}$, but the effect decreased and eventually disappeared as the animals grew to adulthood.

Ozone-induced changes in a number of other components with potential pro-inflammatory properties have also been reported in animals. These changes include increases in IL-6 (Pino *et al.*, 1992), histamine (Kleeberger *et al.*, 1988), procoagulant and fibrinolytic activities (Shima and Adachi, 1991), fibronectin (Pino *et al.*, 1992), elastin (Damji and Sherwin, 1989), lysozyme (Shelley *et al.*, 1991), pyridine nucleotides (Montgomery *et al.*, 1991), mitochondrial enzymes (Bassett *et al.*, 1988a), and proteinase–antiproteinase levels (Pickrell *et al.*, 1987).

The time course of the inflammatory reaction in animals exposed to ozone has also been studied. Bassett *et al.* (1988b) exposed rats to 1.8 ppm ozone for 2 or 4 hr, followed by BAL 0, 1, 3, and 8 days later. In animals lavaged immediately after exposure, these researchers found increased LDH activity, decreased numbers of macrophages, but no change in albumin or PMN content. BAL fluid taken from rats 1 day after ozone exposure contained substantial elevations of both PMNs and albumin, but by 3 days only albumin levels remained elevated, and by 8 days albumin levels had also returned to control values. These data demonstrate different time courses of response for LDH, macrophage number, PMNs, and albumin, and suggest that the inflammatory response to ozone may be mediated by different factors at various times after an acute exposure.

Hotchkiss *et al.* (1989) compared the inflammatory response in the nose and lungs of rats exposed acutely to ozone. Animals exposed to low concentrations of ozone (0.12 ppm) had elevated levels of PMNs in NAL fluid immediately after exposure, but no change in PMNs in BAL fluid. Rats exposed to 0.8 ppm ozone initially had more PMNs in NAL fluid but, 42 hr after exposure, the number of BAL fluid PMNs reached a peak whereas NAL fluid PMNs had diminished. Rats exposed to high ozone concentrations (1.5 ppm) had significant elevations of BAL fluid PMNs but no increases in NAL fluid PMNs. The results of Hotchkiss *et al.* (1989) suggest that, at high ozone concentrations, the acute nasal inflammatory response is attenuated by a competing response in the alveolar region of the lung.

2. Inflammatory Effects of Repeated Ozone Exposures

Stokinger *et al.* (1956) originally showed that a 6-hr exposure of exercising rats to 1 ppm ozone was lethal, but that animals pre-exposed to a nonlethal dose of 1 ppm at rest were not killed even after several successive days of exposure with exercise. This phenomenon, termed "tolerance," suggested that animals could be conditioned to high ozone exposure by pre-exposure to lower ozone levels. Several subsequent studies have shown that human volunteers exposed to ozone for several consecutive days have decrements in pulmonary function performance after the first and second day of exposure, but that succeeding exposures attenuate these effects (Hackney *et al.*, 1977; Farrell *et al.*, 1979; Folinsbee *et al.*, 1980). This "adaptation" to ozone persists for several days afterward (Horvath *et al.*, 1981; Kulle *et al.*, 1982; Linn *et al.*, 1982). However, determining whether "adaptation" is restricted to pulmonary function parameters, or whether the inflammatory response seen after an acute exposure to ozone can also be diminished by repeated exposures, is important. Schwartz *et al.* (1976) exposed rats to 0.5 ppm ozone for 7 days (6 hr per day) and reported thickened terminal bronchioles that were attributed to accumulation of eosinophilic hyaline material and mononuclear cells. Similarly, Brummer *et al.* (1977) found increased macrophages in rats exposed to 0.5 ppm ozone for 7 days (4 hr per day). These early studies suggest that tissue damage and inflammation may progress in rats even while pulmonary function "adaptation" occurs.

Tepper *et al.* (1989) exposed Fischer rats to different levels of ozone (0.35–1.0 ppm) for 2.25 hr on each of 5 consecutive days. As expected, decrements in pulmonary function response occurred after the first and second day of exposure to ozone, but these decrements diminished with each succeeding day and were attenuated by the fifth day. In contrast, BAL fluid protein was elevated after the first day of exposure and remained elevated at the same level for the remaining 4 days of exposure. Light microscopic examination of fixed lung sections also showed progressive inflammation and tissue damage in the terminal bronchiolar region. These data suggest that attenuation of the pulmonary function response occurs in rats after repeated exposure to ozone, but that cell damage and inflammatory changes become increasingly worse.

Van Bree *et al.* (1989) exposed Wistar rats to 0.4 ppm ozone for 1, 2, or 3 consecutive days (12 hr/day). BAL fluid protein and PMN levels were assessed as markers of inflammation and permeability. Rats exposed for only 1 day had a substantial elevation in BAL fluid PMNs and protein compared with air-exposed controls; the increase peaked at 24 hr and returned to baseline levels by 3 days. Comparison of the PMN response after 1 day with the response after 2 or 3 days of exposure showed that these last 2 days of exposure did not contribute at all above the increase in PMNs seen after a single day of exposure. Similar results were reported when BAL fluid protein levels were measured. However, when LDH activity in BAL fluid was measured as an indicator of cell damage and repair, the results were different. LDH activity in BAL fluid after a single day of ozone exposure peaked between 2 and 3 days after exposure but remained elevated for at least 7–8 days. Rats exposed to ozone for 2 or 3 days had elevated LDH levels compared with rats exposed only a single day, and LDH activity did not return to baseline even after 9 days. These data suggest that, although indices of inflammation and permeability were primarily induced by the first day of ozone exposure and showed full reversibility even with continued exposure, indices of cell damage or repair increased with continued exposures and did not return to baseline values on the same time course as indices in rats exposed for only a single day.

Van Bree et al. (1993) also exposed Wistar rats to 0.4 ppm (8 hr) ozone for 5 consecutive days, with BAL performed before and after the exposure. Similar levels of PMNs were found in the BAL fluid of animals exposed to ozone for 5 days and in those exposed to filtered air for 5 days, suggesting that the inflammatory response seen after a single exposure was attenuated after 5 days of exposure. Similar results were seen with BAL fluid protein, IL-6, and fibronectin. Some rats were exposed to ozone for 5 days, held in clean air for various times up to 26 days, and then challenged with a single acute exposure to 0.4 ppm ozone to determine the duration of the "adaptive" response. The inflammatory response (as measured by PMNs, protein, IL-6, and fibronectin) to a single exposure gradually began to return, but even after 26 days in clean air, the inflammatory response of "adapted" rats to an acute ozone exposure was less than that of naive rats.

Collectively, these three studies suggest that, in animals, ozone-induced decrements in pulmonary function and the inflammatory response measured by analysis of BAL fluid components are attenuated with repeated ozone exposures. This "adaptation" lasts for several days for pulmonary function performance, and considerably longer for BAL fluid inflammatory components. However, indicators of cell damage and inflammation measured by microscopic analysis of lung sections become progressively worse with repeated ozone exposure.

Several studies have been reported in which rats and monkeys were exposed repeatedly to low levels of ozone for periods of up to 18 mo. The principal lesions resulting from such long-term exposures are low grade inflammation with increased numbers of PMNs and macrophages at the junction between the conducting airways and alveolar gas exchange region. Changes in the type and volume of airway and alveolar epithelial cells are also seen in the centriacinar region of the lung (Gross and White, 1987; Moffatt et al., 1987; Barr et al., 1988, 1990; Barry et al., 1988; Tyler et al., 1988; Hiroshima et al., 1990; Hyde et al., 1989). Increased lung collagen content (Last et al., 1984), as well as changes in the type of collagen cross-linking to a type characteristic of fibrosis (Reiser et al., 1987), have also been reported, as have restricted changes in lung ventilatory parameters (Gross and White, 1987; Grose et al., 1989). The ventilatory changes and much of the inflammation observed are reversed if the animals are placed in clean air for 3 mo (Gross and White, 1987), but some of the epithelial cell abnormalities (Gross and White, 1987; Gross et al., 1990) as well as the deposition of collagen (Reiser *et al.*, 1987) were still evident some months after ozone exposure was ended.

3. *Inflammation and Airway Hyperreactivity*

An inherent feature of asthma and other bronchorespiratory diseases is increased airway sensitivity to a variety of physical and pharmacological stimuli such as cold air and acetylcholine. The mechanisms underlying this nonspecific airway hyperreactivity are not well understood. However, an acute exposure to ozone (1.0–3.0 ppm) has been used to induce a rapid and transient increase in airway reactivity in various animal species, including dogs (Holtzman *et al.*, 1983a; Fabbri *et al.*, 1984) and guinea pigs (Murlas and Roum, 1985a). Ozone was also shown to induce a rapid inflammatory response in dogs, as evidenced by increased levels of PMNs found in the upper (Holtzman *et al.*, 1983a) and lower (Fabbri *et al.*, 1984) airways. Because a temporal association was reported between the onset of ozone-induced hyperresponsiveness and the influx of PMNs into the upper and lower airways, these authors suggested that the inflammatory response may be required for the development of airway hyperreactivity. In support of this idea, O'Byrne *et al.* (1984a) reported that dogs depleted of neutrophils failed to develop ozone-induced airway hyperreactivity. O'Byrne *et al.* (1984b) also reported that indomethacin, an inhibitor of pro-inflammatory cyclooxygenase products of arachidonic acid, inhibited ozone-induced hyperresponsiveness without altering the influx of neutrophils into the upper airways. These investigators suggested that neutrophils release eicosanoids that act on airway smooth muscle or its nerves to bring about hyperreactivity. However, Murlas and Roum (1985a) failed to find a similar temporal linkage between ozone-induced inflammation and airway hyperreactivity in guinea pigs, although they did report a high correlation between the amount of epithelial cell damage induced by ozone and the degree of airway hyperreactivity. Murlas and Roum (1985b) also found that neutrophil depletion in guinea pigs inhibited the development of ozone-induced airway hyperreactivity. Subsequently, Evans *et al.* (1988) reported that rats exposed to 4.0 ppm ozone for 2 hr developed airway hyperreactivity without an accompanying increase in neutrophils into the upper airways. Aizawa *et al.* (1985) reported that OKY-046, an inhibitor of TxA_2, could inhibit the airway hyperreactivity associated with ozone exposure without diminishing the PMN influx. Chitano *et al.* (1989) also reported that ambroxol, an inhibitor of arachidonic acid release from cell membranes, inhibited the ozone-induced increase in airway reactivity to acetylcholine without decreasing the influx of neutrophils into the lungs. Similarly, Okazawa *et al.* (1990) reported that guinea pigs exposed to 2.9 ppm ozone for 30 min developed airway hyperresponsiveness within 1 hr with no increase in PMNs in the BAL fluid, but that pretreatment with a specific inhibitor of TxA_2 synthetase or a leukotriene C_4/D_4 receptor agonist prevented the increase in airway hyperreactivity. Collectively, these studies suggest that inflammation as measured by increased airway PMNs is not required for the development of airway hyperreactivity and imply that a cellular source other than PMNs is responsible, as least in part, for the production of compounds, likely to be cyclooxygenase products, that play a role in the development of airway hyperreactivity after ozone exposure.

C. Variability among Individuals and Animal Strains in Response to Ozone

A wide variability exists in human responses to ozone exposure. Decrements in pulmonary function can vary by more than an order of magnitude among humans exposed to ozone (Horvath *et al.*, 1981; McDonnell *et al.*, 1983). However, the response of each individual is reproducible over time (Gliner *et al.*, 1983; McDonnell *et al.*, 1985). Also, large individual variations are seen in accumulation of inflammatory mediators such as PMNs, IL-6, and PGE_2 in the BAL fluid of humans exposed to ozone (Devlin *et al.*, 1991; Koren *et al.*, 1989). Interestingly, those individuals with the largest decrements in pulmonary function do not necessarily have the largest increases in inflammatory mediators, suggesting that separate mechanisms underlie these two responses to ozone (Devlin *et al.*, 1991).

Identification of susceptibility or risk factors that may predispose individuals to harmful effects of pollutants have received great interest. These risk factors include nutritional factors, antioxidants, trace minerals, age, and sex of the individual. Kleeberger *et al.* (1990) exposed nine strains of inbred mice to ozone and identified a susceptible (C57BL/6J) and a resistant (C3H/HeJ) strain. A 22-fold difference in PMNs present in the BAL fluid was seen in the two strains exposed to ozone. BAL fluid protein was also significantly higher in the susceptible strain. The phenotype of backcross progeny of the two strains suggested that a single autosomal recessive gene, termed the *inf* locus, conferred susceptibility to the ozone-induced influx of PMNs. However, another as yet unidentified locus is likely to be responsible for the increase in BAL fluid protein. The ability to segregate genetically the loci involved in the inflammatory response to ozone provides a powerful tool with which to identify and characterize the mechanisms responsible for susceptibility to ozone-induced inflammation.

Two studies have compared the inflammatory responses of different rat strains to ozone. In one study (Pino *et al.*, 1991), the influx of PMNs and BAL fluid protein were measured in Wistar and Sprague–Dawley rats exposed to 1.0 ppm ozone for 8 hr. Wistar rats had a larger PMN influx than Sprague–Dawley rats; histological examination confirmed this finding. However, no differences were seen in BAL fluid protein of the two strains. Another study (Costa *et al.*, 1992) compared the response of three rat strains to ozone: Wistar, Sprague–Dawley, and Fischer 344. Several inflammatory mediators were measured, including PMNs, IL-6, protein, and fibronectin. The results of this study demonstrated that, in general, Wistar rats are most sensitive and Fischer 344 least sensitive to ozone, although this overall hierarchy was not true for all end points, ozone concentrations, or time points examined. These studies emphasize the importance of choosing, even within a species, appropriate animal strains when trying to compare the results with human data.

III. *In Vitro* Studies of Pulmonary Cells after Exposure to Ozone

Although much is known about the manifestation of ozone effects as lung inflammation and injury *in vivo*, little is known about the involvement of the various lung cells in these ozone-induced processes. The alveolar macrophage is the cell type that first comes to mind as the cell responsible for recruitment of inflammatory PMNs into the lung. These cells produce a variety of protein and lipid mediators that are chemotactic to granulocytes, among them chemokines IL-8 (Rankin *et al.*, 1990), GROα, GROβ, and GROγ (Becker *et al.*, 1994) and various arachidonic acid metabolites with PMN stimulatory activity (Brown *et al.*, 1988). Further, the cells produce several complement components including C3 and C5, fibronectin (Fels and Cohn, 1986), IL-6 (Becker *et al.*, 1991a), and tissue factor and factor VII (Chapman *et al.*, 1984; McGee *et al.*, 1990), all of which were found to be elevated in BAL fluid after exposure of humans to ozone (Koren *et al.*, 1990; Devlin *et al.*, 1991). In various animal studies, alveolar macrophages have been found to be affected by ozone since they show decreased production of reactive oxygen species (Amuroso *et al.*, 1981) and decreased phagocytosis (Driscoll *et al.*, 1987), and produce lower amounts of lysozyme (Kimura and Goldstein, 1981) when tested *in vitro*.

The role of epithelial cells in inflammatory responses has been realized as well. Airway epithelial cells were shown to produce eicosanoids generated by both cyclooxygenase and lipoxygenase pathways (Henke *et al.*, 1988; Churchill *et al.*, 1989; Salari *et al.*, 1989). These cells also produce IL-6 and IL-8 (Standiford *et al.*, 1990; Noah and Becker, 1993) and fibronectin (Shoji *et al.*, 1990). Since injury to airway epithelium is evident in morphological studies of ozone exposure, these cells are likely to produce inflammatory products including chemotactic factors and mediators involved in tissue repair.

To try to unravel the contribution of each cell type to the inflammatory response after ozone exposure, experiments with alveolar macrophages from human subjects and animals exposed to ozone *in vivo*, as well as with macrophages or airway epithelial cells exposed to ozone *in vitro*, have been performed. Much of the data on inflammatory mediators produced by these cells after ozone exposure have been accumulated recently and have not yet been published. In this section, current knowledge of the inflammatory products of ozone-exposed macrophages and airway epithelial cells is summarized based on both published and unpublished data.

A. *In Vitro* Studies of *in Vivo* Exposed Cells

1. *Responses of Human Alveolar Macrophages*

To elucidate the contribution of alvelor macrophages (AM) to the inflammatory events associated with ozone exposure and indicated by the increase in various inflammatory mediators in lavage fluids of ozone-exposed individuals (see Section II,A), the possible release of these proteins and lipid mediators was studied by studying AMs *in vitro* that were previously exposed to ozone *in vivo* and then subsequently harvested by BAL. Two-dimensional gel analysis comparing AMs from ozone (0.4 ppm/2 hr)-exposed and control subjects indicated that the rate of synthesis of a large number of proteins had been altered after ozone exposure (Devlin and Koren, 1990). Of nearly 900 proteins analyzed, 78 proteins were synthesized at a reduced rate, whereas 45 proteins were synthesized at a significantly higher rate. Some of these proteins may be inflammatory mediators regulating PMN influx and tissue repair. Particular attention has been paid to the possible production and release of the cytokines IL-1, TNF, IL-6, IL-8, and transforming growth factor (TGF) by ozone-exposed AMs. Comparing the molecular sizes and isoelectric points of the proteins showing increased synthesis after ozone exposure with properties of proteins such as IL-1, TNF, IL-6, and TGF suggested that these cytokines were not induced by ozone *in vivo*. IL-8 does not contain methionine and, thus, was not detected by the [^{35}S]methionine labeling method used for the two-dimensional gel analysis (Yoshimura *et al.*, 1987). As described in Section II,A, IL-6 was the only cytokine consistently increased in lavage fluid of ozone-exposed subjects, whereas TNF, IL-1, and IL-8 levels, if detectable, were similar in control and ozone-exposed subjects.

To assess whether ozone inhalation altered the ability of AMs to produce cytokines on further stimulation, AMs from ozone- and air-exposed humans (BAL performed either 2 or 18 hr after exposure) were cultured in the presence and absence of endotoxin (1 μg/ml) for 3–24 hr. The supernatants were then tested for the presence of IL-1, IL-6, IL-8, and TNF. Although the cells spontaneously released small amounts of IL-1, IL-6, and TNFα, and somewhat larger amounts of IL-8, no difference was detected in the levels produced by air- or ozone-exposed AMs (S. Becker, unpublished observations). RNA was also purified from the AMs; cytokine mRNA levels were determined by Northern blot hybridization. No differences in cytokine mRNA levels were found between air- and ozone-exposed AMs. BAL fluid from which the AMs had been isolated showed increased levels of IL-6, but not of the other cytokines, after ozone exposure.

PGE$_2$ levels have consistently been found to be elevated in BAL of ozone-exposed humans 1–3 hr and 18 hr after exposure (Seltzer *et al.*, 1986; Koren *et al.*, 1989; Devlin *et al.*, 1990, 1991). Therefore, production of eicosanoids by AMs isolated from air- and ozone-exposed individuals 1 hr after exposure (Devlin *et al.*, 1990) was assessed *in vitro.* The AMs were cultured in the presence or absence of A23187 Ca^{2+} ionophore, and supernatants were collected over a 4-hr time course for assessment of production of arachidonic acid metabolites. Neither spontaneous nor A23187 Ca^{2+} ionophore-induced PGE$_2$, TxB$_4$, and LTB$_4$ production was significantly different in ozone-exposed and air-exposed AMs at any of the time points assayed (M. C. Madden, unpublished observations).

No differences were detected in fibronectin levels in supernatants of air- and ozone-exposed AMs as were found with cytokines and eicosanoids. Thus, based on data from *ex vivo* testing of the macrophage secretory capacity, no indication exists that the increased IL-6, PGE$_2$, and fibronectin levels found in the lavage fluid originate from the AMs. However, mRNA expression and secretory events are transitory and the time of lavage may not coincide with the observed cellular changes in the materials released *in vitro*. Tissue factor mRNA was present in ozone-exposed AMs at 2.4-fold higher levels than in air-exposed AMs (McGee *et al.*, 1990), suggesting that the increased levels of tissue factor in the lavage fluids may indeed originate from the macrophages. Another example of an effect of *in vivo* ozone exposure on human AM function is their decreased ability to phagocytose *C. albicans* microorganisms *in vitro* (Devlin *et al.*, 1991). Similar decreases in phagocytic activity have been observed in rodent species and have been found to correlate with increased microbial burden and mortality rates (Gardner, 1982; Van Louveren *et al.*, 1988).

2. *Responses of Animal Alveolar Macrophages*

Production of some cytokines and arachidonic acid metabolites have been studied in AMs removed from ozone-exposed animals. Cells obtained by BAL from rats exposed to ozone were tested for release of IL-1 (Amoruso *et al.*, 1988). Increased production of IL-1 48 hr after exposure was reported that was, at least in part, caused by the influx of inflammatory monocytes into the lung. Driscoll *et al.* (1988) reported that AMs removed from rabbits exposed to 1.2 ppm ozone for 2 hr were found to release 5- to 6-fold greater levels of PGE$_2$ and PGF$_{2\alpha}$ than AMs from air-exposed rabbits. No effect on the production of these metabolites was seen in cells exposed to 0.12 ppm ozone. No LTB$_4$, LTC$_4$, or TxB$_2$ was detected after ozone exposure.

B. *In Vitro* Ozone Exposure Studies

1. *Responses of Human Alveolar Macrophages*

The *in vivo* ozone exposure experiments certainly suggest that the numerous changes in AM protein metabolism may be involved in the inflammatory response to ozone. To investigate whether these protein changes are the result of a direct effect of ozone on the macrophages or of secondary effects resulting from previous response to injury, two-dimensional gel analysis was performed on *in vitro* ozone-exposed AMs (1.0 ppm/2 hr) in a controlled exposure chamber previously described in detail (Harder *et al.*, 1990). The *in vitro* ozone-exposed cells showed changes in the rate of synthesis of only 11 proteins (Becker *et al.*, 1991b), compared with changes in 123 proteins in AMs removed from ozone-exposed humans (Devlin and Koren, 1990). This result suggested that most of the *in vivo* changes (which amounted to about 10% of the total number of proteins detected) were indeed the results of biological effects secondary to ozone exposure. Note that none of the proteins that had increased in rate of synthesis in response to *in vitro* ozone exposure corresponded to the protein size and isoelectric points of cytokines IL-1, IL-6, TNFα, or TGF.

Human AMs were exposed to ozone *in vitro* to investigate the direct effect of ozone exposure on several functions of macrophages. The cells were exposed either in culture dishes with a thin layer of phosphate buffered saline (PBS, maintaining the humidity) with rocking, or on collagen-coated membranes where humidity was provided by a basolateral source of PBS during the exposure without rocking. Medium was added to the cells immediately after exposure and supernatants were collected at different time points for analysis of cytokines (IL-1, IL-6, IL-8, and TNF) and fibronectin. Exposure to 1 ppm ozone for 2 hr or 4 hr (under PBS) or to 0.5 ppm for 10–60 min (when exposed on collagen-coated membranes) did not result in induction or increased release of any of these cytokines. However, ozone did affect the ability of the cells to respond subsequently to a signal such as bacterial lipopolysaccharide, showing a decrease in the production of cytokines (Becker *et al.*, 1991b) relative to the air-exposed AMs. The ozone-exposed AMs also showed a number of other defects such as decreased Fc receptor function, phagocytosis, and superoxide production.

A consistent ozone effect on AMs *in vitro*, which correlates with observations in BAL *in vivo*, is an increase in the release of arachidonic acid metabolites such as PGE_2 and TxB_4. Human AMs exposed to air and 0.1, 0.3, and 1.0 ppm ozone for 2 hr showed an ozone concentration-dependent increase in PGE_2 release into the exposure medium (Becker *et al.*, 1991b). No difference was detected in PGE_2 levels in the medium that replaced the exposure medium over the next 2 hr, indicating that the effect of ozone was immediate and not long-term for arachidonic acid metabolism. Rabbit AMs (Driscoll *et al.*, 1988) were exposed to air and 0.1, 0.3, and 1.2 ppm ozone for 2 hr, and supernatants from the exposed cells were collected 2 and 6 hr later. Significantly increased levels of PGE_2 were present in supernatants of cells exposed to 0.3 and 1.2 ppm ozone 6 hr after exposure. At 2 hr, increased levels of PGE_2 were produced only by cells exposed to 1.2 ppm ozone. Madden *et al.* (1991a) exposed rat AMs labeled with [^{3}H]arachidonic acid to ozone (0.1–1.0 ppm) for 2 hr *in vitro* and analyzed eicosanoids in the supernatants. Significantly increased levels of 6-keto-PGF$_{1\alpha}$, TxB$_2$, PGE$_2$, LTB$_4$, LTD$_4$, and 15-hydroxyeicosatetraenoic acid (HETE) were formed by AMs exposed to 1.0 ppm ozone relative to air-exposed cells. Ozone-exposed AMs also released free arachidonic acid which, in the presence of ozone, forms different aldehyde products and hydrogen peroxide. The formation of these aldehydes was demonstrated in a cell-free system (Pryor *et al.*, 1991; Madden *et al.*, 1993). Aldehydes of arachidonic acid induced PMN shape change (polarization), an indication of stimulation and a likely chemotactic response.

The precursor of platelet activation factor (PAF), lysoPAF, and free arachidonic acid are formed simultaneously through activation of phospholipase A$_2$. Friedman *et al.* (1992) demonstrated that human AMs exposed to 1 ppm ozone for 1 hr significantly increased their production of PAF (1.7-fold) relative to air-exposed cells. Phorbol-differentiated HL60 cells were studied in more detail (Samet *et al.*, 1992), and were found to respond to as little as 0.05 ppm ozone for 15 min with significantly elevated levels of PAF. A 3-fold increase in PAF was found after exposure to 1.0 ppm ozone for 1 hr.

2. Responses of Human Lymphocytes

Lymphocytes make up 5–20% of the cells obtained by BAL; the majority of these lymphocytes are T cells. The T cells have been found to be of memory cell phenotype (Becker *et al.*, 1990; Saltini *et al.*, 1990), and may be involved in local immune responses to inhaled antigens. These cells may also play a role in the activation of AMs during antigenic insult by releasing various cytokines including interferon, IL-2, and IL-4. The cytokine profile of lung lymphocytes shows a preferential production of IL-4 and interferon compared with peripheral blood lymphocytes (Holt *et al.*, 1988; S. Becker, unpublished finding). The relatively low and variable number of lymphocytes that can be purified from BAL fluid has precluded *in vitro* ozone exposure studies with these cells, as well as studies of *in vivo* exposed lymphocytes. Instead, as a model, direct effects of ozone on lymphocyte function have been studied using peripheral blood lymphocytes exposed in PBS in *in vitro* exposure chambers, as described earlier. Stimulation of lymphocytes with pokeweed mitogen after exposure to 1 ppm ozone for 2 hr resulted in decreased cell proliferation and production of IL-2, had no effect on interferon production, and increased production of IL-6 (Becker *et al.*, 1989,1991c). Changes in the relative proportions of the different cytokines produced may affect the outcome of the immune response since the cytokines are intimately involved in the development of cytotoxic T cells and in the preferential production of different immunoglobulin subclasses. In a study by Bocci and Paulesu (1990), ozone exposure of human blood mononuclear cells resulted in production of interferon γ in the absence of additional stimulation of the cells. Interferon γ is the primary macrophage stimulatory cytokine for lymphocytes.

3. Responses of Human and Animal Epithelial Cells

As described in Section II,A,3, epithelial cells in the airways are damaged by exposure to low levels of ozone. PMNs can be found in tissue lining the airways and can also be recovered by nasal and bronchial lavage. Contribution of airway epithelium to the inflammatory reaction is likely since airway epithelial cell cultures of human and several animal species have been shown to secrete 12-HETE, 15-HETE, PGE_2, $PGF_{2\alpha}$, and LTB_4 (Hunter et al., 1985; Henke et al., 1988; Churchill et al., 1989; Duniec et al., 1989; Hansbrough et al., 1989). Airway epithelial cells also produce PAF (Salari and Wong, 1989). All these lipid metabolites have been implicated in airway inflammation and hyperreactivity. Further, airway epithelial cells have been shown to be capable of secreting cytokines IL-6 and IL-8, as well as hematopoietic growth factors such as granulocyte (G), granulocyte–macrophage (GM), and macrophage (M) colony stimulating factors (CSF) (Smith et al., 1990; Standiford et al., 1990; Ohtoshi et al., 1991).

To study ozone effects on human airway epithelium, a model system has been established in which the immortalized bronchial epithelial cell line BEAS-2B was grown to confluence on collagen-impregnated millipore filters (transwells) and differentiated to form tight junctions under the influence of calcium. Before exposure to ozone or air, the medium in the apical compartment was removed to allow direct interaction of the oxidant with the cells. Exposure time courses with different concentrations of ozone established that the epithelial cells responded to ozone exposure by the release of increased levels of eicosanoids PGE_2, TxB_2, LTC_4, and LTD_4 (McKinnon et al., 1992a,b) as well as PAF (Samet et al., 1992). BEAS cells also released aldehyde products derived from arachidonic acid (Madden et al., 1993). Decreased cell viability did not account for these releases. BEAS-2B supernatants collected at various times after ozone exposure contained increased levels of IL-6 and IL-8 (R. Devlin, unpublished observations). Although the cytokines were released apically, the lipid mediators, with the exception of PAF, were preferentially found in the basolateral compartment. Fibronectin levels were also increased in the supernatants of ozone-exposed cells; this molecule was increased in both the apical and basolateral compartments.

In a study by Leikauf et al. (1988) primary cultures of bovine tracheal epithelium were exposed to ozone (0.1–10 ppm) in vitro, and eicosanoid production was measured in the cell supernatants. The ozone-exposed cells showed significant ozone dose-dependent increase in PGE_2, $PGF_{2\alpha}$, and LTB_4 compared with the air-exposed cells. Ozone concentrations as low as 0.1 ppm produced increase in $PGF_{2\alpha}$ levels.

Samet *et al.* (1992) studied the production of PAF in primary cultures of human airway epithelium and in the BEAS-S6 cell line. Both cell types responded to 1 ppm for ozone exposure 15 min by an increased production of PAF (4- versus 8-fold) compared with the air-exposed controls.

IV. Discussion and Conclusions

The findings reviewed in this chapter illustrate that ozone, a major air pollutant, is capable of inducing an inflammatory response in the lung. The data are based on *in vivo* human and animal studies and on *in vitro* studies. The importance and relevance of inflammation is that it can impair host defenses after acute exposure. Inflammation can also cause tissue damage in excess of the tissue damage associated with the induction of the inflammatory response, especially when the condition is perpetuated and becomes chronic, which could also lead to irreversible fibrotic changes in the lung. No doubt ozone is capable of inducing an inflammatory response; however, whether ozone, even under chronic exposure conditions, can lead to a clear fibrotic state in the lung is less clear.

The other issue relative to inflammation is its relationship to lung function and, in particular, to its ability to cause airway hyperreactivity, which has also been established as one of the effects of exposure to ozone. Although this effect has not been the major focus of this review, data presented in this chapter indicate that the relationship between inflammation, as evidenced by the presence of PMNs in the lung, and hyperreactivity has not been clearly established. In fact, the current weight of evidence would suggest that the two phenomena are not mechanistically linked (see Section II,B,3).

Because of the continuous interest in ozone as a potential risk to the public, comparing its effects on lung cells relative to those of other materials including gaseous and particulate pollutants seems important.

Sulfur dioxide has drawn a lot of attention and concern since the middle of the century because of the London "fogs," of which SO_2 was a major component. Several investigators were able to demonstrate that SO_2 caused changes in respiratory patterns and that the effect was concentration dependent (Amdur *et al.*, 1953). Sulfur dioxide by itself, however, has not been shown to be a potent inducer of an inflammatory response in humans or in animal model systems. Sulfuric acid is also thought to be one of the main components of the London "killer fogs" of the 1950s. The most sensitive biological end point for effects of sulfuric acid in healthy adults is a change in mucociliary clearance (Leikauf *et al.*, 1981), apparently by increased airway acidity. Neither sulfur dioxide nor sulfuric acid aerosol has been shown to induce this type of response in animals.

Studies of human exposure to HNO_3 vapor have been performed only recently (Koenig *et al.*, 1989; Becker *et al.*, 1992a), and suggest possible pulmonary function responses in asthmatics. BAL studies (Becker *et al.*, 1992a) of subjects who were exposed to 0.08 ppm HNO_3 for 2 hr with moderate exercise have shown no significant increase in protein concentration, LDH, fibronectin, PGE_2, LTB_4, C3a, α_1-antitrypsin, or neutrophils, indicating that this acid does not cause the permeability changes, cell damage, or inflammatory events in the lungs found with ozone. On the other hand, although superoxide production was decreased after HNO_3 exposure, a significant increase in phagocytic activity of AMs was observed. Further, HNO_3-exposed AMs showed increased resistance to infection with respiratory syncytial virus. Thus, HNO_3 does not appear to cause the damaging effects that ozone does; instead, phagocytic and antiviral activities of AMs appear to be stimulated after HNO_3 inhalation. Additional investigations into the generality of these observations with HNO_3 and other acid air pollutants deserve further attention.

Nitrogen dioxide is the main precursor of ozone and, as such, is a major component of oxidant air pollution. Mice exposed to NO_2 show greater mortality from induced bacterial or viral infections than control mice. These effects may be associated with impaired mucociliary clearance mechanisms and depression of AM functions (Schlesinger, 1987). In humans, some evidence exists of impairment of host defense properties of AMs *in vitro*, including their ability to resist infection to viruses (Frampton *et al.*, 1989). In one study (Devlin *et al.*, 1992a), a significant increase in neutrophils (3.7-fold) was observed in the bronchial washes (but not in the alveolar region) conducted 18 hr after exposure to 2.0 ppm NO_2 for 4 hr. Also, a decrease was seen in phagocytic activity and superoxide release. However, other indicators of inflammation such as PGE_2, fibronectin, and IL-6, which are significantly changed by ozone, were not affected by NO_2. Therefore, NO_2 seems to cause significantly fewer detectable health effects in humans than ozone in controlled chamber studies. However, NO_2 can have synergistic effects when combined with other air pollutants such as ozone (Hazucha *et al.*, 1992).

These comparisons of the effects induced by ozone relative to other air pollutants demonstrate that ozone is probably one of the most .potent gaseous air pollutants with respect to pro-inflammatory response. On a relative scale, however, some inhaled particulate matter seems to be quite potent in its ability to induce an inflammatory response and fibrogenic changes in the lung. Chapter 10 discussed the role of several particles in the induction of fibrosis. In the context of this chapter, a brief comparison of the pro-inflammatory and fibrogenic potential of some of these particles with that of ozone seems useful.

Airway inflammation and fibrosis are common features of prolonged exposure to mineral particles such as silica and asbestos, known to cause a group of diseases commonly referred to as pneumoconioses. Although many studies have documented the etiopathogenesis, the exact mechanism by which these particles can induce inflammatory and fibrogenic lung disease remains to be elucidated. Increasing evidence suggests that AMs play a key role in the onset and development of inflammatory and fibrogenic lung disease through their ability to release potent inflammatory and fibrogenic mediators including IL-1, TNFα, and lipoxygenase metabolites such as LTB$_4$ (Dubois *et al.*, 1989). In fact, in animal studies, TNFα has been shown to be required for silica-induced fibrosis (Piguet *et al.*, 1990). In contrast, studies with humans have shown that exposure to ozone does not cause the release of IL-1 or TNFα. In addition, several studies have shown that silica particles can cause the release of various eicosanoids. Studies with AMs from normal human subjects stimulated with silica particles *in vitro* have shown that eicosanoids associated with fibroblast growth and inflammation (e.g., lipoxygenase metabolites) are increased, whereas those products associated with suppression of fibroblast growth (e.g., PGE$_2$) are decreased (Koren *et al.*, 1992). In a clinical study of nonsmoking subjects with clinically apparent pneumoconiosis, Rom and colleagues (Kelley, 1990) documented elevated levels of insulin-like growth factor (IGF; produced by the AMs obtained by BAL from these patients), which acts as a progression factor and thus complements platelet-derived growth factor (PDGF) in stimulating mitosis in a wide variety of cell types including fibroblasts. Similar results were found in patients with asbestosis.

Asbestosis is an inflammatory and fibrotic process of the alveolar structures that is mediated, at least in part, by cytokines released by activated AMs. The development of pulmonary fibrosis (asbestosis) is characterized by the accumulation of fibroblasts and connective tissue matrix in lung interstitium. The fibrosis causes alterations in the architecture of the lung parenchyma, resulting in abnormal gas exchange and hypoxia. The AM can play a critical role in the pathogenesis of asbestosis that is similar to its putative role in silicosis. Animal studies have demonstrated the production of PDGF, a cytokine that has potent chemotactic and mitogenic effects on mesenchymal cells, can also cause the proliferation of cells such as fibroblasts and muscle cells (Schapira *et al.*, 1991). In addition, an increased number of PMNs and increased levels of TNFα and LTB$_4$ can be found in the BAL fluid of asbestos-exposed rats (Dubois *et al.*, 1989). A very similar profile of mediators and cytokines is found in the BAL fluid of patients with asbestosis (Rom, 1991). Specifically, their BAL fluid contains an increased number of PMNs; the AMs demonstrate high levels of spontaneously released superoxide anion and hydrogen peroxide, increased levels of fibronectin production, and increased release of progression factors such as IGF and PDGF.

These observations suggest a common mechanism by which asbestos and silica modulate the production of inflammatory and fibrogenic mediators and cytokines. Also, a similarity may exist between these occupational diseases and interstitial pulmonary fibrosis (IPF) in terms of the cytokines produced by their AMs.

Various other lung diseases can cause fibrosis, some of which are caused by known etiologic agents such as organic dusts (silica, asbestos) and others of which are caused by unknown etiologic agents (e.g., sarcoidosis). To review the fibrogenic processes in each of these diseases is beyond the scope of this chapter (for review, see Crystal *et al.*, 1984). However, mentioning that fibroid lung disorders are chronic inflammatory processes in the lower respiratory tract that injure the lung and modulate the proliferation of mesenchymal cells that form the basis for fibrotic scar is appropriate. Consistent with the concept that inflammation drives the process of fibrosis, the basis for the differences among the fibrotic lung disorders centers on the differences in the type of inflammation that characterizes each disorder. In this regard, inflammation of some interstitial lung disorders is dominated by AMs, whereas in others the inflammation has major components of PMNs, lymphocytes, and/or eosinophils.

The preceding discussion reveals that the inflammatory responses caused by exposure to organic materials such as silica or asbestos or to the cause of IPF are different than those caused by ozone. One of the major differences is that cells or fluid obtained from BAL fluids of ozone-exposed subjects do not contain demonstrable levels or elevated levels (compared with control exposures) of cytokines such as IL-1, TNFα, or PDGF, which have been shown to be critical for the development of fibrotic lung disease. The controlled human exposures do, however, demonstrate that acute ozone exposure induces the transient increase in cell types (primarily PMNs) and in some materials (e.g., fibronectin, PGE$_2$) that are also known to be associated with inflammation. Particulate matter such as silica and asbestos is much more pro-inflammatory and fibrogenic than the previously mentioned gaseous pollutants.

The type of mechanistic studies that can be done *in vitro* with isolated cells are important and complement the *in vivo* data. The significance of and the conclusions drawn from *in vitro* ozone exposure studies will be briefly discussed. Based on *in vitro* experiments using AMs exposed to ozone *in vivo*, these cells are not directly responsible for recruiting inflammatory cells into the airways since AMs produce neither chemotactic mediators nor inflammatory cytokines (see Section III,A,1). However, the AMs are no doubt altered as a result of *in vivo* ozone exposure, as revealed by two-dimensional gel analysis of these cells, as far as some of their functions related to host defenses are concerned. The *in vitro* exposure studies of AMs from unexposed subjects support the contention that production of cytokines by ozone-exposed AMs is not a mechanism of ozone-induced inflammatory response. Moreover, the two-dimensional gel analysis of *in vitro*-exposed AMs revealed only minor changes in protein synthesis (Becker *et al.*, 1991b) relative to the changes observed in *in vivo*-exposed AMs (Devlin and Koren, 1990).

As described in Section II, epithelial cells in the centriacinar region are most heavily damaged by ozone exposure, but cell damage and effects on ciliary function are also found in the bronchial region. The potential of bronchial epithelial cells to induce inflammatory events has only recently been realized. Brush scrapings or biopsy techniques can be used to obtain these cells for two-dimensional gel and PCR analysis of the various inflammatory mediators. Bronchial epithelium has been found to express mRNA for IL-8 and IL-1. *In vitro*, these cells can be induced to express and produce IL-6 and GM-CSF also (Becker *et al.*, 1992b). Using such techniques, key questions related to the response of respiratory epithelium to ozone exposure can be addressed. In addition, the human BEAS-2B bronchial epithelial cell line can be used as a model to study the effects of ozone on epithelial cells *in vitro*. The findings with the BEAS-2B cell line model for epithelial cell injury indicate that this cell type may be the target and the effector cell in the inflammatory response to ozone, since these cells release arachidonic acid metabolites, PAF, IL-8, IL-6, and fibronectin on exposure to ozone under exposure conditions that cause no changes in the levels of cytokines and eicosanoids in human AMs. These findings, combined with the results presented earlier that were obtained with the two-dimensional gel technique, strongly indicate that the observed effects of ozone exposure on AMs are secondary in nature. Model systems designed to assess the temporal relationship and interactive events leading to the changes in biomarker expression that are detected after exposure to ozone will need to employ co-culture techniques of epithelial cells, inflammatory cells, and fibroblasts.

To understand better the effects of ozone on the lung, new methodologies will need to be explored that will provide better insight into the role epithelial cells play in the response to ozone. NAL is a noninvasive technique that has been used to assess the inflammatory response of the upper airways to various materials including ozone (Graham and Koren, 1990). In the case of ozone, NAL can be used as a surrogate for the more invasive BAL technique, with some assurance that inflammation seen in nasal passages mirrors inflammation present in the alveolar region of the lung. In addition to measuring NAL fluid for the presence of mediators, nasal brush scrapings or biopsies in which several thousands of cells are removed can also be performed. These cells can then be analyzed by novel techniques such as RNA *in situ* hybridization and PCR. This approach may extend the sensitivity and the range of end points that can be assayed. This newly emerging area of study is likely eventually to provide us with a better understanding of the health effects of oxidant pollutants. Clearly much more research in the clinical, epidemiological, and animal toxicology arenas is needed to determine the potential significance and risk associated with the inflammatory response seen after exposure to ozone.

Acknowledgments

The authors thank L. Folinsbee and M. Madden for their critical review, and V. Worrell for excellent secretarial assistance. The authors also recognize the invaluable assistance provided by the Center for Environmental Medicine and Lung Biology (EPA cooperative agreement #CR812738) and its Pulmonary Fellows in performing the bronchoscopies and bronchoalveolar lavages related to the studies mentioned in this chapter.

References

Aizawa, H., Chung, K. F., Leikauf, G. D., Ueki, I., Bethel, R. A., O'Byrne, P. M., Hirose, T., and Nadel, J. A. (1985). Significance of thromboxane generation in ozone-induced airway hyperresponsiveness in dogs. *J. Appl. Physiol.* **59**, 1918–1923.

Amdur, M. O., Melvin, W. W., and Drinker, P. (1953). Effects of inhalation of sulfur dioxide by man. *Lancet* **2**, 758–759.

Amoruso, M. A., Witz, G., and Goldstein, B. D. (1981). Decreased superoxide anion radical production by rat alveolar macrophages following inhalation of ozone or nitrogen dioxide. *Life Sci.* **28**, 2215–2221.

Amoruso, M., Laskin, D., Liesch, J., Goldstein, B., and Robertson, F. (1988). Alteration in rat alveolar macrophage production of interleukin-1 following inhalation of ozone. *Toxicologist* **8**, 196.

Barr, B. C., Hyde, D. M., Plopper, C. G., and Dungworth, D. L. (1988). Distal airway remodeling in rats chronically exposed to ozone. *Am. Rev. Resp. Dis.* **137**, 924–938.

Barr, B. C., Hyde, D. M., Plopper, C. G., and Dungworth, D. L. (1990). A comparison of terminal airway remodeling in chronic daily versus episodic ozone exposure. *Toxicol. Appl. Pharmacol.* **106**, 384–407.

Barry, B. E., Mercer, R. R., Miller, F. J., and Crapo, J. D. (1988). Effects of inhalation of 0.25 ppm ozone on the terminal bronchioles of juvenile and adult rats. *Exp. Lung Res.* **14**, 225–245.

Bascom, R., Naclerio, R. M., Fitzgerald, T. K., Kagey-Sobotka, A., and Proud, D. (1990). Effect of ozone inhalation on the response to nasal challenge with antigen of allergic subjects. *Am. Rev. Resp. Dis.* **142**, 594–601.

Bassett, D. J., Bowen-Kelly, E., Elbon, C. L., and Reichenbaugh, S. S. (1988a). Rat lung recovery from 3 days of continuous exposure to 0.75 ppm ozone. *J. Toxicol. Environ. Health* **25**, 329–347.

Bassett, D. J., Bowen-Kelly, E., Brewster, E. L., Elbon, C. L., Eichenbaugh, S. S., Bunton, T., and Kerr, J. S. (1988b). A reversible model of acute injury based on ozone exposure. *Lung* **166**, 355–369.

Becker, S., Jordan, R. L., Orlando, G. S., and Koren, H. S. (1989). In vitro ozone exposure inhibits mitogen-induced lymphocyte proliferation and IL-2 production. *J. Toxicol. Environ. Health* **26**, 469–483.

Becker, S., Harris, D. T., and Koren, H. S. (1990). Characterization of normal human lung lymphocytes and interleukin-2 induced Lung T cell lines. *Am. J. Resp. Cell. Mol. Biol.* **3**, 441–448.

Becker, S., Quay, J., and Soukup, J. (1991a). Cytokine (tumor necrosis factor, IL-6, and IL-

8) production by respiratory syncytial virus-infected human alveolar macrophages. *J. Immunol.* **147,** 4307–4312.

Becker, S., Madden, M. C., Newman, S. L., Devlin, R. B., and Koren, H. S. (1991b). Modulation of human alveolar macrophage properties by ozone exposure *in vitro. Toxicol. Appl. Pharmacol.* **110,** 403–415.

Becker, S., Quay, J., and Koren, H. S. (1991c). Effect of ozone on immunoglobulin production by human B cells *in vitro. J. Toxicol. Environ. Health* **34,** 353–366.

Becker, S., Roger, L. J., Devlin, R. B., and Koren, H. S. (1992a). Increased phagocytosis and antiviral activity of alveolar macrophages from humans exposed to nitric acid. *Am. Rev. Resp. Dis.* **145,** A429.

Becker, S., Henke, D., and Koren, H. S. (1992b). Expression of inflammatory cytokines in normal and stimulated airway epithelium. *Am. Rev. Resp. Dis.* **145,** A831.

Becker, S., Koren, H. S., and Henke, D. C. (1993). Interleukin-8 expression in normal nasal epithelium and its modulation by infection with respiratory syncytial virus and cytokines tumor necrosis factor, interleukin-1, and interleukin-6. *Am. J. Respir. Cell Mol. Biol.* **8,** 20–27.

Becker, S., Quay, J., Koren, H. S., and Haskill, J. S. (1994). Constitutive and stimulated MCP-1, GROα, β, and γ expression in human airway epithelium and bronchoalveolar macrophages. *Am. J. Physiol. (Lung Cell. Mol. Physiol.)* in press.

Beutler, B., and Cerami, A. (1986). Cachectin: More than a tumor necrosis factor. *N. Engl. J. Med.* **316,** 379–385.

Bocci, V., and Paulesu, L. (1990). Studies on the biological effects of ozone. 1. Induction of interferon gamma in human leucocytes. *Haematologica* **75,** 510–515.

Brown, G. P., Monick, M. M., and Hunninghake, G. W. (1988). Human alveolar macrophage arachidonic acid metabolism. *Am. J. Physiol.* **245,** C809–815.

Brummer, M. E. G., Schwartz, L. W., and McQuillen, N. K. (1977). A quantitative study of lung damage by scanning electron microscopy: Inflammatory cell response to high-ambient levels of ozone. *Scan. Electron Microsc.* **2,** 513–518.

Chapman, H. A., Allen, C. L., Stone, O. L., and Fair, D. S. (1984). Human alveolar macrophages synthesize factor VII *in vitro:* Possible role in interstitial lung disease. *J. Clin. Invest.* **75,** 2030–2038.

Chitano, P., Di-Stefano, A., Finotto, S., Zavattini, G., Mapp, C., Fabbri, L. M., and Allegra, L. (1989). Ambroxol inhibits airway hyperresponsiveness induced by ozone in dogs. *Respiration* **55,** 74–78.

Churchill, L., Chilton, F. H., Resau, J. H., Bascom, R., Hubbard, W. C., and Proud, D. (1989). Cyclooxygenase metabolism of endogenous arachidonic acid by cultured human tracheal epithelial cells. *Am. Rev. Resp. Dis.* **140,** 449–459.

Costa, D. L., Tepper, J. S., Lehmann, J. R., Weber, M. F., Winsett, D. W., Hatch, G. E., and Devlin, R. B. (1992). Strain as a factor in the magnitude and time-course of response to acute ozone (03): A study of lung dysfunction and injury in Wistar, Fischer, and Sprague–Dawley rats. *Am. Rev. Resp. Dis.* **145,** A96.

Crystal, R. G., Bitterman, P. B., Rennard, S. I., Hance, A., and Keogh, B.A. (1984). Interstitial lung disease of unknown cause: Disorders characterized by chronic inflammation of the lower respiratory tract. *N. Engl. J. Med.* **310,** 154–166, 235–244.

Damji, K. S., and Sherwin, R. P. (1989). The effect of ozone and simulated high altitude on murine lung elastin: Quantitation by image analysis. *Toxicol. Ind. Health* **5,** 995–1003.

Deuel, T. F., Senior R. M., Huang, J. S., and Griffin, G. L. (1982). Chemotaxis of monocytes and neutrophils to platelet-derived growth factor. *J. Clin. Invest.* **69,** 1046–1049.

Devlin, R. B., and Koren H. S. (1990) The use of quantitative two-dimensional gel electrophoresis to analyze changes in alveolar macrophage proteins in human exposed to ozone. *Am. J. Resp. Cell Mol. Biol.* **2,** 281–288.

Devlin, R. B., McDonnell, W. F., Perez, R., Becker, S., and Koren, H. S. (1990). Humans exposed to 0.4 ppm ozone exhibit cellular and biochemical changes in the lung one hour following exposure. *Am. Rev. Resp. Dis.* **141**, A71.

Devlin, R. B., McDonnell, W. F., Perez, R., Becker, S., House, D. E., and Koren, H. S. (1991). Prolonged exposure of humans to ambient levels of ozone causes cellular and biochemical changes in the lung. *Am. Rev. Resp. Dis.* **4**, 72–81.

Devlin, R. G., Horstman, D., Becker, S., Gerrity, T., Madden, M., and Koren, H. S. (1992a). Inflammatory response in humans exposed to 2.0 ppm NO_2. *Am. Rev. Resp. Dis.* **145**, A456.

Drazen, J. M., and Austen, K. F. (1987). Leukotrienes and airway responses. *Am. Rev. Resp. Dis.* **135**, 1176–1185.

Dubois, C. M., Bissonette, E., and Rona-Pleszczynski, M. (1989). Asbestos fibers and silica particles stimulate rat alveolar macrophages to release tumor necrosis factor. *Am. Rev. Resp. Dis.* **139**, 1257–1264.

Duniec, Z. M., Eling, T. E., Jetten, A. M., Gray, T. E., and Nettesheim, P. (1989). Arachidonic acid metabolism in normal and transformed rat tracheal epithelial cells and its possible role in regulation of cell proliferation. *Exp. Lung Res.* **15**, 391–408.

Driscoll, K. E., Vollmuth, T. A., and Schlesinger, R. B. (1987). Acute and subchronic ozone inhalation in the rabbit: Response of alveolar macrophages. *J. Toxicol. Environ. Health* **21** 27–43.

Driscoll, K. E., Leikauf, G. D., and Schlesinger, R. B. (1988). Effects of *in vitro* and *in vivo* ozone exposure on eicosanoid production by rabbit alveolar macrophages. *Inhalation Toxicol.* **1**, 109–122.

Eschenbacher, W. L., Ying, R. L., Kreit, J. W., and Gross, K. B. (1989). Ozone-induced lung function changes in normal and asthmatic subjects and the effect of indomethacin. In "Atmospheric Ozone Research and Its Policy Implications" (T. Schneider, S. D. Lee, G. J. R. Wolters, and L. D. Grant, eds.), pp. 493–499. Elsevier Science Publishers, Amsterdam.

Evans, T. W., Brokaw, J. J., Chung, K. F., Nadel, J. A., and McDonald, D. M. (1988). Ozone-induced bronchial hyperresponsiveness in the rat is not accompanied by neutrophil influx or increased vascular permeability in the trachea. *Am. Rev. Resp. Dis.* **138**, 140–144.

Fabbri, L. M., Aizawa, H., Alpert, S. E., Walters, E. H., O'Byrne, P. M., Gold, B. D., Nadel, J. A., and Holtzman, M. J. (1984). Airway hyperresponsiveness and changes in cell counts in bronchoalveolar lavage after ozone exposure in dogs. *Am. Rev. Resp. Dis.* **129**, 288–291.

Fantone, J. C., and Ward, P. A., III (1984). Mechanisms of lung parenchymal injury. *Am. Rev. Resp. Dis.* **130**, 484–491.

Farrell, B. P., Kerr, H. D., Kulle, T. J., Sauder, L. R., and Young, J. L. (1979). Adaptation in human subjects to the effects of inhaled ozone after repeated exposure. *Am. Rev. Resp. Dis.* **119**, 725–730.

Fels, A. O., and Cohn, Z. A. (1986). The alveolar macrophage. *J. Appl. Physiol.* **60**, 353–369.

Folinsbee, L. J., Bedi, J. F., and Horvath, S. M. (1980). Respiratory responses in humans repeatedly exposed to low concentrations of ozone. *Am. Rev. Resp. Dis.* **121**, 431–439.

Frampton, M. W., Smeglin, A. M., Roberts, N. J., Finkelstein, J. N., Morrow, P. E., and Utell, M. J. (1989). Nitrogen dioxide exposure *in vivo* and human alveolar macrophage inactivation of influenza virus *in vitro*. *Environ. Res.* **48**, 179–192.

Friedman, M., Madden, M. C., Samet, J. M., and Koren, H. S. (1992). Effects of ozone exposure on lipid metabolism in human alveolar macrophages. *Environ. Health Perspect.* **97**: 95–101.

Garcia, J. G. N., Noonan, T. C., Jubiz, W., and Malik, A. B. (1987). Leukotrienes and the pulmonary microcirculation. *Am. Rev. Resp. Dis.* **136**, 161–169.

Gardner, D. E. (1982). Effect of gases and airborne particles on lung infections. *In* "Air Pollution" (J. McGrath and C. O. Barnes, eds.), pp. 47–79. Academic Press, New York.

Gliner, J. A. Horvath, S. M., and Folinsbee, L. J. (1983). Pre-exposure to low ozone concentrations does not diminish the pulmonary function response on exposure to higher ozone concentration. *Am. Rev. Resp. Dis.* **127**, 51–55.

Graham, D. E., and Koren, H. S., (1990). Biomarkers of inflammation in ozone-exposed humans. *Ann. Rev. Respir. Dis.* **142**, 152–156.

Graham, D. E., Henderson, F., and House, D. E. (1988). Neutrophil influx measured in nasal lavages of humans exposed to ozone. *Arch. Environ. Health* **43**, 229–233.

Grose, E. C., Stevens, M. A., Hatch, G. E., Jaskot, R. H., Selgrade, M. J. K., Stead, A. G., Costa, D. L., and Graham, J. A. (1989). The impact of a 12-month exposure to a diurnal pattern of ozone on pulmonary function, antioxidant biochemistry, and immunology. *In* "Atmospheric Ozone Research and Its Policy Implications" (T. Schneider, S. D. Lee, G. J. R. Wolters, and L. D. Grant, eds.), pp. 535–544. Elsevier Science Publishers, Amsterdam.

Gross, K. B., and White, H. J. (1987). Functional and pathologic consequences of a 52-week exposure to 0.5 PPM ozone followed by a clean air recovery period. *Lung* **165**, 283–295.

Gross, T. J., Simon, R. H., and Sitrin, R. G. (1990). Expression of urokinase-type plasminogen activator by rat pulmonary alveolar epithelial cells. *Am. J. Resp. Cell Mol. Biol.* **3**, 449–456.

Gunnison, A. F., Finkelstein, I., Weidman, P., Su, W. Y., Sobo, M., and Schlesinger, R. B. (1990).Age-dependent effect of ozone on pulmonary eicosanoid metabolism in rabbits and rats. *Fund. Appl. Toxicol.* **15**, 779–790.

Guth, D. J., Warren, D. L., and Last, J. A. (1986). Comparative sensitivity of measurements of lung damage made by bronchoalveolar lavage after short-term exposure of rats to ozone. *Toxicology* **40**, 131–143.

Hackney, J. D., Linn, W. S., Mohler, J. G., and Collier, C. R. (1977). Adaptation to short-term respiratory effects of ozone in men exposed repeatedly. *J. Appl. Physiol. Resp. Environ. Exercise Physiol.* **43**, 82–85.

Hansbrough, J. R., Atlas, A. B., Turk, J., and Holtzman, M. J. (1989). Arachidonate 12-lipoxygenase and cyclooxygenase: PGE isomerase are predominant pathways of oxygenation in bovine tracheal epithelium. *Am. J. Resp. Cell. Mol. Biol.* **1**, 237–244.

Harder, S. D., Harris, D. T., House, D., and Koren, H. S. (1990). Inhibition of human antureal killer activity following *in vitro* exposure to ozone. *Inhal. Toxicol.* **2**, 161–173.

Hazucha, M., Pape, G., Madden, M., Koren, H., Kehrl, H., and Bromberg, P. (1991). Effects of cyclooxygenase inhibition on ozone-induced respiratory inflammation and lung function. *Am. Rev. Resp. Dis.* **143**, A701.

Hazucha, M. J., Seal, E., Folinsbee, L. J., and Bromberg, P. A. (1992). Lung function response of healthy subjects following sequential exposures to NO_2 and O_3. *Am. Rev. Resp. Dis.* **145**, A456.

Henderson, W. R., Jr. (1987). Eicosanoids and lung inflammation. *Am. Rev. Resp. Dis.* **135**, 1176–1185.

Henke, D., Danilowicz, R. M., Curtis, J. F., Boucher, R. C., and Eling, T. E. (1988). Metabolism of arachidonic acid by human nasal and bronchial epithelial cells. *Arch. Biochem. Biophys.* **267**, 426–436.

Hiroshima, K., Kohno, T., Ohwada, H., and Hayashi, Y. (1990). Morphological study of the effects of ozone on rat lung. II. Long term exposure. *Exp. Mol. Pathol.* **50**, 270–280.

Holt, P. G., Kees, U. R., Shon-Hegrad, M. A., Rose, A., Bilkyd, N., Bowman, R., and Robinson, B. W. (1988). Limiting dilution analysis of T cells extracted from solid human lung tissue: Comparison of precursor frequencies for proliferative responses and lymphokine production between lung and blood T cells from individual donors. *Immunology* **64**, 649–654.

Holtzman, M. J. (1991). Arachidonic acid metabolism. *Am. Rev. Resp. Dis.* **143**, 188–203.

Holtzman, M. J., Fabbri, L. M., O'Byrne, P. M., Gold, B. D., Aizawa, H., Walters, E. H., Apert, S. E., and Nadel, J. A. (1983a). Importance of airway inflammation for hyperresponsiveness induced by ozone. *Am. Rev. Resp. Dis.* **127,** 686–690.

Holtzman, M. J., Aizawa, H., Nadel, J. A., and Goetzl. (1983b). Selective generation of LTB4 by tracheal epithelial cells from dogs. *Biochem. Biophys. Res. Commun.* **114,** 1071–1076.

Horvath, S. M., Gilner, J. A., and Folinsbee, L. J. (1981). Adaptation to ozone: Duration of effect. *Am. Rev. Resp. Dis.* **123,** 496–499.

Hotchkiss, J. A., Harkema, J. R., Sun, J. D., and Henderson, R. F. (1989). Comparison of acute ozone-induced nasal and pulmonary inflammatory responses in rats. *Toxicol. Appl. Pharmacol.* **98,** 289–302.

Hunninghake, G. W. (1984). Release of interleukin-1 by alveolar macrophages of patients with active pulmonary sarcoidosis. *Am. Rev. Resp. Dis.* **129,** 569–572.

Hunter, J. A., Finkbeiner, W. E., Nadel, J. A., Goetzl, E. J., and Holtzman, M. J. (1985). Predominant generation of 15-lipoxygenase metabolites of arachidonic acid by epithelial cells from human trachea. *Proc. Natl. Acad. Sci. USA* **82,** 4633–4637.

Hyde, D. M., Plopper, C. G., Harkema, J. R., St. George, J. A., Tyler, W. S., and Dungworth, D. L. (1989). Ozone-induced structural changes in monkey respiratory system. *In* "Atmospheric Ozone Research and Its Policy Implications" (T. Schneider, S. D. Lee, G. J. R. Wolters, and L. D. Grant, eds.), pp. 523–532. Elsevier Science Publishers, Amsterdam.

Kelley, J. (1990). Cytokines in the lung. *Am. Rev. Resp. Dis.* **141,** 765–788.

Kimura, A., and Goldstein, E. (1981). Effect of ozone on concentration of lysozyme in phagocytizing alveolar macrophages. *J. Infect. Dis.* **143,** 241–251.

Kleeberger, S. R., Kolbe, J., Adkinson, N. F., Jr., Peters, S. P., and Spannhake, W. E. (1988). The role of mediators in the response of the canine peripheral lung to 1 ppm ozone. *Am. Rev. Resp. Dis.* **137,** 321–325.

Kleeberger, S. R., Kleeberger, S. R., Bassett, D. J., Jakab, G. J., and Levitt, R. C. (1990). A genetic model for evaluation of susceptibility to ozone-induced inflammation. *Am. J. Physiol.* **258,** L313–320.

Koenig, J. Q., Covert, D. S., and Pierson, W. E. (1989). Effects of inhalation of acidic compounds on pulmonary function in allergic adolescent subjects. *Environ. Health Perspect.* **79,** 173, 178.

Koren, H. S., Devlin, R. B., Graham, D. E., Mann, R., McGee, M. P., Horstman, D. H., Kozumbo, W. S., Becker, S., House, D. E., McDonnell, W. F., and Bromberg, P. A. (1989). Ozone induced inflammation in the lower airways of human subjects. *Am. Rev. Resp. Dis.* **139,** 404–415.

Koren, H. S., Hatch, G. E., and Graham, D. E., (1990). Nasal lavage as a tool in assessing acute inflammation in response to inhaled pollutants. *Toxicology* **60,** 15–25.

Koren, H. S., Devlin, R. B., Becker, S., Perez, R., and McDonnell, W. F. (1991). Time-dependent changes of markers associated with inflammation in the lungs of humans exposed to ambient levels of ozone. *Toxicol. Pathol.* **19,** 406–411.

Kulle, T. J., Sauder, L. R., Kerr, H. D., Farrell, B. P., Bermel, M. S., and Smith, D. (1982). Duration of pulmonary function adaptation to ozone in humans. *Am. Ind. Hyg. Assoc. J.* **43,** 832–837.

Last, J. A., Reiser, K. M., Tyler, W. S., and Rucker, R. B. (1984). Long-term consequences of exposure to ozone. I. Lung collagen content. *Toxicol. Appl. Pharmacol.* **72,** 111–119.

Le, J., and Vilcek, J. (1987). Tumor necrosis factor and interleukin 1: Cytokines with multiple overlapping biological activities. *Lab. Invest.* **56,** 234–248.

Leikauf, G., Yeates, D. B., Wales, K. A., Spektor, D., Albert, R. E., and Lippmann, M. (1981). Effects of sulfuric acid aerosol on respiratory mechanics and mucociliary particle clearance in healthy nonsmoking adults. *Am. Ind. Hyg. Assoc. J.* **42,** 273–282.

Leikauf, G. D., Driscoll, K. E., and Wey, H. E. (1988). Ozone-induced augmentation of eicosanoid metabolism in epithelial cells from bovine trachea. *Am. Rev. Resp. Dis.* **137**, 435–442.

Linn, W. S., Medway, D. A., Anzar, U. T., Valencia, L. M., Spier, C. E., Tsao, F. S. O., Fischer, D. A., and Hackney, J. D. (1982). Persistence of adaptation to ozone in volunteers exposed repeatedly over six weeks. *Am. Rev. Resp. Dis.* **125**, 491–495.

Lippmann, M. (1989). Health effects of ozone. *JAPCA* **39**, 672–695.

Madden, M. C., Eling, T. E., Dailey, L. A., and Friedman, M. (1991). The effect of ozone exposure on rat alveolar macrophage arachidonic acid metabolism. *Exp. Lung Res.* **17**, 47–63.

Madden, M. C., Hazucha, M., Devlin, R. B., Harder, S. D., Cole, L. E., Pape, G., Becker, S., and Koren, H. S. (1991b). Effects of ibuprofen administration on cellular and biochemical lung lavage parameters in ozone-exposed subjects. *Am. Rev. Resp. Dis.* **143**, A699.

Madden, M. C., Friedman, M., Hanley, N., Siegler, E., Quay, J., Becker, S., Devlin, R., and Koren, H. S. (1993). Chemical nature and immunotoxicological properties of arachidonic acid degradation products formed by exposure to ozone. *Environ. Health Perspect.* **101**, 154–164.

McDonnell, W. F., Horstman, D. H., Hazucha, M. J., Seal, E., Haak, E. D., Salaam, S., and House, D. E. (1983). Pulmonary effects of ozone exposure during exercise: dose-response characteristics. *J. Appl. Physiol. Resp. Environ. Exercise Physiol.* **54**, 1345–1352.

McDonnell, W. F., Horstman, D. H., Abdul-Salaam, S., and House, D. E. (1985). Reproducibility of individual responses to ozone exposure. *Am. Rev. Resp. Dis.* **131**, 36–40.

McGee, M., Devlin, R. B., Saluta, G., and Koren, H. S. (1990). Tissue factor and factor VII mRNAs in human alveolar macrophages: Effects of breathing ozone. *Blood* **75**, 122–27.

McKinnon, K., Noah, T., Madden, M., Koren, H., and Devlin, R. (1992a). Cultured bronchial epithelial cells produce eicosanoids, cytokines, and fibronectin in response to ozone exposure. *Chest* **101**, 22 (S).

McKinnon, K., Madden, M. C., Noah, T. L., and Devlin, R. B. (1992b). *In vitro* ozone exposure increases release of arachidonic acid products from a human bronchial epithelial cell line. *J. Toxicol. Appl. Pharmacol.* **118**, 215–223.

Moffatt, R. K., Hyde, D. M., Plopper, C. G., Tyler, W. S., and Putney, L. F. (1987). Ozone-induced adaptive and reactive cellular changes in respiratory bronchioles of bonnet monkeys. *Exp. Lung Res.* **12**, 57–74.

Montgomery, M. R., Raska-Emery, P., and Balis, J. U. (1991). Recovery of lung pyridine nucleotides following acute exposure of adult and aged rats to ozone. *J. Toxicol. Environ. Health* **34**, 115–126.

Murlas, C. G., and Roum, J. H. (1985a). Sequence of pathologic changes in the airway mucosa of guinea pigs during ozone-induced bronchial hyperreactivity. *Am. Rev. Resp. Dis.* **131**, 314–320.

Murlas, C. G., and Roum, J. H. (1985b). Bronchial hyperreactivity occurs in steroid-treated guinea pigs depleted of leukocytes by cyclophosphamide. *J. Appl. Physiol.* **58**, 1630–1637.

Noah, T. L., and Becker, S., (1993). Respiratory syncytial virus-induced cytokine production by human bronchial epithelial cell line. *Am. J. Physiol. (Lung Cell. Mol. Physiol.)* **265**, L472–L478.

O'Byrne, P. M., Walters, E. H., Gold, B. D., Aizawa, H., Fabbri, L. M., Alpert, S. E., and Nadel, J. A., (1984a). Neutrophil depletion inhibits airway hyperresponsiveness induced by ozone exposure. *Am. Rev. Resp. Dis.* **130**, 214–219.

O'Byrne, P. M., Walters, E. H., Aizawa, H., Fabbri, L. M., Holtzman, M. J., and Nadel, J. A. (1984b). Indomethacin inhibits the airway hyperresponsiveness but not the neutrophil influx induced by ozone in dogs. *Am. Rev. Resp. Dis.* **130**, 220–224.

Ohtoshi, T., Vanchieri, C., Cox, G., Gauldie, J., Dolovich, J., Denburg, J. A., and Jordana,

M. (1991). Monocyte-macrophage differentiation induced by human upper airway epithelial cells. *Am. J. Cell. Mol. Biol.* **4**, 255–263.

Okazawa, A., Kobayashi, H., Adachi, M., Takahashi, T., and Misawa, M. (1990). [The effect of leukotriene C_4/D_4 receptor antagonist (ONO-1078) and thromboxane A2 synthetase inhibitor (OKY-046) on airway hyperresponsiveness induced by ozone exposure in guinea pigs.] *Nippon-Kyobu-Shikkan-Gakkai-Zasshi* **28**, 293–299.

Pickrell, J. A., Gregory, R. E., Cole, D. J., Hahn, F. F., and Henderson, R. F. (1987). Effect of acute ozone exposure on the proteinase-antiproteinase balance in the rat lung. *Exp. Mol. Pathol.* **46**, 168–179.

Piguet, P. F., Collart, M. A., Grau, G. G., Sappino, A. P., and Vassalli, P. (1990). *Nature (London)* **344**, 245–247.

Pino, M. V., Hyde, D. M., and Stovall, M. Y. (1991). Strain differences in the response of the rat lung to an acute ozone exposure. *Am. Rev. Resp. Dis.* **143**, A698.

Pino, M., Stovall, M. Y., Levin, J. R., Devlin, R. B., Koren, H. S., and Hyde, D. M. (1992). Acute ozone-induced injury in neutrophil-depleted rats. *Tox. Appl. Pharm.* **114**, 268–276.

Pryor, W. A., Das, B., and Church, D. F. (1991). The ozonation of unsaturated fatty acids: Aldehydes and hydrogen peroxide as products and possible mediators of ozone toxicity. *Chem. Res. Toxicol.* **4**, 341–348.

Rankin, J. A., Sylvester, I., Smith, S., Yoshimura, T., and Leonard, E. J. (1990). Macrophages cultured *in vitro* release leukotriene B4 and neutrophil attractant protein (interleukin-8) sequentially in response to stimulation with lipopolysaccharide and zymosan. *J. Clin. Invest.* **86**, 1556–1561.

Reiser, K. M., Tyler, W. S., Hennessy, S. M., Dominguez, J. J., and Last, J. A. (1987). Long-term consequences of exposure to ozone. II. Structural alterations in lung collagen of monkeys. *Toxicol. Appl. Pharmacol.* **89**, 314–322.

Reynolds, H. Y. (1987). Bronchoalveolar lavage. *Am. Rev. Resp. Dis.* **135**, 250–263.

Rom, W. N. (1991). Relationship of inflammatory cell cytokines to disease severity in individuals with occupational inorganic dust exposure. *Am. J. Ind. Med.* **19**, 15–27.

Salari, H., and Wong, A. (1989). Generation of platelet activating factor (PAF) by a human lung epithelial cell line. *Eur. J. Pharmacol.* **175**, 253–259.

Saltini, C., Kirby, M., Trapnell, B. C., Tamura, N., and Crystal, R. G. (1990). Biasad accumulation of T lymphocytes with memory-type CD45 leukocyte common antigen gene expression on the epithelial surfaces of human lung. *J. Exp. Med.* **171**, 1123–1140.

Samet, J. M., Noah, T. L., Devlin, R. B., Yankaskas, J. R., McKinnon, K., Dailey, L. A., and Friedman, M. (1992). Effect of ozone on platelet activating factor production in phorbol-differentiated HL60 cells, a human bronchial epithelial cell line (BEAS S6) and primary human bronchial epithelial cells. *Am. J. Resp. Cell. Mol. Biol.* **7**, 514–522.

Schapira, R. M., Osornio-Vargas, A., and Brody, A. R. (1991). Inorganic particles induce secretion of a macrophage homologue of platelet-derived growth factor in a density and time-dependent manner *in vitro*. *Exp. Lung Res.* **17**, 1011–1024.

Schelegle, E. S., Adams, W. C., and Siefkin, A. D. (1987). Indomethacin pretreatment reduces ozone-induced pulmonary function decrements in human subjects. *Am. Rev. Resp. Dis.* **136**, 1350–1354.

Schelegle, E. S., Siefkin, A. D., and McDonald, R. J. (1991). Time course of ozone-induced neutrophilia in normal humans. *Am. Rev. Resp. Dis.* **143**, 1353–1358.

Schlesinger, R. B. (1987). Effects of intermittent inhalation exposures to mixed atmospheres of NO_2 and H_2SO_4 on rabbit alveolar macrophages. *J. Toxicol. Environ. Health* **22**, 301–312.

Schlesinger, R. B., Driscoll, K. B., Gunnison, A. F., and Zelikoff, J. T. (1990). Pulmonary arachidonic metabolism following acute exposure to ozone and nitrogen dioxide. *J. Toxicol. Environ. Health* **31**, 275–290.

Schwartz, L. W., Dungworth, D. L., Mustafa, M. G., Tarkington, B. K., and Tyler, W. S.

(1976). Pulmonary responses of rats to ambient levels of ozone: Effects of 7-day intermittent or continuous exposure. *Lab. Invest.* **34,** 565–578.

Seltzer, J., bigby, B. G., Stulbarg, M., Holtzman, M. J., Nadel, J. A., Ueki, I. F., Leikauf, G. D., Goetzl, E. J., and Boushey, H. A. (1986). Ozone-induced change in bronchial reactivity to methacholine and airway inflammation in humans. *J. Appl. Physiol.* **60,** 1321–1326.

Shelly, S. A., Paciga, J. E., and Balis, J. U. (1991). Lysozyme is an ozone-sensitive component of alveolar type II cell lamellar bodies. *Biochim. Biophys. Acta* **1096,** 338–344.

Shima, M., and Adachi, M. (1991). Changes of procoagulant and fibrinolytic activities in the alveoli of rats exposed to ozone. *Nippon-Eiseigaku Zasshi* **46,** 724–733.

Shoji, S., Ertl, R. F., Liner, J., Romberger, D. J., and Rennard, S. I. (1990). Bronchial epithelial cells produce chemotactic activity for bronchial epithelial cells. *Am. Rev. Resp. Dis.* **141,** 218–225.

Slauson, D. O. (1982). The mediation of pulmonary inflammatory injury. *Adv. Vet. Sci. Comp. Med.* **26,** 99–154.

Smith, S. M., Lee, D. K. P., Lacy, J., and Coleman, D. L. (1990). Rat tracheal epithelial cells produce granulocyte-macrophage colony stimulating factor. *Am. J. Resp. Cell. Mol. Biol.* **2,** 59–68.

Standiford, T. J., Kunkel, S. L., Basha, M. A., Chensue, S. W., Lynch, J. P., III, Toews, G. B., Westwick, J., and Strieter, R. M. (1990). Interleukin-8 gene expression by a pulmonary epithelial cell line. A model for cytokine networks in the lung. *J. Clin. Invest.* **86,** 1945–1953.

Stevens, R. J., Sloan, M. F., Evans, M. J., and Freeman, G. (1974a). Early response of lung to low levels of ozone. *Am. J. Pathol.* **74,** 31–58.

Stevens, R. J., Sloan, M. F., Evans, M. J., and Freeman, G. (1974b). Alveolar type 1 cell response to exposure to 0.5 ppm ozone for short periods. *Exp. Mol. Pathol.* **20,** 11–23.

Stokinger, H. E., Wagner, W. D., and Wright, P. G. (1956). Studies on ozone toxicity. I. Potentiating effects of exercise and tolerance development. *Am. Med. Assoc. Arch. Ind. Health* **14,** 158–162.

Tepper, J. S., Costa, D. L., Lehmann, J. R., Weber, M. F., and Hatch, G. E. (1989). Unattenuated structural and biochemical alterations in the rat lung during functional adaptation to ozone. *Am. Rev. Resp. Dis.* **140,** 493–501.

Tyler, W. S., Tyler, N. K., Last, J. A., and Gillespie, M. J. (1988). Comparison of daily and seasonal exposures of young monkeys to ozone. *Toxicology* **50,** 131.

United States Environmental Protection Agency (1986). Air quality criteria for ozone and other photochemical oxidants. EPA/600/8-84/020af-ef. U.S. Government Printing Office, Washington, D.C.

Van Bree, L., Rombout, P. J. A., Rietjens, I. M. C. M., Dormans, J. A. M. A., and Marra, M. (1989). Pathobiochemical effects in rat lung related to episodic ozone exposure. *In* "Atmospheric Ozone Research and Its Policy Implications" (T. Schneider, S. D. Lee, G. J. R. Wolters, and L. D. Grant, eds.), pp. 723–732. Elsevier Science Publishers, Amsterdam.

Van Bree, L, Koren, H. S., Devlin, R. B., and Rombout, P. J. A. (1993). Recovery from attenuated inflammation in lower airways of rats following repeated exposure to ozone. *Am. Rev. Resp. Dis.* **147,** A633.

Van Louveren, H. Rombout, P. J., Wagenaar, S. S., Walvoort, H. C., and Vos, J. G. (1988). Effect of ozone on the defense to a respiratory *Listeria monocytogenes* infection in the rat. Suppression of macrophage function an cellular immunity and aggravation of histopathology in lung and liver during infection. *Toxicol. Appl. Pharmacol.* **94,** 374–393.

Wahl, S. M., Hunt, D. A., Wakefield, L. M., McCartney, F. N., Wahl, L. M., Roberts, A. B., and Sporn, M. B. (1987). Transforming growth factor type-beta induces monocyte chemotaxis and growth factor production. *Proc. Natl. Acad. Sci. USA* **84,** 5788–5792.

Wright, E. S., Dziedzic, D., and Wheeler, C. S. (1990). Cellular, biochemical and functional effects of ozone: new research and perspectives on ozone health effects. *Toxicol. Lett.* **51,** 125–145.

Yoshimura, T., Matsushima, K., Tanaka, S., Robinson, E. A., Appella, E., Oppenheim, J. J., and Leonard, E. J. (1987). Purification of a human monocyte-derived neutrophil chemotactic factor that has peptide sequence similarity to other host defense cytokines. *Proc. Natl. Acad. Sci. USA* **84,** 9233–9237.

12

Pulmonary Fibrosis Induced by Silica, Asbestos, and Bleomycin

Pierre F. Piguet

I. Introduction

Numerous pulmonary diseases are associated with fibrosis evolving to respiratory insufficiency. Among the etiologies are the inhalation of nondegradable particles or drugs, pulmonary hypertension, and autoimmune diseases (Colby and Churg, 1986). Pulmonary fibrosis is characterized by an alteration of the alveolar septa associated with the growth of interstitial cells and the accumulation of various proteins of the extracellular matrix (Bowden, 1987). Such tissue remodeling implies complex interactions between cells of the alveolar septa (i.e., endothelial, epithelial, and interstitial cells) and leukocytes that are mediated by cytokines. In this chapter, the role of cytokines in bleomycin and dust particle-induced pulmonary fibrosis and their pathogenesis is reviewed.

II. Bleomycin-Induced Fibrosis

A. Clinical Observations

Bleomycin belongs to a family of glycopeptides derived from *Streptomyces verticillatus;* this drug is widely used in the treatment of some tumors (Umezawa, 1980). The main clinical advantage of this class of antitumor agents is the absence of hematotoxicity. However, the occurrence of pulmonary fibrosis in about 10% of the patients is a serious limitation to use of this drug (Blum, 1973).

After systemic administration, bleomycin is rapidly (>99% within 24 hr) degraded (reviewed by Hay *et al.*, 1991). The drug is preferentially retained in the skin and the lung (Umezawa *et al.*, 1968), particularly within alveolar epithelium (Adamson and Bowden, 1979). Bleomycin is degraded by BLM

Xenobiotics and Inflammation

hydrolases, but no correlation is evident between the BLM hydrolase activity of a particular tissue and its susceptibility to bleomycin (Hay *et al.*, 1991).

Bleomycin exhibits toxicity to various cell lines *in vitro*. The drug exerts its toxicity by cleaving DNA in a process dependent on both oxygen and a metal ion (reviewed by Hay *et al.*, 1991). *In vitro*, the toxicity of bleomycin is inversely related to the efficacy of BLM hydrolases (Lazo and Pham, 1984; Sebti *et al.*, 1989). Bleomycin toxicity is associated with the generation of superoxide anion and can be attenuated by oxygen radical scavengers (Galvan *et al.*, 1981).

B. Pulmonary Fibrosis in Animal Models

Bleomycin has been used extensively in experimental animals as a model of pulmonary fibrosis (reviewed by Bowden, 1984). Pulmonary fibrosis can be induced in about 15 days by either a single intratracheal (it) dose or repeated doses administered iv or ip (Bowden, 1990). Histologically, the lesions are characterized by thickening of the alveolar septa, infiltration by leukocytes, transformation of the alveolar epithelium into a cuboidal layer, and growth of interstitial cells associated with the deposition of proteins of the extracellular matrix (Aso *et al.*, 1976; Jones and Reeve, 1978; Table I). An inflammatory reaction becomes evident only 2–3 days after it instillation. The rate of collagen synthesis is increased between 3 and 13 days after it instillation. Total lung collagen increases between days 7 and 15, and thereafter remains stable (Phan *et al.*, 1980).

In mice, the susceptibility to pulmonary fibrosis varies widely among strains and is influenced by genes from various chromosomes, including those of the major histocompatibility complex (MHC) (Schrier *et al.*, 1983a; Rossi *et al.*, 1987; Table II). Clearance of bleomycin also varies among various mouse strains, but high susceptibility to fibrosis is not correlated with a slow clearance of the drug, that is, the strains that retain a higher level of bleomycin within their lungs are not those with the most severe fibrotic reaction (Table II).

Several types of treatment that can influence the development of bleomycin-induced fibrosis are summarized in Table III.

C. Involvement of the Immune Response

An important role of the immune response, particularly of T lymphocytes, in pulmonary fibrosis is supported by the following observations: (1) administration of bleomycin induces an influx of lymphocytes into the lung (Jones and Reeve, 1978), (2) the fibrotic reaction is markedly attenuated in athymic mice or in T lymphocyte-depleted mice (Schrier *et al.*, 1983b; Piguet *et al.*, 1989), (3) full expression of the fibrotic reaction requires T lymphocytes of both the CD4 and CD8 subsets, as indicated by *in vivo* deletion with mono-

Table I   Morphological Alterations Associated
with Fibrosis

	Silicosis	Bleomycin
Growth of fibroblast	+	+
Endothelial damage	+	+
Epithelial damage	+	+
Alveolar exudate	+	+
Platelet sequestration	+	+
Lymphocytic infiltration	+	+
Leukocyte exudate	+	+

clonal antibodies (Piguet *et al.*, 1989), and (4) MHC is involved in the
expression of the susceptible/resistant phenotype (Rossi *et al.*, 1987; see
Table II).

III. Pulmonary Dust Diseases

Pulmonary fibrosis may result from the inhalation of nondegradable
particles by humans or laboratory animals. Morphologically, pneumoconiosis is characterized by nodules, formations of fibroblasts and dust-
containing cells, in a rich network of collagen fibrils (Figure 1). Interstitial
macrophages containing silica particles are obviously damaged when examined by electron microscopy (Figure 1). Particles are deposited along the
bronchial tree and are subsequently taken in by the alveolar macrophages
as well as by other cells such as epithelial and endothelial cells (Adamson
and Bowden, 1987). Particles are, in general, toxic to the cells that host
them. Silicosis is associated with long-lasting alveolar damage (Bowden
and Adamson, 1984). This cellular damage is associated with an acceleration
of the turnover rate of various cells including those of monocytic origin
(Adamson and Bowden, 1987; Brody and Overby, 1989).

A. Particle Clearance

Several physicochemical parameters of the particles affect the ultimate
lung response (reviewed by Bowden, 1987). In general, clearance of particles
can occur through the mucociliary escalator or the lymphatic drainage, the
latter leading to systemic dissemination. Neither method is very efficient,
however, since the half-life of a single dose of silica particles administered
it is about 4 mo in rodents (Adamson *et al.*, 1989).

Table II   Role of the Major Histocompatibility
Complex in Bleomycin Retention and Fibrosis
and Absence of Correlation between Pulmonary
Retention and Fibrosis

Strain	H-prol[a]	Co-Bleo[b]
C57Bl/10 (H-2[b])	132 (13)	1.2 (0.7)
C57Bl/10 D2 (H-2[d])	135 (22)	6.4 (2.4)**
C57Bl/10 BR (H-2[k])	91 (10)*	2.0 (0.8)

[a] Mean ($\pm$ SD) of lung hydroxyproline measured
15 days after instillation of bleomycin. Values for
saline injected controls: 93 (12).
[b] cpm from lung 48 hr after ip injection of ^{60}Cobalt-
labeled bleomycin as % of the injected dose/mg
tissue $\times 10^{-4}$.
* $p < .05$.
** $p < .01$.

B. Interaction between Particles and Various Cell Types *in Vitro*

In vitro, nondegradable particles such as asbestos or silica, are toxic for
macrophages since their uptake results in the death of macrophages in a
few hours; these properties are therefore commonly used to rid the body
of these particles (Piguet *et al.*, 1981). Cell death can, however, be preceded
by a short burst of cellular activity, including the secretion of various mediators (Englen *et al.*, 1990). Toxicity is also evident for nonphagocytic cells
such as endothelial cells (Garcia *et al.*, 1989) and epithelial cells (Mossman

Table III   Modulation of Bleomycin-Induced Pulmonary Fibrosis by Various Treatments

Treatments[a]	Effect	References
Steroid	Prevention	Phan *et al.* (1981)
Indomethacin	Prevention	Thrall *et al.* (1979)
NDGA	Prevention	Phan and Kunkel (1986)
LPS	Prevention	Phan and Fantone (1984)
Athymic mice	Prevention	Schrier *et al.* (1983a), Piguet *et al.* (1989)
Fish and coconut oil	Prevention	Kennedy *et al.* (1987, 1989)
Dietetary antioxidants	Prevention	Wang *et al.* (1989, unpublished observations)
Complement depletion	Prevention	Thrall *et al.* (1981)
Depletion of polymorphic leukocytes	Aggravation	Thrall *et al.* (1981)
Alkylating agents	Aggravation	Schrier and Phan (1984)
beige mutations	Aggravation	Schrier *et al.* (1983b)

[a] Abbreviations: LPS, lipopolysaccharide.

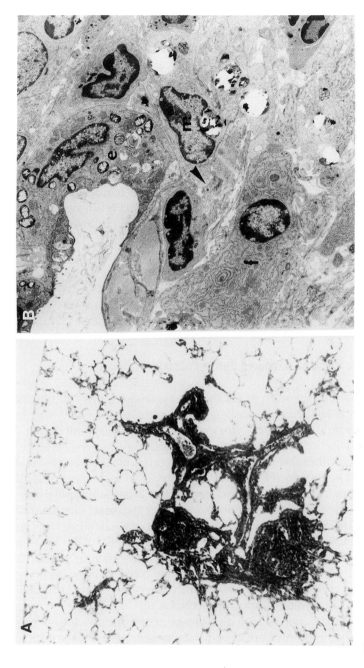

Fig. 1 Silicosis. (A) A nodular formation is evident near a main bronchus 15 days after silica instillation (hematoxylin and eosin, 40×). (B) By transmission electron microscopy, the nodules are seen to be surrounded by an epithelium made of type-2 cells (e) and to contain fibroblast-like cells (f) and macrophages (m) containing silica. Intercellular space is rich in collagen fibrils (arrow) (2800×).

et al., 1986). Toxicity is associated with the generation of oxygen radicals and can be, to some extent, attenuated by oxygen radical scavengers (Garcia *et al.*, 1989; Mossman *et al.*, 1986). The toxicity observed *in vitro* is the probable explanation for the acceleration of the turnover rate (and a reduced life expectancy) of various pulmonary cells that are susceptible to taking up particles, such as macrophages and epithelial cells (Adamson and Bowden, 1987; Brody and Overby, 1989).

C. Involvement of the Immune Response

An involvement of the immune system in the expression of the pneumoconioses is suggested by (1) an influx of T and B lymphocytes following instillation of particles (Kumar, 1989); (2) a less severe silicosis in athymic nude mice than in the euthymic *nu/+* control mice (Hubbard, 1989; P. F. Piguet, unpublished observation), a difference that is, however, not as pronounced as with bleomycin; (3) various humoral manifestations such as production of auto-antibodies (Doll, 1983); and (4) the presence of particle-specific CD4 T lymphocytes within the lung (Saltini *et al.*, 1989). The role and importance of the immune response in pneumoconioses is likely to be dependent on the type of particle and on host factors.

IV. Fibrogenic Cytokines Produced during Pulmonary Fibrosis

Fibrogenesis can result from (1) an increase in the growth of fibroblasts, (2) an increase in the rate of collagen synthesis, or (3) a decrease in the rate of collagen degradation. Cytokines that are known to modulate these responses *in vitro* or *in vivo* are listed in Table IV.

The study of fibroblasts *in vitro* is complicated by the heterogeneity of fibroblast cell lines, which exhibit opposite types of responsiveness. These differences might correspond to different fibroblast subpopulations that exist *in vivo*, which have been reported to express distinct surface proteins (Phipps *et al.*, 1990), alpha-actin content (Sappino *et al.*, 1990), and responses to growth factors (Goldring *et al.*, 1990). Thus, interstitial cells that accumulate during bleomycin- or silica-induced fibrosis differ in their content of alpha actin, being alpha actin-positive in bleomycin-induced fibrosis (Mitchell *et al.*, 1989) but negative in silicosis (P. F. Piguet, unpublished observations). In addition, opposing conclusions might emerge from the exploration of cytokines *in vitro* and *in vivo*. For example, tumor necrosis factor (TNF) is commonly considered to be antifibrogenic since it increases the collagenolytic activity of cell lines (Dayer *et al.*, 1985). However, after infusion into mice, TNF is strongly fibrogenic, increasing both the growth of fibroblasts and the collagen deposition, either locally or within the lung (Piguet *et al.*, 1990a,b).

Table IV   Cytokines That Influence Growth of Fibroblasts and Collagen Secretion

Cytokine[a]	Fibroblast proliferation	Collagen secretion	Fibrogenesis *in vivo*
IL-1	+/−	+/−	
TNF-α	+/−	+/−	+
TGF-β	+/−	+	+
FGF	+		+
PDGF	+	+	+
IFN-γ	−	−	−

[a] Abbreviations: IL-1, interleukin 1; TNF-α, tumor necrosis factor α; TGF-β, transforming growth factor β; FGF, fibroblast growth factor; PDGF, platelet-derived growth factor; IFNγ, interferon γ.

Several cytokines are known or suspected to be fibrogenic, including interleukin 1 (IL-1), TNFα, transforming growth factor beta (TGFβ), platelet-derived growth factor (PDGF), and fibroblast growth factor (FGF).

IL-1 is a highly pleiotropic cytokine that exists in two forms: IL-1α and IL-1β. IL-1 is 17 kDa (reviewed by Dinarello, 1989). IL-1 is mitogenic for some fibroblast cell lines (Schmidt *et al.*, 1982; Thornton *et al.*, 1990) and can, depending on the cell line, increase the synthesis or the degradation of collagen (Postlethwaite *et al.*, 1983; Matsushima *et al.*, 1985).

TNF is a pleiotropic cytokine initially isolated on the basis of its capacity to induce tumor necrosis (Beutler and Cerami, 1988). This protein exists in two forms, TNFα and TNFβ, and is around 17 kDa. TNF has a wide range of biological activities, including a fibrogenic activity. *In vitro*, TNF enhances the proliferation of some fibroblast lines and inhibits others (Sugarman *et al.*, 1985), and inhibits collagen secretion (Dayer *et al.*, 1985). *In vivo*, TNF is strongly fibrogenic (Piguet *et al.*, 1990a,b).

TGF corresponds to a family of disulfide-linked homodimers (Wahl *et al.*, 1989), and is produced by many cell types. TGF might be involved in a variety of biological processes, notably development, wound healing, and immune responses. TGF may enhance the proliferation of some fibroblast lines *in vitro*, but inhibits others (Thornton *et al.*, 1990). TGF increases the rate of collagen secretion (Roberts *et al.*, 1986) and is fibrogenic *in vivo* (Roberts *et al.*, 1986; Sprugel *et al.*, 1987; Roberts and Sporn, 1989).

PDGF was initially isolated from platelets but is now known to be produced by various cells (Ross *et al.*, 1986). PDGF exists in various forms of homo- and heterodimers of about 30 kDa. PDGF has been reported to enhance the replication of fibroblasts, the rate of collagen secretion, and the rate of fibrogenesis *in vivo* (Thornton *et al.*, 1990). Production of this cytokine has been reported in association with idiopathic pulmonary fibrosis (Antoniades *et al.*, 1990).

FGF comprises a family of peptides with a potent fibrogenic activity *in vitro* and *in vivo* (Sprugel *et al.*, 1987), but with biological roles that are poorly understood (reviewed by Klagsbrun and Edelman, 1989; Rifkin and Moscatelli, 1989). These molecules are present in a wide variety of cell types, but whether their synthesis and secretion are regulated and/or whether they are released only by damaged cells has not been established (D'Amore, 1990).

The potency of all these fibrogenic agents has not yet been precisely compared. Their respective roles are, therefore, not defined. On the other hand, interferon γ (IFNγ) is known to inhibit the growth of various cells (including fibroblasts), as well as collagen secretion (Rosenbloom *et al.*, 1984). IFNγ is an antifibrogenic agent used successfully *in vivo* (Hyde *et al.*, 1988).

A. Methodological Considerations in the Evaluation of Cytokine Production

The involvement of a cytokine in a given process is suggested by a positive correlation, that is, an increase in the production of that cytokine during the fibrotic reaction. This possibility can be explored using different methods. (1) Tissue extraction is obviously the most direct approach and has been performed successfully for TGFβ during bleomycin-induced pulmonary fibrosis (Khalil *et al.*, 1989). (2) RNA extraction and evaluation of the mRNA content by Northern blotting has been performed successfully for several cytokines, including IL-1, TNF, TGF, PDGF. The primary limitation of this method is the possibility that changes (or absence of change) in the mRNA levels do not necessarily correlate with changes in the amount of protein produced, particularly if posttranscriptional regulation of protein production takes place. (3) Isolation and exploration of a cellular component, in this case alveolar leukocytes and macrophages freshly prepared or after culture, have been done extensively in the context of pulmonary fibrosis. This approach is based on the assumption, most likely incorrect (see subsequent discussion), that these cells are representative, quantitatively or qualitatively, of cytokine production within the lung.

B. Correlations between Pulmonary Fibrosis and the Production of Fibrogenic Cytokines

Findings of a correlation (or absence thereof) between cytokine production and pulmonary fibrosis are summarized in Table V. In several studies, based on the evaluation of the mRNA levels of various cytokines (Figure 2), the best correlations are observed with TNFα, the message of which shows a 10- to 80-fold lasting increase in correlation with either bleomycin-

Table V   Correlation between Pulmonary Fibrosis and Cytokine Overproduction

Model	Cytokine[a]	Method[b]	Correlation[c]	Reference
Bleomycin-induced fibrosis	TGF	TE	+	Khalil *et al.* (1989)
	TGF	RNA	+	Piguet *et al.* (1989)
	PDGF	RNA	+	See Figure A
	IL-1	RNA, AM	−	Piguet *et al.* (1989)
			+	Suwabe *et al.* (1988)
	TNF	RNA	+	Piguet *et al.* (1989)
Silicosis	TGF-β	RNA	−	Piguet *et al.* (1990a)
	PDGF	RNA	−	See Figure 2B
	IL-1	RNA	−	Piguet *et al.* (1990a)
	TNF	RNA, AM	+	Piguet *et al.* (1989)
			+	Bissonnette and Rola-Pleszczynski (1989)
Asbestosis	PDGF	AM	+	Bauman *et al.* (1987)
	IL-1	AM	+	Lemaire (1991)
	TNF-α	AM	+	Bissonnette and Rola-Pleszczynski (1989)
Pneumoconiosis (human)	TNF-α	AM	+	Lassalle *et al.* (1990)
	IL-1	AM	+	Lassalle *et al.* (1990)

[a] For abbreviations, see Table IV.
[b] TE, Tissue extraction; RNA, RNA extraction; AM, alveolar leukocyte and macrophage preparation.
[c] + indicates a positive correlation, − a negative, or an absence of, correlation.

or silica-induced fibrosis. The mRNAs of other fibrogenic cytokines show only a transient and moderate (2- to 3-fold) change during these reactions (Figure 2).

C. Effect of Cytokine or Anticytokine Agents

Correlations do not establish a causal relationship between cytokine overproduction and fibrogenic reaction, but this relationship can be demonstrated by modulating the reaction with specific inhibitors. Table VI summarizes studies performed *in vivo* using cytokine or anticytokine agents. Evidently this type of evaluation is incomplete at this time, since potent inhibitors are not available for all potentially fibrogenic cytokines. This situation might change rapidly since soluble inhibitors, composed of the extracellular part of the cytokine receptor, are now available for IL-1 (Fanslow *et al.*, 1990), TNF (Lesslauer *et al.*, 1991), and other cytokines.

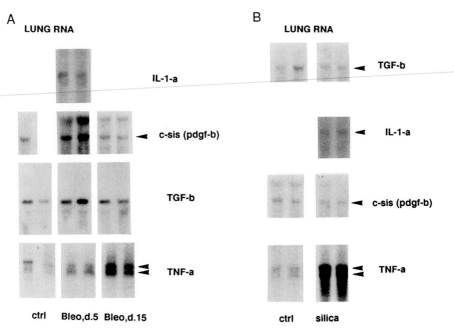

Fig. 2 Northern blot analysis of the mRNA for various cytokines during (A) bleomycin- and (B) silica-induced pulmonary fibrosis. Mice instilled with bleomycin (0.08 mg) or silica (1.5 mg) were sacrificed on days 5 and 15 (bleomycin) or day 15 (silica) after instillation. The lung RNA was extracted and studied by Northern blotting.

V. Is Tumor Necrosis Factor the Main Effector of Pulmonary Fibrosis?

A. Evidence for a Key Role for TNFα

A major role for TNFα in pulmonary fibrosis is supported by the following evidence obtained in mice treated with fibrinogenic doses of bleomycin or silica particles. (1) These diseases are associated with a marked and lasting increase of TNFα mRNA within the lung (Piguet et al., 1989,1990a). (2) They can be prevented by treatment with anti-TNF antibody or aggravated by perfusion with mouse recombinant TNFα (Piguet et al., 1989,1990a,1991c). (3) An infusion of TNFα can reproduce the alterations observed during pulmonary fibrosis, such as growth of fibroblasts, collagen deposition, and cell necrosis (Tracey et al., 1986; Piguet et al., 1991c).

B. Cellular Origin of TNF and Mechanism of Activation

TNF is generally considered to be produced by macrophages (Beutler and Cerami, 1989) but other observations have demonstrated that several

Table VI   Modulation of Pulmonary Fibrosis by Cytokines or Anticytokines

Cytokine or inhibitor[a]	Model	Effect	Reference
TNF	Bleomycin	Aggravation	Piguet et al. (1991c)
TNF	Silicosis	Aggravation	Piguet et al. (1990a)
Anti-TNF	Bleomycin	Protection	Piguet et al. (1989)
Anti-TNF	Silicosis	Protection	Piguet et al. (1990a)
IFN-γ	Bleomycin	Protection	Hyde et al. (1988)
Anti-GM-CSF	Bleomycin	Aggravation	Piguet et al. (1993b)
Anti-GM-CSF	Silicosis	Aggravation	Piguet et al. (1993b)

[a] Abbreviations: See Table IV. GM-CSF, Granulocyte–macrophage colony stimulating factor.

cell types are also capable of TNF production, including neutrophils (Dubravec et al., 1990), mastocytes (Gordon and Galli, 1990), and keratinocytes (Kock et al., 1990; Piguet et al., 1991b). The cellular origin of pulmonary TNF during bleomycin- and silica-induced pulmonary fibrosis has been examined by in situ hybridization to detect its mRNA or by histochemistry to detect the protein. The results indicate that, although TNF mRNA accumulates in damaged areas (e.g., the silicotic nodule; Piguet et al., 1990a) and is detectable in macrophages and neutrophils (Figure 3), TNF protein in contrast is most abundant in (or on) alveolar and bronchial epithelial cells (P. Piguet, unpublished observations). In cases of idiopathic pulmonary fibrosis, TNFα is most abundant in the alveolar epithelium (Piguet et al., 1993).

TNF mRNA accumulation induced by silica or bleomycin is markedly decreased in T lymphocyte-depleted mice (Piguet et al., 1989). Similar observations have been made in several other immunopathological reactions associated with TNF overproduction, where T lymphocytes have been found to increase TNF production in other cells, notably macrophages, by the secretion of cytokines such as GM-CSF, IL-2, and IFNγ (reviewed by Piguet et al., 1991c). A role for GM-CSF in the expression of TNF within the lung is evident in the bleomycin model, but not in silicosis, since in the former case administration of anti-GM-CSF antibody decreases the TNF mRNA level within the lung (Piguet et al., 1991a).

C. Negative Correlations between TNF Overproduction and Fibrosis

If a strikingly positive correlation between TNF mRNA accumulation and fibrosis is evident in bleomycin- or silica-induced pulmonary fibrosis, cases of negative correlations have also been observed. Several chronic infectious diseases are associated with TNF overproduction but, whereas some are associated with fibrotic reactions (e.g. schistosomiasis), others are not (e.g., BCG infections). On the other hand, modulation of GM-CSF by administra-

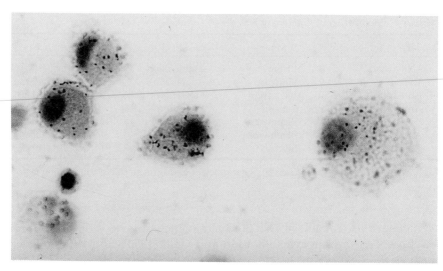

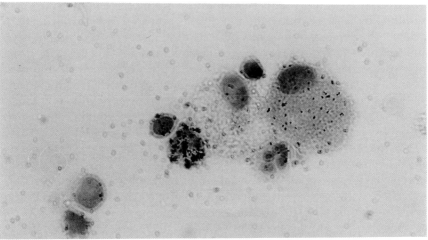

Fig. 3 Cellular origin of the TNF mRNA among the cells from the bronchoalveolar lavage, detected by *in situ* hybridization. (*Top*) Mice instilled with bleomycin, showing four large mononuclear cells bearing autoradiographic grains. (*Bottom*) Mice instilled with silica, showing one heavily labeled cell, presumably a polymorphonuclear leukocyte, a moderately labeled large mononuclear leukocyte, and other unlabeled cells.

tion of anti-GM-CSF antibody markedly aggravates the bleomycin-induced pulmonary fibrosis, but studies of the TNF mRNA level indicate that TNF is not increased but decreased by this treatment (Piguet *et al.*, 1993b).

In conclusion, the radical abrogation of bleomycin- or silica-induced pulmonary fibrosis with anti-TNF antibody indicates that TNF is, in some cases, a decisive factor in fibrogenesis. However, evidence also exists that this correlation might not be a general rule and that, under other circumstances, other fibrogenic cytokines may predominate.

VI. Conclusions: Pathogenesis and Outlook

A. Bleomycin

Evidently bleomycin is toxic, that is, it can kill various cell types directly. This toxicity also explains its pharmacological toxicity. However, the pulmonary reaction that occurs at sublethal doses cannot be explained by toxicity alone. (1) Its occurrence is rather delayed after drug administration. (2) It is evident only in some strains of mice or in some of the treated patients. (3) It requires T lymphocytes. (4) Macrophages or fibroblasts cannot be directly stimulated by bleomycin *in vitro*, for either growth factor production or proliferation. These observations strongly argue in favor of an autoimmune type of alveolitis, in addition to the toxic effects of bleomycin. Thus, injury induced by the toxicity of bleomycin (for example, DNA alterations) might induce antigenic alterations of tissues, notably of the alveolar epithelium. In susceptible individuals, particularly those bearing permissive MHC molecules, these changes will induce an autoimmune alveolitis. The recognition of an antigen on the alveolar epithelium is indeed known to lead to a fibrosing alveolitis (Stein-Streilein *et al.*, 1987). Activation of T lymphocytes will result, either directly or via the activation of other cells, in the overproduction of several cytokines within the lung, particularly TNF and perhaps other fibrogenic cytokines, as discussed in Section V,B. A central role for T lymphocytes in the fibrogenic process has also been reported in others types of fibrosis. For example, athymic nude mice infected with *Schistosoma* spp. are unable to produce a fibrogenic granuloma (Prakash *et al.*, 1990). After a single injection of bleomycin, the reaction will decrease after about 3 wk, leaving inactive scars as a consequence of the rapid degradation of the bleomycin and the subsequent turnover of the alveolar epithelium.

B. Dust Diseases

A simple pathogenic interpretation of pneumoconiosis has been proposed, in which phagocytosis of particles by macrophages leads to the production of fibrogenic factors (Heppleston and Styles, 1967). However, the production of fibrogenic factors by macrophages exposed to nondegradable particles is difficult to demonstrate (Bowden, 1987), perhaps because these particles are generally toxic. Further, *in vivo* the macrophages loaded with silica do not contain detectable TNF mRNA. These observations argue for more complex interactions involving the immune system, as discussed earlier. The presence of intracellular particles leads to antigenic alterations recognized by the immune response system, thus leading to further amplification of cytokine production. TNF mRNA accumulates in silicotic nodules (Piguet *et al.*, 1990a), but mainly in young monocytes or in monocytes containing a small load of particles. TNF overproduction within alveolar interstices leads to growth of fibroblasts, collagen deposition, and further alveolar damage. Because of the slow clearance of the particles, these alterations persist for months after a single exposure.

C. Outlook

The characterization of cytokines involved in fibrotic reactions is important for understanding pathogenesis and for therapy. Several fibrogenic cytokines have been characterized but their respective roles in pulmonary fibrosis cannot be ascertained at this time. Information concerning cytokine production during the development of fibrosis is incomplete. The exploration of their roles with inhibitors is only beginning, but this gap in current knowledge should soon be filled.

Implications for therapy are of two kinds. First, several of the drugs commonly used in the treatment of pulmonary fibrosis diseases, such as steroids and cyclosporin, act by inactivating cytokines, particularly TNF, among other effects. Second, the inhibition of experimental bleomycin-induced fibrosis or silicosis with infusions of IFNγ or anti-TNF antibodies presents new opportunities for therapy.

Acknowledgments

This work was performed in collaboration with colleagues to whom I am indebted: Y. Kapanci, P. Vassalli, and G. Grau. I am also grateful to A. F. Rochat and C. Vesin for their technical collaboration. This work is supported by a grant from the Swiss National Science Foundation No. 31-28855.90.

References

Adamson, I. Y. R., and Bowden, D. H. (1979). Bleomycin-induced injury and metaplasia of alveolar type 2 cells. *Am. J. Pathol.* **96**, 531–544.
Adamson, I. Y. R., and Bowden, D. H. (1987). Response of mouse lung to crocidolite asbestos. 1. Minimal fibrotic reaction to short fibres. *J. Pathol.* **152**, 99–107.
Adamson, I. Y. R., Letourneau, H. L., and Bowden, D. H. (1989). Enhanced macrophage-fibroblast interactions in the pulmonary interstitium increases fibrosis after silica injection to monocyte-depleted mice. *Am. J. Pathol.* **134**, 411–418.
Antoniades, H. N., Bravo, M. A., Avila, R. E., *et al.* (1990). Platelet-derived growth factor in idiopathic pulmonary fibrosis. *J. Clin. Invest.* **86**, 1055–1064.
Aso, Y., Yoneda, K., and Kikkawa, Y. (1976). Morphologic and biochemical study of pulmonary changes induced by bleomycin in mice. *Lab. Invest.* **35**, 558–568.

Bauman, M. D., Jetten, A. M., and Brody, A. R. (1987). Biolological and biochemical character-ization of a macrophage-derived growth factor for rat lung fibroblasts. *Chest* **91**, 15s–16s.

Beutler, B., and Cerami, A. (1988). The history, properties and biological effects of cachectin. *Biochem.* **27**, 7575–7582.

Beutler, B., and Cerami, A. (1989). The biology of cachectin/TNF—A primary mediator of the host response. *Ann. Rev. Immunol.* **7**, 625–655.

Bissonnette, E., and Rolapleszczynski, M. (1989). Pulmonary inflammation and fibrosis in a murine model of asbestosis and silicosis—Possible role of tumor necrosis factor. *Inflamma-tion* **13**, 329–339.

Blum, R. H. (1973). A clinical review of bleomycin. *Cancer* **31**, 903–914.

Bowden, D. H. (1984). Unraveling pulmonary fibrosis: The bleomycin model. *Lab. Invest.* **50**, 487–488.

Bowden, D. H. (1987). Macrophages, dust and pulmonary diseases. *Exp. Lung Res.* **12**, 89–107.

Bowden, D. H. (1990). Experimental induction of pulmonary fibrosis. In "Models of Lung Disease" (J. Gil, ed.), Marcel Dekker, New York.

Bowden, D. H., and Adamson, I. Y. R. (1984). The role of cell injury and the continuing inflammatory response in the generation of silicotic pulmonary fibrosis. *J. Pathol.* **144**, 149–161.

Brody, A. R., and Overby, L. H. (1989). Incorporation of triated thymidine by epithelial and intestinal cells in bronchiolar-alveolar regions of asbestos-exposed rats. *Am. J. Pathol.* **134**, 133–140.

Colby, T. V., and Churg, A. C. (1986). Patterns of pulmonary fibrosis. *Pathol. Ann.* **21**, 277–309.

D'Amore, P. A. (1990). Modes of FGF release *in vivo* and *in vitro*. *Cancer Metastasis Rev.* **9**, 227–238.

Dayer, J. M., Beutler, B., and Cerami, A. (1985). Cachectin/tumor necrosis factor stimulates collagenase and prostaglandin E2 production by human synovial cells and dermal fibro-blasts. *J. Exp. Med.* **162**, 2163–2168.

Dinarello, C. A. (1989). Interleukin-1 and its biologically related cytokines. *Adv. Immunol.* **44**, 153–204.

Doll, N. J. (1983). Immunopathogenesis of asbestosis, silicosis and coal worker's pneumoconio-sis. *Clin. Chest Med.* **4**, 3.

Dubravec, D. B., Spriggs, D. R., Mannick, J. A., and Rodrick, M. L. (1990). Circulating human peripheral blood granulocytes synthesize and secrete tumor necrosis factor-alpha. *Proc. Natl. Acad. Sci. USA* **87**, 6758–6761.

Englen, M. D., Taylor, S. M., Laegreid, W. W., Silflow, R. M., and Leid, R. W. (1990). The effects of different silicas on arachidonic acid metabolism in alveolar macrophages. *Exp. Lung Res.* **16**, 691–709.

Fanslow, W. C., Sims, J. E., Sassenfeld, H., *et al.* (1990). Regulation of alloreactivity *in vivo* by a soluble form of the interleukin-1 receptor. *Science* **248**, 739–741.

Galvan, L., Huang, C. H., Prestakyo, A. W., Stout, J. T., Evans, J. E., and Crooke, S. T. (1981). Inhibition of Bleomycin-induced DNA breakage by superoxide dismutase. *Cancer Res.* **41**, 5103–5106.

Garcia, J. G. N., Dodson, R. F., and Callahan, K. S. (1989). Effect of environmental particulates on cultured human and bovine endothelium. Cell injury via an oxidant-dependant path-way. *Lab. Invest.* **61**, 53–61.

Goldring, S. R., Stephenson, M. L., Downie, E., Krane, S. M., and Korn, J. (1990). Heterogene-ity in hormone response and patterns of collagen synthesis in cloned dermal fibroblasts. *J. Clin. Invest.* **85**, 798–803.

Gordon, J. R., and Galli, S. J. (1990). Mast cells as a source of both preformed and immunologically-inducible TNF-alpha/cachectin. *Nature (London)* **346**, 274–276.

Hay, J., Shahzeidi, S., and Laurent, G. (1991). Mechanism of bleomycin-induced lung damage. *Arch. Toxicol.* **65**, 81–94.

Heppleston, A. G., and Styles, J. A. (1967). Activity of a macrophage factor in collagen formation by silica. *Nature (London)* **214**, 521–522.

Hubbard, A. K. (1989). Role for T lymphocytes in silica-induced pulmonary inflammation. *Lab. Invest.* **61**, 46–52.

Hyde, D. M., Henderson, T. S., Giri, S. N., Tyler, N. K., and Stovall, M. Y. (1988). Effect of murine gamma interferon on the cellular responses to bleomycin in mice. *Exp. Lung Res.* **14**, 687–704.

Jones, A. W., and Reeve, N. L. (1978). Ultrastructural study of bleomycin-induced pulmonary changes in mice. *J. Pathol.* **124**, 227–233.

Kennedy, J. I., Chandler, D. B., Fulmer, J. D., Wert, M. B., and Grizzle, W. E. (1987). Effects of dietary fats on bleomycin-induced pulmonary fibrosis. *Exp. Lung Res.* **12**, 149–161.

Kennedy, J. I., Chandler, D. B., Fulmer, J. D., Wert, M. B., and Grizzle, W. E. (1989). Dietary fish oil inhibits bleomycin-induced pulmonary fibrosis in the rat. *Exp. Lung Res.* **15**, 315–329.

Khalil, N., Bereznay, O., Sporn, M., and Greenberg, A. H. (1989). Macrophage production of transforming growth factor-beta and fibroblast collagen synthesis in chronic pulmonary inflammation. *J. Exp. Med.* **170**, 727–737.

Klagsbrun, M., and Edelman, E. R. (1989). Biological and Biochemical properties of fibroblast growth factors. *Arteriosclerosis* **9**, 269–278.

Kock, A., Schwarz, T., Kirnbauer, R., *et al.* (1990). Human Keratinocytes are a source for tumor necrosis factor alpha: Evidence for synthesis and release upon stimulation with endotoxin or ultraviolet light. *J. Exp. Med.* **172**, 1609–1614.

Kumar, R. K. (1989). Quantitative immunohistologic assessment of lymphocyte populations in the pulmonary inflammatory response to intratracheal silica. *Am. J. Pathol.* **135**, 605–614.

Lassalle, P., Gosset, P., Aerts, C., *et al.* (1990). Abnormal secretion of interleukin-1 and tumor necrosis factor-alpha by alveolar macrophages in coal worker's pneumoconiosis: Comparison between simple pneumoconiosis and progressive massive fibrosis. *Exp. Lung Res.* **16**, 73–80.

Lazo, J. S., and Pham, E. T. (1984). Pulmonary fate of ^{3}H-bleomycin A2 in mice. *J. Pharmacol. Exp. Ther.* **228**, 13–18.

Lemaire, I. (1991). Selective differences in macrophage populations and monokine production in resolving pulmonary granuloma and fibrosis. *Am. J. Pathol.* **138**, 487–495.

Lesslauer, W., Tabuchi, H., Gentz, R., *et al.* (1991). Recombinant soluble TNF receptor proteins protect mice from LPS-induced lethality. *Eur. J. Immunol.* **21**, 2883–2886.

Matsushima, K., Bano, M. J., Kidwell, W. R., and Oppenheim, J. J. (1985). Interleukin 1 increases collagen type IV production by murine mammary epithelial cells. *J. Immunol.* **134**, 904–909.

Mitchell, J., Woodcok-Mitchell, J., Reyolds, S., *et al.* (1989). Alpha-smooth muscle actin in parenchymal cells of bleomycin-injured rat lung. *Lab. Invest.* **60**, 643–650.

Mossman, B. T., Marsh, J. P., and Shatos, M. A. (1986). Alteration of superoxise dismutase activity in tracheal epithelial cells by asbestos and inhibition of cytotoxicity by antioxidants. *Lab. Invest.* **54**, 204–212.

Phan, S. H., and Fantone, J. C. (1984). Inhibition of bleomycin-induced pulmonary fibrosis by lipopolysaccharide. *Lab. Invest.* **50**, 587–591.

Phan, S. H., and Kunkel, S. L. (1986). Inhibition of bleomycin-induced pulmonary fibrosis by Nordihydroguiaretic acid. *Am. J. Pathol.* **124**, 343–352.

Phan, S. H., Thrall, R. S., and Ward, P. A. (1980). Bleomycin-induced pulmonary fibrosis in rats: Biochemical demonstration of increased rate of collagen synthesis. *Am. Rev. Resp. Dis.* **121**, 501–506.

Phan, S. H., Thrall, R. S., and Williams, C. (1981). Bleomycin-induced pulmonary fibrosis. Effects of steroid on Lung collagen metabolism. *Am. Rev. Resp. Dis.* **124**, 428–434.

Phipps, R. P., Baecher, C., Frelinger, J. G., Penney, D. P., Keng, P., and Brown, D. (1990). Differential expression of interleukin 1-alpha by Thy-1[+] and Thy-1[-] lung fibroblast subpopulations: Enhancement of interleukin 1-alpha production by tumor necrosis factor-alpha. *Eur. J. Immunol.* **20**, 1723–1727.

Piguet, P. F., Irle, C., and Vassalli, P. (1981). Immunosuppressor cells from newborn spleen are macrophages differentiating *in vitro* from monoblastic precursors. *Eur. J. Immunol.* **11**, 56–61.

Piguet, P. F., Collart, M. A., Grau, G. E., Kapanci, Y., and Vassalli, P. (1989). Tumor necrosis factor/cachectin plays a key role in bleomycin-induced pneumopathy and fibrosis. *J. Exp. Med.* **170**, 655–663.

Piguet, P. F., Collart, M. A., Grau, G. E., Sappino, A. P., and Vassalli, P. (1990a). Requirement of tumor necrosis factor for development of silica-induced pulmonary fibrosis. *Nature (London)* **344**, 245–247.

Piguet, P. F., Grau, G. E., and Vassalli, P. (1990b). Subcutaneous perfusion of tumor necrosis factor induces local proliferation of fibroblasts, capillaries, and epidermal cells, or massive tissue necrosis. *Am. J. Pathol.* **136**, 103–110.

Piguet, P. F., Grau, G. E., Hauser, C., and Vassalli, P. (1991b). Tumor necrosis factor is a critical mediator in hapten-induced irritant and contact hypersensitivity reactions. *J. Exp. Med.* **173**, 673–679.

Piguet, P. F., Grau, G. E., and Vassalli, P. (1991c). Tumor necrosis factor (TNF) and immunopathology. *Immunol. Res.* **10**, 122–140.

Piguet, P. F., Ribaux, C., Karpuz, V., Grau, G. E., and Kapanci, Y. (1993b). Expression and localization of tumor necrosis factor α and its mRNA in idiopathic pulmonary fibrosis. *Am. J. Pathol.* **143**, 1–5.

Piguet, P. F., Grau, G. E., and de Kossodo, S. (1993b). Role of Granulocyte-macrophage colony stimulating factor (GM-CSF) in pulmonary fibrosis induced by bleomycin. *Exp. Lung Res.* **19**, 579–582.

Postlethwaite, A. E., Lachman, L. B., Mainardi, C. L., and Kang, A. H. (1983). Interleukin-1 stimulation of collagenase production by cultured fibroblasts. *J. Exp. Med.* **157**, 801–805.

Prakash, S., Postlethwaite, A. E., Stricklin, G. P., and Wyler, D. J. (1990). Fibroblast stimulation in schistosomiasis. IX. Schistosomal egg granulomas from congenitally athymic mice are deficient in production of fibrogenic factors. *J. Immunol.* **144**, 317–322.

Rifkin, D. B., and Moscatelli, D. (1989). Recent developments in the cell biology of basic fibroblast growth factor. *J. Cell Biol.* **109**, 1–6.

Roberts, A. B., and Sporn, M. B. (1989). Regulation of endothelial cell growth, architecture, and matrix synthesis by TGF-beta. *Am. Rev. Resp. Dis.* **140**, 1126–1128.

Roberts, A. B., Sporn, M. B., Assoian, R. K., *et al.* (1986). Transforming growth factor type beta: Rapid induction of fibrosis and angiogenesis *in vivo* and stimulation of collagen formation *in vitro*. *Proc. Natl. Acad. Sci. USA* **83**, 4167–4171.

Rosenbloom, J., Feldman, G., Freundlich, B., and Jimenez, S. A. (1984). Transcriptional control of human diploid fibroblast collagen synthesis by gamma interferon. *Biochem. Biophys. Res. Commun.* **123**, 365–372.

Ross, R., Raines, E. W., and Bowen-Pope, D. F. (1986). The biology of platelet-derived growth factor. *Cell* **46**, 155–169.

Rossi, G. A., Szapiel, S., Ferrans, V. J., and Crystal, R. G. (1987). Susceptibility to experimental interstitial lung disease is modified by immune and non immune-related genes. *Am. Rev. Resp. Dis.* **135**, 448–455.

Saltini, C., Winestock, K., Kirby, M., Pinkston, P., and Crystal, R. G. (1989). Maintenance of alveolitis in patients with chronic beryllium disease by beryllium-specific helper T cells. *N. Engl. J. Med.* **320**, 1103–1109.

Sappino, A. P., Schurch, W., and Gabbiani, G. (1990). Biology of disease. Differentiation repertoire of fibroblastic cells: Expression of cytoskeletal proteins as marker of phenotypic modulations. *Lab. Invest.* **63**, 144–161.

Schmidt, J. A., Mizel, S. B., Cohen, D., and Green, I. (1982). Interleukin 1, a potential regulator of fibroblast proliferation. *J. Immunol.* **128**, 2177–2182.

Schrier, D. J., and Phan, S. H. (1984). Modulation of bleomycin-induced pulmonary fibrosis in the BALB/c mouse by cyclophosphamide-sensitive T cells. *Am. J. Pathol.* **116**, 270–278.

Schrier, D. J., Kunkel, R. G., and Phan, S. H. (1983a). The role of strain variation in murine bleomycin-induced pulmonary fibrosis. *Am. Rev. Resp. Dis.* **127,** 63–66.

Schrier, D. J., Phan, S. H., and McGary, M. (1983b). The effects of the nude (nu/nu) mutation on bleomycin-induced pulmonary fibrosis. *Am. Rev. Resp. Dis.* **127,** 614–617.

Sebti, S. M., DeLeon, J. C., Mai, L. T., Hecht, S. M., and Lazo, J. S. (1989). Substrate specificity of bleomycin hydrolase. *Biochem. Pharmacol.* **38,** 141–147.

Sprugel, K. H., McPherson, J. M., Clowes, A. W., and Ross, R. (1987). Effects of growth factors *in vivo.* 1 Cell ingrowth into porous subcutaneous chambers. *Am. J. Pathol.* **129,** 601–613.

Stein-Streilein, J., Lipscomb, M. F., Fisch, H., and Whitney, P. L. (1987). Pulmonary interstitial fibrosis induced in hapten-immune hamsters. *Am. Rev. Resp. Dis.* **136,** 119–123.

Sugarman, B. J., Aggarwal, B. B., Hass, P. E., Figari, I. S., Palladino, M. A., and Shepard, M. H. (1985). Recombinant human tumor necrosis factor-alpha: Effects on proliferation of normal and transformed cells *in vitro. Science* **230,** 943–945.

Suwabe, A., Takahashi, K., Yasui, S., Arai, S., and Sendo, F. (1988). Bleomycin-stimulated hamster alveolar macrophages release interleukin-1. *Am. J. Pathol.* **132,** 512–520.

Thornton, S. C., Por, S. B., Walsh, B. J., Penny, R., and Breit, S. N. (1990). Interaction of immune and connective tissue cells. 1 Effects of lymphokines and monokines on fibroblast growth. *J. Leuk. Biol.* **47,** 312–320.

Thrall, R. S., McCormick, J. R., Jack, R. M., McReynolds, R. A., and Ward, P. A. (1979). Bleomycin-induced pulmonary fibrosis in the rat. *Am. J. Pathol.* **95,** 117–130.

Thrall, R. S., Phan, S. H., McCormick, J. R., and Ward, P. A. (1981). The development of bleomycin-induced pulmonary fibrosis in neutrophil-depleted and complement-depleted rats. *Am. J. Pathol.* **105,** 76–81.

Tracey, K. J., Beutler, B., Lowry, S. F., Merryweather, J., Wolpe, S., Milsark, I. W., Hariri, R. J., Fahey, T. J., Zentella, A., Albert, J. D., Shires, G. T., and Cerami, A. (1986). Shock and tissue injury induced by recombinant human cachectin. *Science* **234,** 470.

Umezawa, H. (1980). Recent progress in bleomycin studies. *In* "Anticancer Agents Based upon Natural Product Models" (J. M. Cassady and J. D. Douros, eds.), Academic Press, New York.

Umezawa, H., Ishizuka, M., Maeda, K., and Takeuchi, T. (1968). The distribution of ^{3}H bleomycin in mouse tissue. *J. Antibiot.* **21,** 638–649.

Wahl, S. M., McCartney-Francis, N., and Mergenhagen, S. E. (1989). Inflammatory and immunomodulatory roles of TGF-beta. *Immunol. Today* **10,** 258–261.

Wang, Q., Giri, S. N., Hyde, D. M., and Nakashima, J. M. (1989). Effects of taurine on bleomycin-induced lung fibrosis in hamsters. *Proc. Soc. Exp. Biol. Med.* **190,** 330–338.

13

Nonparenchymal Cells, Inflammatory Mediators, and Hepatotoxicity

Debra L. Laskin

I. Introduction

Treatment of experimental animals with toxic doses of xenobiotics such as acetaminophen or carbon tetrachloride results in hepatic necrosis and/ or fibrosis. This effect is associated with infiltration of inflammatory cells into the liver (Laskin and Pilaro, 1986; Geerts et al., 1988). Tissue injury in response to these toxicants is predominantly localized in centrilobular regions of the liver, presumably because of high levels of cytochrome P450 mixed function oxidases (MFO) in these regions that metabolically activate these agents to toxic intermediates (Mitchell et al., 1973). Reactive metabolites can bind to cellular macromolecules, initiating a variety of reactions including lipid peroxidation and changes in cellular energy stores (Jollow et al., 1973; Gillette, 1974; Moldeus, 1978). Several studies have suggested that the toxicity of agents such as acetaminophen, carbon tetrachloride, and allyl alcohol is not limited to a direct effect on hepatocytes. Other cell types, particularly sinusoidal cells including Kupffer cells, endothelial cells, and fat-storing cells as well as inflammatory leukocytes, participate in the pathogenesis of tissue injury. For example, treatment of rats with hepatotoxic doses of acetaminophen results in an increase in the number of macrophages and endothelial cells in the liver (Laskin and Pilaro, 1986; Laskin, 1990). These cells release reactive mediators that may be inflammatory, cytotoxic, and/or vasoactive (Nathan, 1987; Decker, 1990) and have been implicated in liver injury (Table I). When animals are treated with agents that activate hepatic macrophages, acetaminophen hepatotoxicity is enhanced. In contrast, hepatoprotective effects are observed following treatment of animals with gadolinium chloride or dextran sulfate, both of which block Kupffer cell function and/or mediator release (Laskin, 1989; Nakae et al., 1990). Thus, in this example, inflammatory macrophages and resident

Kupffer cells appear to play a critical role in liver parenchymal cell damage. This cytotoxic process most likely involves extracellular mediators such as reactive oxygen intermediates and reactive nitrogen intermediates, lysosomal enzymes, leukotrienes, tumor necrosis factor α (TNFα), platelet activating factor (PAF), and interleukins (ILs) released by hepatic macrophages as well as by other nonparenchymal cells (Table I). This chapter reviews studies implicating hepatic macrophages, endothelial cells, and fat-storing cells, as well as inflammatory mononuclear phagocytes, in chemically induced hepatotoxicity.

II. Hepatic Sinusoidal Cells

Approximately 30–35% of the cells in the liver reside within the hepatic sinusoids. Most of these cells are Kupffer cells, endothelial cells,

Table I Nonparenchymal Cell-Derived Mediators Implicated in Hepatotoxicity

Mediator	Reference
Reactive oxygen intermediates (superoxide anion, hydrogen peroxide)	Arthur et al. (1985), Laskin et al. (1986a, 1988), Sugino et al. (1989), Bautista et al. (1990), Mochida et al., (1990), Nakae et al. (1990), Shiratori et al. (1990a), El Sisi et al. (1993b), Gunawardhana et al. (1993)
Reactive nitrogen intermediates (nitric oxide, peroxynitrite)	Billiar et al. (1989, 1990), Gardner et al. (1992), Harbrecht et al. (1992), Beckman and Crow (1993)
Proteolytic enzymes	Ferluga and Allison (1978), Tanner et al. (1981, 1983)
Leukotrienes	Hagmann et al. (1984), Keppler et al. (1985), Tiegs and Wendel (1988), Rodriguez de Turco and Spitzer (1990), Shiratori et al. (1990b)
Tumor necrosis factor α	Freudenberg et al. (1986), Lehman et al. (1987), McClain and Cohen (1989), Thiele (1989), Tiegs et al. (1989), Hishinuma et al. (1990), Larrick and Wright (1990), Chensue et al. (1991), Monden et al. (1991), Shinagawa et al. (1991)
Interleukins (IL-1, IL-6)	Sipe et al. (1979), Sztein et al. (1981), Filkins (1985), West et al. (1989), Monden et al. (1991), Chensue et al. (1991), Hirano (1992), Feder et al. (1993)
Interferon γ	Shinagawa et al. (1991), Silva and Cohen (1992)
Platelet activating factor	Caramelo et al. (1987), Guarner et al. (1989), Crespo and Fernandez-Gallardo (1991)

and fat-storing cells or Ito cells. A small number of pit cells is also found in the hepatic sinusoids. These large granular lymphocytes are the resident natural killer cells of the liver (Kaneda *et al.*, 1983; Bouwens *et al.*, 1987).

A. Kupffer Cells

Kupffer cells represent the most abundant population of macrophages in the body (80–90%). These mononuclear phagocytes, which constitute approximately 29% of the sinusoidal cells in the liver, are predominantly localized in the lumen of the sinusoids and are anchored to the endothelium by long cytoplasmic processes (Bouwens *et al.*, 1986). Like other tissue macrophages, Kupffer cells are characterized by an enlarged horseshoe-shaped nucleus, abundant rough endoplasmic reticulum, prominent cytoplasmic vesicles and vacuoles, and long stellate processes (DeLeeuw *et al.*, 1983; Pilaro and Laskin, 1986). However, considerable heterogeneity in Kupffer cell size and function has been described that appears to be related to their distribution in the liver lobule. Thus, larger more activated Kupffer cells are found in periportal regions of the liver, whereas smaller less phagocytic cells are predominantly located in central zones.

The major function of Kupffer cells is to clear particulate and other foreign materials from the portal circulation. This goal is accomplished primarily through the process of phagocytosis. Kupffer cells are known to possess Fc and C_3 receptors (Munthe-Kaas, 1976) and to phagocytize both opsonized and nonopsonized particles (Pilaro and Laskin, 1986). In addition, these cells release superoxide anion, hydrogen peroxide, and nitric oxide as well as various hydrolytic enzymes and eicosanoids that aid in antigen destruction (Decker, 1990; Laskin, 1990). Kupffer cells also play a central role in the uptake and detoxification of endotoxin (Mathison and Ulevitch, 1979; Praaning-van Dalen *et al.*, 1981). In fact, the sensitivity of animals to endotoxin has been directly correlated with the number of functionally active Kupffer cells in the liver (Nolan, 1981).

Although researchers initially believed that Kupffer cells primarily served as scavenger cells, more recent data indicate that these cells also have the capacity to act as antigen presenting cells for the induction of T lymphocyte responses (Rogoff and Lipsky, 1980). Kupffer cells express major histocompatibility complex (MHC) class II molecules (Ia antigens), process and present antigen to sensitized lymphocytes, and release a number of different cytokines with immunoregulatory and pro-inflammatory activity including IL-1, IL-6, transforming growth factor β (TGFβ), PAF, interferon γ (IFNγ), and TNFα (Decker, 1990; Laskin, 1990). Some of these mediators also have significant effects on hepatocytes. For example, IL-6 alone, or in combination with IL-1 and TNFα, has been reported to stimulate hepatocyte protein production, fibronectin, and DNA synthesis, as well as glucose and lipid metabolism (Feingold and Grunfield, 1987; Darlington et al., 1989; Whicher and Evans, 1990; Hirano, 1992). IL-1 and TNFα also depress cytochrome P450 activity and albumin synthesis (Hooper et al., 1981; Ghezzi et al., 1986; Peterson and Renton, 1986). Thus, alterations in the release of these mediators by Kupffer cells after hepatotoxicant exposure may have significant effects on liver functioning.

B. Endothelial Cells

The major nonparenchymal cell population (approximately 48%) consists of endothelial cells. These cells, which form the walls of the liver sinusoids, are long slender cells with extended processes. Unlike vascular endothelial cells, hepatic endothelial cells are essentially devoid of basement membrane (Hahn et al., 1980). In addition, they possess pores or fenestrae that are arranged in clusters or sieve plates (Wisse and Knook, 1979). These plates allow direct contact between the plasma and its solutes and the cells located behind the endothelial cell barrier. Hepatic endothelial cells are also unique because they possess "bristle-coated" membrane invaginations and vesicles and lysosome-like vacuoles (Hahn et al., 1980). These features indicate that these cells have a well-developed endocytotic capacity. In this regard, hepatic endothelial cells are known to endocytose a variety of particles and are important in the turnover and catabolism of glycoproteins, as well as of lactoferrin, lipoproteins, albumin, and hyaluronic acid (DeLeeuw et al., 1989). Endocytosis is accomplished through pinocytotic vesicles and lysosomes as well as through Fc receptors (Smedstod et al., 1985). Endothelial cells have been reported to display higher phagocytic capacity than Kupffer cells toward certain types of particles (Praaning-van Dalen et al., 1987; DeLeeuw et al., 1989). In addition, their phagocytic capacity is enhanced when Kupffer cell function is impaired (Steffan et al., 1986).

Endothelial cells primarily function as a selective or semi-accessible barrier between the blood and liver parenchyma. These cells block the passage of chylomicrons into the liver, because these particles must first be metabolized in the blood and reduced in size before they can enter the space of Disse. Thus, endothelial cells act as a mechanical sieve that protects the liver from exposure to large quantities of triglycerides. Hepatic endothelial cells also release various mediators that regulate the function of other nonparenchymal cells as well as hepatocytes. These mediators include IL-1, IL-6, IFN, eicosanoids, lysosomal enzymes, nitric oxide and its oxidation products, and reactive oxygen intermediates (Knook and Sleyster, 1980; Laskin, 1990; Gardner et al., 1992; McCloskey et al., 1992; Feder et al., 1993). Thus, endothelial cells, like Kupffer cells, appear to be important in immunological, inflammatory, and regulatory activities in the liver.

C. Fat-Storing Cells

Fat-storing cells, also called perisinusoidal cells, Ito cells, lipocytes, or stellate cells, are located between the endothelial cells and hepatocytes, or between the hepatocytes, and represent approximately 20% of the hepatic sinusoidal cells. Morphologically, fat-storing cells resemble fibroblasts. These cells possess numerous extensions and dilated rough endoplasmic reticulum. Fat-storing cells are the major site in the body for storage of vitamin A, which is localized in intracellular lipid droplets in the form of retinyl esters (Hendriks et al., 1985). These lipid droplets, which also contain triglycerides, cholesterol, and proteins, function to supply free fatty acids for retinol esterification and storage. Fat-storing cells are also known to synthesize extracellular matrix proteins including collagen types I, III, and IV. Evidence suggests that these cells play a role in collagen synthesis in both normal and fibrotic liver (Friedman et al., 1985; Blomhoff and Wake, 1991; Ramadori, 1991). Studies have demonstrated that fat-storing cells also release proteins and inflammatory mediators that may contribute to liver injury, including fibronectin, gelatinase, nitric oxide, and reactive oxygen intermediates, as well as TGFβ and colony stimulating factor 1 (CSF-1; Ramadori, 1991; Pinzani et al., 1992; Helyar et al., 1993).

III. Role of Hepatic Macrophages and Their Mediators in Hepatotoxicity

Treatment of experimental animals with a number of different hepatotoxicants including acetaminophen, endotoxin (lipopolysaccharide, LPS), carbon tetrachloride, phenobarbital, allyl alcohol, or galactosamine is associated with the accumulation of inflammatory macrophages in the liver (Laskin and Pilaro, 1986; Pilaro and Laskin, 1986; MacDonald et al., 1987; Geerts et al., 1988; Laskin et al., 1988; Przybocki et al., 1992). All these hepatotoxicants induce relatively rapid accumulation, typically occurring within 24–48 hr. However, the localization of these infiltrated cells within the liver varies with the xenobiotic. Thus, treatment of rats with acetaminophen or carbon tetrachloride results in the accumulation of macrophages in centrilobular regions of the liver (Thompson et al., 1980; Laskin and Pilaro, 1986; Geerts et al., 1988). In contrast, examination of histological sections of livers of rats treated with phenobarbital, endotoxin, or galactosamine reveals that the infiltrated macrophages are grouped in clusters and/ or scattered throughout the liver lobule (Pilaro and Laskin, 1986; MacDonald et al., 1987; Laskin et al., 1988). These patterns of macrophage localization appear to be correlated with areas of the liver that subsequently exhibit signs of injury (Shiratori et al., 1986; Hendriks et al., 1987). Macrophages isolated from livers of treated animals have been reported to display morphological and functional properties of activated mononuclear phagocytes. These cells are larger and more stellate than resident Kupffer cells, are highly vacuolated, and display an increased cytoplasm:nucleus ratio (Earnst et al., 1986; Laskin and Pilaro, 1986; Pilaro and Laskin, 1986). In addition, macrophages from treated animals exhibit enhanced phagocytic, chemotactic, cytotoxic, and metabolic activity, as well as increased release of superoxide anion, hydrogen peroxide, nitric oxide and its oxidation products, proteolytic enzymes, IL-1, IL-6, and TNFα (Lloyd and Triger, 1975; Tanner et al., 1981; Laskin and Pilaro, 1986; Pilaro and Laskin, 1986; Shiratori et al., 1986; Gardner et al., 1987,1992; Laskin et al., 1988; Abril et al., 1989). Several studies have suggested that activated Kupffer cells and infiltrated macrophages promote hepatic damage through the release of these toxic secretory products (Ferluga and Allison, 1978; Tanner et al., 1981; Arthur et al., 1985; Chojkier and Fierer, 1985; Laskin et al., 1986a; Lehman et al., 1987; Laskin, 1990; ElSisi et al., 1993b).

Reactive oxygen intermediates have been implicated as the primary mediators of macrophage-induced cytotoxicity, of reperfusion and ischemic tissue injury, and of tissue injury in acute and chronic inflammation (McCord, 1974; Sacks et al., 1977; DelMaestro et al., 1980; Fantone and Ward, 1982; Babior, 1984; Henson and Johnston, 1987; Black, 1989). After stimulation, activated macrophages release superoxide anion, which breaks down generating hydroperoxy and hydroxyl radicals. These radicals are even more toxic than superoxide anion and have been linked to membrane, protein, and DNA damage, lipid peroxidation reactions, and induction of hepatocyte killing (DelMaestro et al., 1980; Fantone and Ward, 1982; Babior, 1984; Halliwell and Gutteridge, 1984; Rubin and Farber, 1984; Sevamian and Hochstein, 1985). When macrophages are recruited to the liver after hepatotoxicant exposure, these cells are activated to release hydrogen peroxide and superoxide anion (Laskin and Pilaro, 1986; McCloskey et al., 1992). Stimulation of these cells to produce additional reactive oxygen intermediates has been reported to augment hepatic injury induced by agents such as Corynebacterium parvum, galactosamine, and carbon tetrachloride, whereas administration of antioxidants such as superoxide dismutase, catalase, or allopurinol is hepatoprotective (Arthur et al., 1985; Sugino et al., 1989; Shiratori et al., 1990a; Gunawardhana et al., 1993; ElSisi et al., 1993b). These studies support the hypothesis that oxygen-derived free radicals produced by macrophages in the liver contribute to the pathogenesis of hepatic injury (Arthur et al., 1985; Laskin, 1990; Shiratori et al., 1988).

Other studies have also implicated reactive nitrogen intermediates, in particular nitric oxide, in macrophage-mediated cytotoxicity, in intracellular destruction of pathogens, and in the regulation of cellular proliferation (Billiar et al., 1989; Stuehr and Nathan, 1989; Heck et al., 1992; Punjabi et al., 1992). Nitric oxide and its oxidation products, nitrate and nitrite, are produced by activated hepatic macrophages, endothelial cells, and fat-storing cells as well as by hepatocytes and are hypothesized to be involved in alterations in hepatic functioning after sepsis or trauma (Kilbourn et al., 1990; Stark and Szurszewski, 1992). Nitric oxide may also contribute to tissue injury induced by certain xenobiotics, and has also been discovered to be involved in the regulation of hepatic DNA synthesis and in apoptosis (Laskin et al., 1993a). Nitric oxide is known to react with superoxide anion to form peroxynitrite, a relatively long-lived cytotoxic oxidant that has been implicated in stroke, heart disease, and immune complex-mediated pulmonary edema (Beckman, 1991; Beckman and Crow, 1993). Peroxynitrite may also initiate lipid peroxidation and can react directly with sulfhydryl groups in cell membranes. Paradoxically, the reaction of superoxide anion and nitric oxide may also function as a defense against oxidant stress by reducing intracellular levels of these reactive intermediates (Beckman and Crow, 1993). In this regard, inhibition of nitric oxide synthesis has been reported to augment oxidant-dependent tissue injury induced by C. parvum and has been proposed to play a protective role in the hepatotoxicity of endotoxin (Billiar et al., 1990; Harbrecht et al., 1992; Frederick et al., 1993). Thus, nitric oxide or secondary oxidants generated from nitric oxide may be cytotoxic or hepatoprotective, depending on levels of superoxide anion present and the extent to which tissue injury is mediated by reactive oxygen intermediates (Beckman and Crow, 1993). Nitric oxide may also modulate drug-induced hepatotoxicity by altering cytochrome P450 MFO activity. Nitric oxide binds to heme-containing proteins, which may result in inhibition or activation of various enzymes (Moncada et al., 1991).

Peroxidation of membrane lipids by reactive oxygen intermediates may also induce the formation and release of a number of other vasoactive agents including prostaglandins, thomboxanes, and leukotrienes by macrophages. These mediators are known to be released by activated hepatic macrophages as well as by endothelial cells (Decker, 1990; Laskin, 1990). The precise role of these reactive species in hepatotoxicity is unknown. Leukotrienes and prostaglandins are generated in acute allergic reactions and have been shown to contribute to persistent and late-onset responses to allergens (Brain et al., 1984). In addition, leukotriene B_4 is known to be a potent polymorphonuclear leukocyte (PMN) chemoattractant and to induce monocyte IL-1, TNFα, and hydrogen peroxide production (Goetzl and Pickett, 1981; Gagnon et al., 1989). Thus, release of leukotriene B_4 in the liver may constitute a local control mechanism for recruitment and activation of inflammatory cells. In this regard, studies have demonstrated that administration of lipoxygenase inhibitors or antagonists to mice protected against galactosamine-induced liver injury (Keppler et al., 1985; Shiratori et al., 1990b). These data suggest that leukotrienes may be involved in inflammatory liver disease.

Proteolytic and lysosomal enzymes released from macrophages and Kupffer cells may also contribute to hepatotoxicity. Enzymes such as plasminogen activator, collagenase, elastase, gelatinase, acid phosphatase, and cathepsin D can act directly on hepatocyte membranes to induce damage. Some of these proteases have been shown to play a role in macrophage-mediated target cell destruction, as well as in altered hepatocyte functioning (Williams et al., 1978; Seglen et al., 1980).

Kupffer cells and inflammatory macrophages are known to release a number of different cytokines that may also contribute to hepatotoxicity. These mediators can act directly on hepatocytes or may indirectly activate other nonparenchymal cells as well as leukocytes that migrate into the liver, thus amplifying the inflammatory response (Shedlofsky and McClain, 1991). TNFα is a secretory product of activated macrophages (Tracey et al., 1986; Beutler and Cerami, 1987) that has been implicated not only in the pathogenesis of septic shock and inflammation, but also in the regulation of acute-phase gene expression, cytochrome P450 activity, cellular proliferation, and apoptosis (Ghezzi et al., 1986; Perlmutter et al., 1986; Tracey et al., 1986; Beutler and Cerami, 1987; Larrick and Wright, 1990). TNFα also stimulates the release of other immune mediators including IL-1, IL-6, CSFs, PAF, and prostaglandins from parenchymal and/or nonparenchymal cells (Dinarello et al., 1986; Munkee et al., 1986; Beutler and Cerami, 1989). TNFα can act in concert with these mediators to augment injury to the liver. For example, in alcoholic cirrhosis in which endotoxemia is present, TNFα is thought to be a major mediator of liver damage (McClain and Cohen, 1989). TNFα has also been implicated in the hepatotoxicity of acetaminophen, galactosamine, and endotoxin (Hishinuma et al., 1990; Shedlofsky and McClain, 1991; Laskin et al., 1993b). TNFα is also known to have deleterious effects on endothelial cells (Sato et al., 1986). In addition, this mediator primes neutrophils and monocytes to produce reactive oxygen intermediates (Klebanoff et al., 1986; Beutler and Cerami, 1987).

IL-1 is a low molecular weight protein that mediates a wide variety of biological effects including induction of proliferation and activation of B and T lymphocytes, synovial cells, endothelial cells, and epithelial cells (Dinarello, 1989). IL-1 also acts on the liver in conjunction with IL-6 to induce and regulate hepatocyte production of acute-phase proteins, and on macrophages and natural killer cells to augment cytotoxicity (Onozaki et al., 1985; Darlington et al., 1989; Dinarello, 1989; Whicher and Evans, 1990; Hirano, 1992). Reports have been made of the synthesis of IL-1, as well as IL-6, by cells other than macrophages including hepatic fat-storing cells and endothelial cells, as well as fibroblasts, epidermal cells, and glial cells (reviewed by Oppenheim et al., 1986; Dinarello, 1989; Hirano, 1992). The fact that these cytokines can affect so many different target tissues, and are produced by a variety of cell types, suggests that these proteins are major mediators of inflammation and immune responses.

A. Mechanisms of Macrophage Accumulation and Activation in the Liver

The mechanisms underlying the increase in the number of macrophages in the liver after hepatotoxicant exposure and their subsequent activation are unknown. Damaged tissues and cells release chemotactic and activating factors for phagocytes that may be important in the recruitment of inflammatory macrophages into the liver. These factors bind to specific receptors on phagocytic cells and induce directed cell movement. Several mediators have been reported to induce chemotaxis of phagocytes including complement fragments, products involved in the kinin and coagulation pathways, collagen and tissue breakdown products, arachidonic acid metabolites (particularly leukotriene B_4), synthetic peptides related to bacteria-derived products, and a variety of cell-derived chemotactic proteins (Ward and Newman, 1969; Kaplan et al., 1972; Schiffman et al., 1975; Goetzl and Pickett, 1981; Laskin et al., 1986b; Matsushima and Oppenheim, 1989). Hepatocytes treated with acetaminophen were found also to release a factor that is chemotactic for Kupffer cells as well as blood monocytes (Laskin et al., 1986a). Similarly, Perez et al. (1984) reported that hepatocytes treated with ethanol release a neutrophil chemotactic factor. These investigators provided preliminary evidence that the chemotactic activity was leukotriene B_4. The monocyte and Kupffer cell chemotactic factor was found to be stable to freeze-thawing, but lost activity after heat or trypsin treatment (Laskin et al., 1986a). In addition, this factor eluted in the void volume after size exclusion chromatography. These results suggest that the factor is a relatively large molecular weight protein. In the past few years, several cell-derived chemotactic factors have been described, all of which belong to a family of phagocyte chemoattractants that include macrophage inflammatory protein 1 (MIP-1), MIP-2, macrophage chemotactic protein (MCP), IL-8, and KC (murine homolog of *gro*) and are thought to participate in early inflammatory responses. The factor released from injured hepatocytes may be similar to one of these chemotactic proteins. In this regard, preliminary studies indicate that acetaminophen treatment of rats causes a time-dependent increase in expression of the KC chemokine in the liver.

Hepatocytes treated with acetaminophen were also found to release factors that activate Kupffer cells (Laskin et al., 1986a). These factors induce morphological changes in Kupffer cells that are characteristic of activated macrophages, including flattening and spreading of the cells on culture dishes and increased vacuolization. This morphology is similar to that of activated macrophages isolated from acetaminophen-treated rats (Laskin and Pilaro, 1986). Culture medium from hepatocytes treated with acetaminophen, but not acetaminophen by itself, also stimulates Kupffer cell phagocytosis, release of superoxide anion, and cytotoxicity toward normal as well as transformed hepatocytes (Laskin *et al.*, 1986a; Laskin and Pilaro, 1988). These data suggest that accumulation and activation of macrophages in the liver after treatment with chemicals such as acetaminophen is mediated, at least in part, by factors released from injured hepatocytes.

Although Kupffer cells, like other mononuclear phagocytes, are generally considered to be derived from bone marrow precursors, these cells also appear to be capable of local proliferation (Bouwens *et al.*, 1986). After partial hepatectomy or under inflammatory conditions, dividing Kupffer cells have been observed *in situ* (Widmann and Fahimi, 1975; Bouwens *et al.*, 1984). Thus, Kupffer cells appear to have a dual origin that involves local proliferation of more mature cells and extrahepatic recruitment from bone marrow precursors. In support of this concept, Kupffer cells isolated from rats treated with endotoxin have been discovered to display a significantly increased proliferative capacity in response to a number of different inflammatory cytokines including IL-1, CSF-1, and granulocyte–macrophage colony stimulating factor (GM-CSF) (Feder *et al.*, 1993).

B. Effects of Modifying Macrophage Function on Hepatotoxicity

Direct evidence in support of the hypothesis that macrophages play a role in tissue injury comes from experiments analyzing the effects of modifying Kupffer cell activity on hepatotoxicity and/or liver function. These data clearly indicate that the degree of hepatic injury induced by a number of different chemicals is directly correlated with macrophage function (reviewed by Laskin, 1990). Lipopolysaccharide and poly-I:C are potent activators of liver macrophages (Peterson and Renton, 1986; Pilaro and Laskin, 1986). Lipopolysaccharide may also activate endothelial cells and fat-storing cells (McCloskey *et al.*, 1992; Helyar *et al.*, 1993). Pretreatment of rats with poly-I:C or lipopolysaccharide has been demonstrated to enhance the hepatotoxicity of acetaminophen, as evidenced by increases in serum transaminase levels and tissue injury. Similarly, lipopolysaccharide pretreatment has been reported to aggravate hepatic injury induced by carbon tetrachloride, as well as by galactosamine and *C. parvum* (Nolan and Leibowitz, 1978; Galanos *et al.*, 1979). Animals made tolerant to lipopolysaccharide or treated with polymyxin B, a positively charged detergent that binds to and neutralizes lipopolysaccharide, are also protected from hepatotoxicity induced by these agents (Nolan and Ali, 1973; Nolan and Leibowitz, 1978). Administration of large doses of vitamin A, which activates Kupffer cells *in vivo* (Abril *et al.*, 1989; Sim *et al.*, 1989), has also been reported to augment the hepatotoxicity of carbon tetrachloride, as well as of allyl alcohol, acetaminophen, and endotoxin (Hendriks *et al.*, 1987; ElSisi *et al.*, 1993a). This effect is thought to be the result of reactive oxygen intermediates released from vitamin A-activated Kupffer cells (ElSisi *et al.*, 1993b). In this regard, methyl palmitate, which blocks Kupffer cell oxidative metabolism, was found to abrogate the enhanced toxicity of carbon tetrachloride induced by vitamin A. Methyl palmitate has also been reported to exert hepatoprotective effects against tissue injury induced by galactosamine as well as 1,2-dichlorobenzene (Al-Tuwaijri et al., 1981; Gunawardhana et al., 1993). In agreement with these studies, the accumulation of macrophages in the liver, and subsequent toxicity of acetaminophen, was found to be blocked by pretreatment of rats with dextran sulfate or gadolinium chloride, agents also known to depress macrophage function (Husztik et al., 1980; Souhami and Bradfield, 1981). Similar hepatoprotective effects of gadolinium chloride have been described for allyl alcohol and carbon tetrachloride (Przybocki et al., 1992; Edwards et al., 1993). Collectively, these data support the hypothesis that macrophages play a role in hepatotoxicity.

C. Role of Endothelial Cells and Fat-Storing Cells in Hepatotoxicity

Other studies suggest that hepatic endothelial cells and fat-storing cells may also contribute to tissue injury induced by hepatotoxicants. For example, after treatment of rats with acetaminophen or lipopolysaccharide, increased numbers of endothelial cells and fat-storing cells are found in the liver (Laskin, 1990; Helyar et al., 1993). As observed for liver macrophages, these cells appear to be "activated." The cells are larger and more granular than cells from untreated animals and produce increased levels of reactive oxygen intermediates and reactive nitrogen intermediates (McCloskey et al., 1992; Helyar et al., 1993). Endothelial cells are also primed after hepatotoxicant exposure to produce increased amounts of IL-1 and IL-6 (Feder et al., 1993). The capacity of hepatic endothelial and fat-storing cells to produce these mediators may represent an important mechanism by which these cells participate in the inflammatory and immune reactions associated with hepatotoxicity. Vascular endothelial cells have been reported to proliferate and to produce increased amounts of superoxide anion, as well as IL-1 and IL-6, in response to macrophage-derived cytokines (Ooi et al., 1983; Matsubara and Ziff, 1986; Jirik et al., 1989). Endothelial cells activated by inflammatory mediators are also known to release eicosanoids, PAF, reactive nitrogen intermediates, plasminogen activator, and lysosomal enzymes (Knook and Sleyster, 1980; Tiku and Tomasi, 1985; Cotran, 1987; Eyhorn et al., 1988). These data indicate that inflammatory cells and their secretory products may play a regulatory role in the growth and integrity of the microvasculature. Similarly, in the liver, cytokines released by nonparenchymal cells and inflammatory macrophages after hepatotoxicant exposure may promote proliferation and reactive oxygen intermediate or hydrolytic enzyme release by endothelial cells and fat-storing cells in a paracrine and/or autocrine manner. In this regard, the proliferation of endothelial cells, as well as of fat-storing cells, in response to inflammatory cytokines and growth factors was found to be significantly augmented after hepatotoxicant treatment of rats (Feder and Laskin, 1993). Reactive mediators released by stimulated endothelial cells and/or fat-storing cells may directly injure the matrix of the vasculature as well as the surrounding hepatic tissue.

D. Model of Hepatotoxicity

Based on current experimental data, a model of xenobiotic-induced hepatic injury has been proposed that includes a role for nonparenchymal cells and inflammatory mediators (Laskin et al., 1986a; Laskin, 1990). According to this model, hepatocytes injured by toxicants as well as activated nonparenchymal cells release factors that attract Kupffer cells to specific regions of the liver. Additional mononuclear phagocytes are also recruited from blood and bone marrow precursors. Once localized in the liver, the macrophages become activated by hepatocyte- and nonparenchymal cell-derived factors and release mediators that induce proliferation and activation of endothelial cells and fat-storing cells. Activated macrophages, endothelial cells, and fat-storing cells also release mediators that promote liver injury initiated by toxicants. This sequence of events eventually leads to cell death and necrosis. Data collected by a number of investigators support this model of hepatotoxicity. Additional studies on the nature of the mediators released from nonparenchymal cells and their effects on hepatocytes will be particularly relevant to understanding mechanisms of liver injury.

IV. Conclusion

Xenobiotic-induced hepatotoxicity involves a variety of cellular and biochemical processes. Although xenobiotics or their metabolites can directly injure hepatocytes, they may also act indirectly on nonparenchymal cells and inflammatory leukocytes, thus augmenting tissue injury. An increase in the content of nonparenchymal cells is a characteristic feature of hepatotoxicant exposure. These cells become activated and release large amounts of inflammatory and cytotoxic mediators, as well as growth- and differentiation-promoting cytokines. These mediators can induce additional nonparenchymal cell proliferation and activation, thus amplifying the toxic response. Understanding the nature of these mediators, their cellular origin, and the mechanism by which they injure hepatocytes and interfere with normal liver functioning represents an important approach to treating hepatotoxicity associated with inflammation.

References

Abril, E. R., Simm, W. E., and Earnest, D. L. (1989). Kupffer cell secretion of cytotoxic cytokines is enhanced by hypervitaminosis A. In "Cells of the Hepatic Sinusoid" (E. Wisse, D. L. Knook, and K. Decker, eds.), Vol. 2, pp. 73–75. Kupffer Cell Foundation, Amsterdam.

Al-Tuwaijri, A., Akdamar, K., and DiLuzio, N. R. (1981). Modification of galactosamine-induced liver injury in rats by reticuloendothelial system stimulation or depression. *Hepatology* **1**, 107–113.

Arthur, M. J. P., Bentley, I. S., Tanner, A. R., Saunders, P. K., Millward-Sadler, G. M., and Wright, R. (1985). Oxygen-derived free radicals promote hepatic injury in the rat. *Gastroenterology* **89**, 1114–1122.

Babior, B. M. (1984). Oxidants from phagocytes: Agents of defense and destruction. *Blood* **64**, 959–966.

Bautista, A. P., Meszaros, K., Bojta, J., and Spitzer, J. J. (1990). Superoxide anion generation in the liver during the early stage of endotoxemia in rats. *J. Leukocyte Biol.* **48**, 123–128.

Beckman, J. S. (1991). The double-edged role of nitric oxide in brain function and superoxide-mediated injury. *J. Dev. Physiol.* **15**, 53–59.

Beckman, J. S., and Crow, J. P. (1993). Pathological implications of nitric oxide, superoxide and peroxynitrite formation. *Biochem. Soc. Trans.* **21**, 330–334.

Beutler, B., and Cerami, A. (1987). Cachectin: More than a tumor necrosis factor. *N. Engl. J. Med.* **316**, 379–385.

Beutler, B., and Cerami, A. (1989). The biology of cachectin/TNF—A primary mediator of the host response. *Annu. Rev. Immunol.* **7**, 625–655.

Billiar, T. R., Curran, R. D., Stuehr, D. J., West, M. A., Bentz, B. G., and Simmons, R. L. (1989). An L-arginine-dependent mechanism mediates Kupffer cell inhibition of hepatocyte protein synthesis *in vitro*. *J. Exp. Med.* **169**, 1467–1472.

Billiar, T. R., Curran, R., Harbrecht, B., Stuehr, D., Demetris, A., and Simmons, R. (1990). Modulation of nitrogen oxide synthesis in vivo: N^G-monomethyl-L-arginine inhibits endotoxin-induced nitrite/nitrate biosynthesis while promoting hepatic damage. *J. Leukocyte Biol.* **48**, 565–569.

Black, H. S. (1989). Role of reactive oxygen species in inflammatory processes. *In* "Nonsteroidal Anti-Inflammatory Drugs. Pharmacology and the Skin," (C. Hensby and N. J. Lowe, eds.), Vol. 2, pp. 1–20. Basel-Karger, Basel.

Blomhoff, R., and Wake, K. (1991). Perisinosoidal stellate cells of the liver: Important roles in retinol metabolism and fibrosis. *FASEB J.* **5**, 271–277.

Bouwens, L., Baekeland, M., and Wisse, E. (1984). Importance of local proliferation in the expanding Kupffer cell population of rat liver after zymosan stimulation and partial hepatectomy. *Hepatology* **4**, 213–219.

Bouwens, L., Baekeland, M., De Zanger, R., and Wisse, E. (1986). Quantitation, tissue distribution and proliferation kinetics of Kupffer cells in normal rat liver. *Hepatology* **6**, 718–722.

Bouwens, L., Remels, L., Baekeland, M., Van Bossuyt, H., and Wisse, E. (1987). Large granular lymphocytes or "pit cells" from rat liver: Isolation, ultrastructural characterization and natural killer activity. *Eur. J. Immunol.* **17**, 37–42.

Brain, S., Camp, R., Greaves, M., Jones, R. R., and Woollard, P. M. (1984). The inflammatory responses of human skin to topical application of leukotriene B$_4$. *Br. J. Clin. Pharmacol.* **17**, 610–611.

Caramelo, C., Fernandez-Gallardo, S., Santos, J. C., Inarrea, P., Sanchez-Crespo, M., Lopez-Novoa, J. M., and Hernando, L. (1987). Increased levels of platelet activating factor in blood from patients with cirrhosis of the liver. *Eur. J. Clin. Invest.* **17**, 7–11.

Chensue, S. W., Terebuh, P. D., Remick, D. G., Scales, W. E., and Kunkel, S. L. (1991). *In vivo* biologic and immunohistochemical analysis of interleukin-1 alpha, beta and tumor necrosis factor during experimental endotoxemia. *Am. J. Pathol.* **138**, 395–402.

Chojkier, M., and Fierer, S. (1985). D-Galactosamine hepatotoxicity is associated with endotoxin sensitivity and mediated by lymphoreticular cells in mice. *Gastroenterology* **88**, 115–121.

Cotran, R. S. (1987). New roles for the endothelium in inflammation and immunity. *Am. J. Pathol.* **129**, 407–413.

Crespo, M. S., and Fernandez-Gallardo, S. (1991). Pharmacological modulation of PAF: A therapeutic approach to endotoxin shock. *J. Lipid Med.* **4**, 127–144.

Darlington, G. J., Wilson, D. R., Revel, M., and Kelly, J. H. (1989). Response of liver genes to acute phase mediators. *Ann. N.Y. Acad. Sci.* **557**, 310–316.

Decker, K. (1990). Biologically active products of stimulated liver macrophages (Kupffer cells). *Eur. J. Biochem.* **192**, 245–261.

De Leeuw, A. M., Brouwer, A., Barelds, R. J., and Knook, D. L. (1983). Maintenance cultures of Kupffer cells isolated from rats at various ages: Ultrastructure, enzyme cytochemistry and endocytosis. *Hepatology* **3**, 497–506.

De Leeuw, A. M., Praaning-Van Dalen, D. P., Brouwer, A., and Knook, D. L. (1989). Endocytosis in liver sinusoidal endothelial cells. *In* "Cells of the Hepatic Sinusoid" (E. Wisse, D. L. Knook, and K. Decker, eds.), Vol. 2, pp. 94–98. Kupffer Cell Foundation, Amsterdam.

DelMaestro, R. F., Thaw, H., Bjork, J., Planker, M., and Arfors, K. E. (1980). Free radicals as mediators of tissue injury. *Acta Physiol. Scand. (Suppl.)* **492**, 43–57.

Dinarello, C. A. (1989). Interleukin-1 and its related cytokines. *In* "Macrophage-Derived Cell Regulatory Factors. Cytokines" (C. Sorg, ed.), Vol. 1, pp. 105–154. Basel-Karger, Basel.

Dinarello, C. A., Cannon, J. G., Wolff, S. M., Bernheim, H. A., Beutler, B., Cerami, A., Figari, I. S., Palladino, M. A., Jr., and O'Connor, J. V. (1986). Tumor necrosis factor (cachectin) is an endogenous pyrogen and induces production of interleukin 1. *J. Exp. Med.* **163**, 1433–1450.

Earnst, D. L., Brouwer, A., Sim, W., Horan, M. A., Hendriks, H. F., de Leeuw, A. M., and Knook, D. L. (1986). Hypervitaminosis A activates Kupffer cells and lowers the threshold for endotoxin liver injury. *In* "Cells of the Hepatic Sinusoid" (A. Kirn, D. L. Knook, and E. Wisse, eds.), Vol. 1, pp. 277–283. Kupffer Cell Foundation, Rijswijk, The Netherlands.

Edwards, M. J., Keller, B. J., Kaufman, F. C., and Thurman, R. G. (1993). The involvement of Kupffer cells in carbon tetrachloride toxicity. *Toxicol. Appl. Pharmacol.* **119**, 275–279.

ElSisi, A. E., Hall, P., Sim, W. W., Earnest, D. L., and Sipes, I. G. (1993a). Characterization of vitamin A potentiation of carbon tetrachloride-induced liver injury. *Toxicol. Appl. Pharmacol.* **119**, 280–288.

ElSisi, A. E., Earnest, D. L., and Sipes, I. G. (1993b). Vitamin A potentiation of carbon tetrachloride hepatotoxicity: Role of liver macrophages and active oxygen species. *Toxicol. Appl. Pharmacol.* **119**, 295–301.

Eyhorn, S., Schlayer, H. J., Henninger, H. P., Dieter, P., Hermann, R., Woort-Menker, M., Becker, H., Schaefer, H., and Decker, K. (1988). Rat hepatic sinusoidal endothelial cells in monolayer culture. Biochemical and ultrastructural characteristics. *J. Hepatol.* **6**, 23–35.

Fantone, J. C., and Ward, P. A. (1982). Role of oxygen-derived free radicals and metabolites in leukocyte-dependent inflammatory reactions. *Am. J. Pathol.* **107**, 397–418.

Feder, L. S., and Laskin, D. L. (1993). Regulation of hepatic endothelial cell proliferation by macrophage derived factors and inflammatory mediators. *In* "Cells of the Hepatic Sinusoid" (D. L. Knook and E. Wisse, eds.), Vol. 4. pp. 33–35. The Kupffer Cell Foundation, Leiden.

Feder, L. S., Todaro, J. A., and Laskin, D. L. (1993). Characterization of interleukin-1 and interleukin-6 production by hepatic endothelial cells and macrophages. *J. Leukocyte Biol.* **53**, 126–132.

Feingold, K. R. and Grunfield, C. (1987). Tumor necrosis factor-alpha stimulates hepatic lipogenesis in the rat in vivo. *J. Clin. Invest.* **80**, 184–190.

Ferluga, J., and Allison, A. (1978). Role of mononuclear infiltrating cells in the pathogenesis of hepatitis. *Lancet* **2**, 610–611.

Filkins, J. P. (1985). Monokines and the metabolic pathophysiology of septic shock. *Fed. Proc.* **44**, 300–305.

Frederick, J., Hasselgren, P., Davis, S., Higashiguchi, T., and Fischer, J. (1993). Nitric oxide upregulates *in vivo* hepatic protein synthesis during endotoxemia. *Arch. Surg.* **128**, 152–157.

Freudenberg, M. A., Keppler, D., and Galanos, C. (1986). Requirement for lipopolysaccharide-responsive macrophages in galactosamine-induced sensitization to endotoxin. *Infect. Immun.* **51**, 891–895.

Friedman, S. L., Roll, F. J., Boyles, J., and Bissell, D. M. (1985). Hepatic lipocytes: The principal collagen-producing cells of normal rat liver. *Proc. Natl. Acad. Sci. USA* **82**, 8681–8685.

Gagnon, L., Filion, L. G., Dubois, C., and Rola-Pleszczynski. (1989). Leukotrienes and macrophage activation: Augmented cytotoxic activity and enhanced interleukin 1, tumor necrosis factor and hydrogen peroxide production. *Agents Actions* **26**, 141–147.

Galanos, C., Freudenberg, M. A., and Reuter, W. (1979). Galactosamine-induced sensitization to the lethal effects of endotoxin. *Proc. Natl. Acad. Sci. USA* **76**, 5939–5943.

Gardner, C. R., Wasserman, A. J., and Laskin, D. L. (1987). Differential sensitivity of tumor targets to liver macrophage-mediated cytotoxicity. *Cancer Res.* **47**, 6686–6691.

Gardner, C. R., Heck, D. E., Feder, L. S., McCloskey, T. W., Laskin, J. D., and Laskin, D. L. (1992). Differential regulation of reactive nitrogen and reactive oxygen intermediate production by hepatic macrophages and endothelial cells. *In* "The Molecular Basis of Oxidative Damage by Leukocytes" (A. J. Jesaitis and E. A. Dratz, eds.), pp. 267–272. CRC Press, Boca Raton, Florida.

Geerts, A., Schellinck, P., Bouwens, L., and Wisse, E. (1988). Cell population kinetics of Kupffer cells during the onset of fibrosis in rat liver by chronic carbon tetrachloride administration. *J. Hepatol.* **6**, 50–56.

Ghezzi, P., Saccardo, B., and Bianchi, M. (1986). Recombinant tumor necrosis factor depresses cytochrome P450-dependent microsomal drug metabolism in mice. *Biochem. Biophys. Res. Commun.* **136**, 316–321.

Gillette, J. R. (1974). A perspective on the role of chemically reactive metabolites of foreign compounds in toxicity. I. Correlation of changes in covalent binding of reactive metabolites with changes in the incidence and severity of toxicity. *Biochem. Pharmacol.* **23**, 2785–2797.

Goetzl, E., and Pickett, W. (1981). Novel structural determinants of the human neutrophil chemotactic activity of leukotriene B. *J. Exp. Med.* **153**, 482–487.

Guarner, F., Wallace, J. L., MacNaughton, W. K., Ibbotson, G. C., Arroyo, V., and Rodes, J. (1989). Endotoxin-induced ascites formation in the rat: Partial mediation by platelet activating factor. *Hepatology* **10**, 788–794.

Gunawardhana, L., Mobley, S. A., and Sipes, I. G. (1993). Modulation of 1,2-dichlorobenzene hepatotoxicity in the Fischer-344 rat by a scavenger of superoxide anions and an inhibitor of Kupffer cells. *Toxicol. Appl. Pharmacol.* **119**, 205–213.

Hagmann, W., Denzlinger, C., and Keppler, D. (1984). Role of peptide leukotrienes and their hepatobiliary elimination in endotoxin action. *Circul. Shock* **14**, 223–235.

Hahn, E., Wick, G., Pencev, D., and Timpl, R. (1980). Distribution of basement membrane proteins in normal and fibrotic human liver: Collagen type IV, laminin and fibronectin. *Gut* **21**, 63–71.

Halliwell, B., and Gutteridge, J. M. C. (1984). Oxygen toxicity, oxygen radicals, transition metals and disease. *Biochem. J.* **219**, 1–14.

Harbrecht, B., Billiar, T., Stadler, J., Demetris, A., Ochoa, J., Curran, R., and Simmons, R. (1992). Inhibition of nitric oxide synthesis during endotoxemia promotes intrahepatic thrombosis and an oxygen radical-mediated hepatic injury. *J. Leukocyte Biol.* **52**, 390–394.

Heck, D. E., Laskin, D. L., Gardner, C. R., and Laskin, J. D. (1992). Epidermal growth factor suppresses nitric oxide and hydrogen peroxide production by keratinocytes. Potential role of nitric oxide in the regulation of wound healing. *J. Biol. Chem.* **267**, 21277–21280.

Helyar, L., Bundschuh, D. S., Laskin, J. D., and Laskin, D. L. (1993). Hepatic fat storing cells produce nitric oxide and hydrogen peroxide in response to bacterially-derived lipopolysaccharide (LPS). *In* "Cells of the Hepatic Sinusoid" (D. L. Knook and E. Wisse, eds.), Vol. 4. pp. 67–69. The Kupffer Cell Foundation, Leiden.

Hendriks, H. F. J., Verhoofstad, W. A. M. M., Brower, A., and Knook, D. L. (1985). Perisinusoidal fat-storing cells are the main vitamin A storage sites in rat liver. *Exp. Cell. Res.* **160**, 138–149.

Hendriks, H. F. J., Horan, M. A., Durham, S. K., Earnest, D. L., Brouwer, A., Hollander,

C. F., and Knook, D. L. (1987). Endotoxin induced liver injury in aged and subacutely hypervitaminotic rats. *Mech. Ageing Dev.* **41**, 241–249.

Henson, P. M., and Johnston, R. B. (1987). Tissue injury in inflammation. Oxidants, proteinases, and cationic proteins. *J. Clin. Invest.* **79**, 669–674.

Hirano, T. (1992). Interleukin-6 and its relation to inflammation and disease. *Clin. Immunol. Immunopathol.* **62**, S60–S65.

Hishinuma, I., Nagakawa, J., Hirota, K., Mityamoto, K., Tsukidate, K., Yamanaka, T., Katayama, K., and Yamatsu, I. (1990). Involvement of tumor necrosis factor-α in development of hepatic injury in galactosamine-sensitized mice. *Hepatology* **12**, 1187–1191.

Hooper, D. C., Steer, C. J., Dinarello, C. A., and Peackock, A. C. (1981). Haptoglobin and albumin synthesis in isolated rat hepatocytes. *Biochim. Biophys Acta* **653**, 118–129.

Husztik, E., Lazar, G., and Parducz, A. (1980). Electron microscopic study of Kupffer cell phagocytosis blockade induced by gadolinium chloride. *Br. J. Exp. Pathol.* **61**, 624–630.

Jirik, F. R., Podor, T. J., Hirano, T., Hirano, T., Kishimoto, T., Loskutoff, D. J., Carson, D. A., and Lotz, M. (1989). Bacterial lipopolysaccharide and inflammatory mediators augment IL-6 secretion by human endothelial cells. *J. Immunol.* **142**, 144–147.

Jollow, D. J., Mitchell, J. R., Potter, W. Z., Davis, D. C., Gillette, J. R., and Brodie, B. B. (1973). Acetaminophen-induced hepatic necrosis. II. Role of covalent binding in vivo. *J. Pharmacol. Exp. Therapeut.* **187**, 195–202.

Kaneda, K., Dan, C., and Wake, K. (1983). Pit cells as natural killer cells. *Biomed. Res.* **4**, 567–576.

Kaplan, A. P., Goetzl, E. J., and Austen, K. F. (1972). The fibrinolytic pathway of human plasma. II. The generation of chemotactic activity by activation of plasminogen activator. *J. Clin. Invest.* **52**, 2591–2595.

Keppler, D., Hagmann, W., Rapp, Denzlinger, C., and Koch, H. K. (1985). The relation of leukotrienes to liver injury. *Hepatology* **5**, 883–891.

Kilbourn, R. G., Jubran, A., Gross, S. S., Griffith, O. W., Levi, R., Adams, J., and Lodato, R. F. (1990). Reversal of endotoxin-mediated shock by N^G-methyl-L-arginine, an inhibitor of nitric oxide synthase. *Biochem. Biophys. Res. Commun.* **172**, 1132–1138.

Klebanoff, S. J., Vadas, M. A., Harlan, J. M., Sparks, L. H., Gamble, J. R., Agosti, J. M., and Waltersdorph, A. M. (1986). Stimulation of neutrophils by tumor necrosis factor. *J. Immunol.* **136**, 4220–4225.

Knook, D. L., and Sleyster, E. Ch. (1980). Isolated parenchymal, Kupffer and endothelial rat liver cells characterized by their lysosomal enzyme content. *Biochem. Biophys. Res. Commun.* **96**, 250–257.

Larrick, J. W., and Wright, S. C. (1990). Cytotoxic mechanism of tumor necrosis factor-α. *FASEB J.* **4**, 3215–3223.

Laskin, D. L. (1989). Potential rule of activated macrophages in chemical and drug induced liver injury. *In* "Cells of the Hepatic Sinusoid" (E. Wisse, D. L. Knook, and K. Decker, eds.), Vol. 2, pp. 284–287. Kupffer Cell Foundation, Amsterdam.

Laskin, D. L. (1990). Nonparenchymal cells and hepatotoxicity. *Sem. Liver Dis.* **10**, 293–304.

Laskin, D. L., and Pilaro, A. M. (1986). Potential role of activated macrophages in acetaminophen hepatotoxicity. I. Isolation and characterization of activated macrophages from rat liver. *Toxicol. Appl. Pharmacol.* **86**, 204–215.

Laskin, D. L., and Pilaro, A. M. (1988). Activation of liver macrophages for killing of hepatocytes following acetaminophen treatment of rats. *Toxicologist* **8**, 32.

Laskin, D. L., Pilaro, A. M., and Ji, S. (1986a). Potential role of activated macrophages in acetaminophen hepatotoxicity. II. Mechanism of macrophage accumulation and activation. *Toxicol. Appl. Pharmacol.* **86**, 216–226.

Laskin, D. L., Kimura, T., Sakakibara, S., Riley, D., and Berg, R. (1986b). Chemotactic activity of collagen-like polypeptides for human peripheral blood neutrophils. *J. Leukocyte Biol.* **39**, 255–266.

Laskin, D. L., Robertson, F. M., Pilaro, A. M., and Laskin, J. D. (1988). Activation of liver macrophages following phenobarbital treatment of rats. *Hepatology* **8**, 1051–1055.

Laskin, D. L., Heck, D. E., Punjabi, C., Pendino, K. J., and Laskin, J. D. (1993a). Role of nitric oxide in chemically induced tissue injury. *Toxicologist* **13**, 25.

Laskin, D. L., Gardner, C. R., Maurer, J. K., and Driscoll, K. E. (1993b). Kupffer cell (KC)-derived tumor necrosis factor-alpha (TNF) as a mediator of hepatotoxicity. *Toxicologist* **13**, 427.

Lehman, V., Freudenberg, M. A., and Galanos, C. (1987). Lethal toxicity of lipopolysaccharide and tumor necrosis factor in normal and D-galactosamine-treated mice. *J. Exp. Med.* **165**, 657–663.

Lloyd, R. S., and Triger, D. R. (1975). Studies on hepatic uptake of antigen. III. Studies of liver macrophage function in normal rats and following carbon tetrachloride administration. *Immunology* **29**, 253–263.

MacDonald, J. R., Beckstead, J. H., and Smuckler, E. A. (1987). An ultrastructural and histochemical study of the prominent inflammatory response in D(+)-galactosamine hepatotoxicity. *Br. J. Exp. Pathol.* **68**, 189–199.

Mathison, J. C., and Ulevitch, R. J. (1979). The clearance, tissue distribution, and cellular localization of intravenously injected lipopolysaccharide in rabbits. *J. Immunol.* **123**, 2133–2143.

Matsubara, T., and Ziff, M. (1986). Increased superoxide anion release from human endothelial cells in response to cytokines. *J. Immunol.* **137**, 3295–3298.

Matsushima, K., and Oppenheim, J. (1989). Interleukin-8 and MCAF: Novel inflammatory cytokines inducible by IL-1 and TNF. *Cytokine* **1**, 2–13.

McClain, C. J., and Cohen, D. A. (1989). Increased tumor necrosis factor production by monocytes in alcoholic hepatitis. *Hepatology* **9**, 349–351.

McCloskey, T. W., Todaro, J. A., and Laskin, D. L. (1992). Effects of lipopolysaccharide treatment of rats on hepatic macrophage and endothelial cell antigen expression and oxidative metabolism. *Hepatology* **16**, 191–203.

McCord, J. M. (1974). Free radicals and inflammation: Protection of synovial fluid by superoxide dismutase. *Science* **185**, 529–531.

Mitchell, J. R., Jollow, D. J., Potter, W. Z., and Davis, D. C., Gillette, J. R., and Brodie, B. B. (1973). Acetaminophen-induced hepatic necrosis. I. Role of drug metabolism. *J. Pharmacol. Exp. Therapeut.* **187**, 185–194.

Mochida, S., Ogata, I., Hirata, K., Ohta, Y., Yamada, S., and Fujiwara, K. (1990). Provocation of massive hepatic necrosis by endotoxin after partial hepatectomy in rats. *Gastroenterology* **99**, 771–777.

Moldeus, P. (1978). Paracetamol metabolism and toxicity in isolated hepatocytes from rat and mouse. *Biochem. Pharmacol.* **27**, 2859–2863.

Moncada, S., Palmer, R., and Higgs, E. (1991). Nitric oxide: Physiology, pathophysiology and pharmacology. *Pharmacol. Rev.* **43**, 109–142.

Monden, K., Arii, S., Itai, S., Sasaoki, T., Adachi, Y., Funaki, N., Higashitsuji, H., and Tobe, T. (1991). Enhancement and hepatocyte-modulating effect of chemical mediators and monokines produced by hepatic macrophages in rats with induced sepsis. *Res. Exp. Med.* **191**, 177–187.

Munkee, R., Gasson, J., Ogawa, M., and Koeffler, H. P. (1986). Recombinant TNF induces production of granulocyte-monocyte colony stimulating factor. *Nature (London)* **323**, 79–82.

Munthe-Kaas, A. C. (1976). Phagocytosis in rat Kupffer cells *in vitro*. *Exp. Cell. Res.* **99**, 319–327.

Nakae, D., Yamamoto, K., Yoshiji, H., Kinugasa, T., Maruyama, H., Farber, J. L., and Konishi, Y. (1990). Liposome-encapsulated superoxide dismutase prevents liver necrosis induced by acetaminophen. *Am. J. Pathol.* **136**, 787–795.

Nathan, C. F. (1987). Secretory products of macrophages. *J. Clin. Invest.* **79**, 319–326.

Nolan, J. P. (1981). Endotoxin, reticuloendothelial function and liver injury. *Hepatology* **1**, 458–465.

Nolan, J. P., and Ali, M. V. (1973). Endotoxin and the liver. II. Effect of tolerance on carbon tetrachloride induced injury. *J. Med.* **4**, 28–38.

Nolan, J. P., and Leibowitz, A. Z. (1978). Endotoxin and the liver. III. Modification of acute carbon tetrachloride injury by polymyxin B, an antiendotoxin. *Gastroenterology* **75**, 445–449.

Onozaki, K., Matsushima, K., Kleinerman, E. S., Saito, T., and Oppenheim, J. J. (1985). The role of interleukin 1 in promoting human monocyte-mediated tumor cytotoxicity. *J. Immunol.* **135**, 314–320.

Ooi, B. S., MacCarthy, E. P., Hsu, A., and Ooi, Y. M. (1983). Human mononuclear cell modulation of endothelial cell proliferation. *J. Lab. Clin. Med.* **102**, 428–433.

Oppenheim, J. J., Kovacs, E. J., Matsushima, K., and Durum, S. K. (1986). There is more than one interleukin 1. *Immunol. Today* **7**, 45–56, 1986.

Perez, H. D., Roll, F. J., Bissell, D. M., Shak, S., and Goldstein, I. M. (1984). Production of chemotactic activity for polymorphonuclear leukocytes by cultured rat hepatocytes exposed to ethanol. *J. Clin. Invest.* **74**, 1350–1357.

Perlmutter, D. H., Dinarello, C. A., Punsal, P. I., and Colten, H. R. (1986). Cachectin/tumor necrosis factor regulates hepatic acute-phase gene expression. *J. Clin. Invest.* **78**, 1349–1354.

Peterson, T. C., and Renton, K. W. (1986). Kupffer cell factor mediated depression of hepatic parenchymal cell cytochrome P-450. *Biochem. Pharmacol.* **35**, 1491–1497.

Pilaro, A. M., and Laskin, D. L. (1986). Accumulation of activated mononuclear phagocytes in the liver following lipopolysaccharide treatment of rats. *J. Leukocyte Biol.* **40**, 29–41.

Pinzani, M., Abboud, H. E., Gesualdo, L., and Abboud, S. L. (1992). Regulation of macrophage colony-stimulating factor in liver fat-storing cells by peptide growth factors. *Am. J. Physiol.* **262**, C876–C881.

Praaning-van Dalen, D. P., Brouwer, A., and Knook, D. L. (1981). Clearance capacity of rat liver Kupffer, endothelial, and parenchymal cells. *Gastroenterology* **81**, 1036–1044.

Praaning-van Dalen, D. P., De Leeuw, A. M., Brouwer, A., and Knook, D. L. (1987). Rat liver endothelial cells have a greater capacity than Kupffer cells to endocytose N-acetylglucosamine- and mannose-terminated glycoproteins. *Hepatology* **7**, 672–679.

Przybocki, J., Reuhl, K., Thurman, R., and Kauffman, F. (1992). Involvement of nonparenchymal cells in oxygen-dependent hepatic injury by allyl alcohol. *Toxicol. Appl. Pharmacol.* **119**, 295–301.

Punjabi, C., Laskin, D. L., Heck, D. E., and Laskin, J. D. (1992). Production of nitric oxide by bone marrow cells: Inverse correlation with proliferation. *J. Immunol.* **149**, 2179–2184.

Ramadori, G. (1991). The stellate cell (Ito cell, fat storing cell, lipocyte, perisinusoidal cell) of the liver. *Virchow's Arch. B Cell Pathol.* **61**, 147–158.

Rodriguez de Turco, E. B., and Spitzer, J. A. (1990). Eicosanoid production in nonparenchymal liver cells isolated from rats infused with E. coli endotoxin. *J. Leukocyte Biol.* **48**, 488–494.

Rogoff, T. M., and Lipsky, P. E. (1980). Antigen presentation by isolated guinea pig Kupffer cells. *J. Immunol.* **124**, 1740–1744.

Rubin, R., and Farber, J. L. (1984). Mechanisms of the killing of cultured hepatocytes by hydrogen peroxide. *Arch. Biochem. Biophys.* **228**, 450–459.

Sacks, T., Malt, C. F., Craddock, P. R., Bowers, T. K., and Jacob, H. S. (1977). Oxygen radicals mediate endothelial cell damage by complement-stimulated granulocytes. An *in vitro* model of immune vascular damage. *J. Clin. Invest.* **61**, 1161–1167.

Sato, N., Goto, T., and Haranaki, K. (1986). Actions of tumor necrosis factor on cultured vascular endothelial cells: Morphologic modulation, growth inhibition, and cytotoxicity. *J. Natl. Cancer Inst.* **76**, 1113–1121.

Schiffman, E., Corcoran, B., and Wahl, S. (1975). N-Formylmethionine peptides as chemoattractants for leukocytes. *Proc. Natl. Acad. Sci. USA* **72**, 1059–1062.

Seglen, P. O., Solheim, A. E., Grinde, B., Gordon, P. B., Schwarze, P. E., Gjessing, R., and

Poli, A. (1980). Amino acid control of protein synthesis and degradation in isolated rat hepatocytes. *Ann. N.Y. Acad. Sci.* **349,** 1–17.

Sevanian, A., and Hochstein, P. (1985). Mechanisms and consequences of lipid peroxidation in biological systems. *Annu. Rev. Nutr.* **5,** 365–390.

Shedlofsky, S. I., and McClain, C. J. (1991). Hepatic dysfunction due to cytokines. In "Cytokines and Inflammation" (E. S. Kimball, ed.), pp. 235–273. CRC Press, Boca Raton, Florida.

Shinagawa, T., Yoshioka, K., Kakumu, S., Wakita, T., Ishikawa, T., Itoh, Y., and Takayanagi, M. (1991). Apoptosis in cultured rat hepatocytes: The effects of tumor necrosis factor-α and interferon-γ. *J. Pathol.* **165,** 247–253.

Shiratori, Y., Takikawa, H., Kawase, T., and Sugimoto, T. (1986). Superoxide anion generating capacity and lysosomal enzyme activities of Kupffer cells in galactosamine-induced hepatitis. *Gastroenterol. Jpn.* **21,** 135–144.

Shiratori, Y., Kawase, T., Shiina, S., Okano, K., Sugimoto, T., Teraoka, H., Matano, S., Matsumoto, K., and Kamii, K. (1988). Modulation of hepatotoxicity by macrophages in the liver. *Hepatology* **8,** 815–821.

Shiratori, Y., Tanaka, M., Hai, K., Kawase, T., Shiina, S., and Sugimoto, T. (1990a). Role of endotoxin-responsive macrophages in hepatic injury. *Hepatology* **11,** 183–192.

Shiratori, Y., Tanaka, M., Umihara, J., Kawase, T., Shiina, S., and Sugimoto, T. (1990b). Leukotriene inhibitors modulated hepatic injury induced by lipopolysaccharide-activated macrophages. *J. Hepatol.* **10,** 51–61.

Silva, A. T., and Cohen, J. (1992). Role of interferon-γ in experimental gram-negative sepsis. *J. Infect. Dis.* **166,** 331–335.

Sim, W. W., Abril, E. R., and Earnest, D. L. (1989). Mechanisms of Kupffer cell activation in hypervitaminosis A. In "Cells of the Hepatic Sinusoid" (E. Wisse, D. L. Knook, and K. Decker, eds.), Vol. 2, pp. 91–93. Kupffer Cell Foundation, Amsterdam.

Sipe, J. D., Vogel, S. N., Ryan, J. L., McAdam, K. P. W. J., and Rosenstreich, D. L. (1979). Detection of a mediator derived from endotoxin-stimulated macrophages that induces the acute phase serum amyloid a response in mice. *J. Exp. Med.* **150,** 597–606.

Smedstod, B., Pertoft, H., Eggertsen, G., and Sundstrom, C. (1985). Functional and morphological characterization of cultures of Kupffer cells and liver endothelial cell prepared by means of density separation in percoll, and selective substrate adherence. *Cell Tissue Res.* **241,** 639–649.

Souhami, R. L., and Bradfield, J. W. (1981). The recovery of hepatic phagocytosis after blockade of Kupffer cells. *J. Reticuloendothel. Soc.* **16,** 75–86.

Stark, M. E., and Szurszewski, J. H. (1992). Role of nitric oxide in gastrointestinal and hepatic function and disease. *Gastroenterology* **103,** 1928–1949.

Steffan, A. M., Gendrault, J. L., McCuskey, R. S., McCuskey, P. A., and Kirn, A. (1986). Phagocytosis, an unrecognized property of murine endothelial liver cells. *Hepatology* **6,** 830–836.

Stuehr, D. J., and Nathan, C. F. (1989). Nitric oxide. A macrophage product responsible for cytostasis and respiratory inhibition in tumor target cells. *J. Exp. Med.* **169,** 1543–1555.

Sugino, K., Dohi, K., Yamada, K., and Kawasaki, T. (1989). Changes in the levels of endogenous antioxidants in the liver of mice with experimental endotoxemia and the protective effects of the antioxidants. *Surgery* **105,** 200–206.

Sztein, M. B., Vogel, S. N., Sipe, J. D., Murphy, P. A., Mizel, S. B., Oppenheim, J. J., and Rosenstreich, D. L. (1981). The role of macrophages in the acute phase response: SAA inducer is closely related to lymphocyte activating factor and endogenous pyrogen. *Cell Immunol.* **63,** 164–176.

Tanner, A., Keyhani, A., Reiner, R., Holdstock, G., and Wright, R. (1981). Proteolytic enzymes released by liver macrophages may promote hepatic injury in a rat model of hepatic damage. *Gastroenterology* **80,** 647–654.

Tanner, A. R., Deyhani, A. H., and Wright, R. (1983). The influence of endotoxin *in vitro* on hepatic macrophage lysosomal enzyme release in different models of hepatic injury. *Liver* **3**, 151–160.

Thiele, D. L. (1989). Tumor necrosis factor, the acute phase response and the pathogenesis of alcoholic liver disease. *Hepatology* **9**, 497–499.

Thompson, W. D., Jack, A. S., and Patrick, R. S. (1980). The possible role of macrophages in transient hepatic fibrogenesis induced by acute carbon tetrachloride injury. *J. Pathol.* **130**, 65–73.

Tiegs, G., and Wendel, A. (1988). Leukotriene-mediated liver injury. *Biochem. Pharmacol.* **37**, 2569–2573.

Tiegs, G., Wolter, M., and Wendel, A. (1989). Tumor necrosis factor is a terminal mediator in galactosamine/endotoxin-induced hepatitis in mice. *Biochem. Pharmacol.* **38**, 627–631.

Tiku, M. L., and Tomasi, T. B. (1985). Enhancement of endothelial plasminogen activator synthesis by lymphokines. *Transplantation* **40**, 293–298.

Tracey, K. J., Beutler, B., Lowry, S. F., Merryweather, J., Wolpe, S., Milsark, I. W., Hariri, R. J., Fahey, T. J., Zentella, A., Albert, J., Shires, G. T., and Cerami, A. (1986). Shock and tissue injury induced by recombinant human cachectin. *Science* **234**, 470–474.

Ward, P. A., and Newman, L. J. (1969). A neutrophil chemotactic factor from C5a. *J. Immunol.* **102**, 93–99.

West, M. A., Billiar, T. R., Curran, R. D., Hyland, B. J., and Simmons, R. L. (1989). Evidence that rat Kupffer cells stimulate and inhibit hepatocyte protein synthesis *in vitro* by different mechanisms. *Gastroenterology* **96**, 1572–1582.

Whicher, J. T., and Evans, S. W. (1990). Cytokines in disease. *Clin. Chem.* **36/7**, 1269–1281.

Widmann, J. J., and Fahimi, H. D. (1975). Proliferation of mononuclear phagocytes (Kupffer cells) and endothelial cells in regenerating rat liver. *Am. J. Pathol.* **80**, 349–366.

Williams, G. M., Bermudez, E., San, R. J. C., Goldblatt, P. J., and Laspia, M. F. (1978). Rat hepatocyte primary cultures. IV. Maintenance of defined medium and the role of production of plasminogen activating factor and other proteases. *In Vitro* **14**, 824–837.

Wisse, E., and Knook, D. L. (1979). The investigation of sinusoidal cells: A new approach to the study of liver function. *Prog. Liver Dis.* **6**, 153–171.

14

Central Nervous System: Viral Infection and Immune-Mediated Inflammation

Georgia Schuller-Levis, Piotr B. Kozlowski, and Richard J. Kascsak

I. Introduction

Because the inflammatory response in the brain differs from the response seen in other organs, the brain was considered to be "immunologically privileged." As knowledge of the immune response in the central nervous system (CNS) accumulated, the concept of "immunological privilege" became largely of historical relevance. It is now recognized that several factors that modify the immune and inflammatory response within the CNS are unique for this organ.

The first factor that contributes to the uniqueness of the CNS immune response is the presence of the blood–brain barrier (BBB). The BBB controls the flow of soluble substances as small as monovalent ions to and from the CNS tissue and, under normal conditions, excludes proteins and other micromolecules (Reese and Karnovsky, 1967; Bradbury, 1979). The BBB is formed by microvascular endothelial cells (ECs), which line the blood vessels and seal the barrier through tight junctional complexes. ECs in the brain, under normal conditions, also lack fenestrae and vesicular channels. Thus, the cytoplasm of ECs is the only route for all micromolecules and macromolecules to enter or leave the bloodstream. The next element of the BBB is the basement membrane lining the extraluminal surface of endothelial cells (Reese and Karnovsky, 1967; Brightman, 1989). The basement membrane is lined on the abluminal side with foot processes of astroglial cells. The effectiveness of the BBB in maintaining CNS homeostasis is enormous. The brain in humans constitutes only about 2% of the total body mass, but it utilizes about 15% of the entire aortal blood output (Brierly and Graham, 1992). The BBB, on the other hand, can easily be broken (or rather, temporarily disabled), and the control of flux of solutes may be locally disabled for long periods of time (Reese and Karnovsky, 1967; Hirano *et al.*, 1970). A peculiarity of the BBB is that it excludes macromolecules from entering the CNS but allows megastructures such as entire hematogenous inflammatory cells to cross the barrier without opening the tight junctions (Hirano *et al.*, 1970; Azarelli *et al.*, 1984; Lossinsky *et al.*, 1989; Raine *et al.*, 1990; Powell, 1991). Nonetheless, the entry of hematogenous inflammatory cells into the CNS appears to be strictly controlled by the ECs.

An initial event in the inflammatory reaction in the CNS is the egress of hematogenous cells into the extravascular milieu of the CNS parenchyma (Figure 1). Only the previously sensitized inflammatory cells, i.e., lymphocytes, can invade the CNS (Raine *et al.*, 1990; Powell, 1991). The prerequisite for transendothelial passage is the attachment of sensitized cells to the luminal surface of endothelial cells. A growing body of evidence suggests that lymphocytes and monocytes (but not neutrophils) attach to parajunctional endothelial cell receptors and subsequently insert pseudopodial projections into tubular, channel-like openings in the endothelial cells (Lossinsky *et al.*, 1989; Powell *et al.*, 1991). These channels serve as eventual conduits for the transendothelial cell passage into the extravascular space. Numerous studies have shown a great variety of specific membrane receptors on endothelial cells that are critical for the binding of hematogenous cells. These highly specific receptors include several distinct classes of adhesion molecules. These receptors include the immunoglobulin super family (ICAM-1 and -2, LFA-3, VCAM-1, ENDOCAM-1, and NCAM-1); the integrins (LFA-1 or CD11a/18, MAC-1, LPAM-1, β1, β2, β3 families); the LEC-CAM family for lectins (ELAM-1, MEL-14); Cadherins (P, N, E-Cadherins), and the Hermes group of antigens (CD-44) (Harlan, 1985; Dustin and Springer, 1988; Lassmann *et al.*, 1991, Staunton *et al.*,1990; Yednock, 1985). The expression of these receptors, also called addressins, on the endothelial surface is under the control of several cytokines, some of which are present only in local inflammatory response and absent under normal conditions. Neutrophils, which also require addressins for adherence, are able to enter the CNS by opening and passing through a tight junction between adjacent endothelial cells (Broadwell, 1989).

Second, there are structural cells of the CNS that, in addition to their "main" roles, may, under certain conditions, play a role in antigen presentation and/or processing. These cells include astrocytes, endothelial cells, and microglial cells (Fontana *et al.*, 1984). Under normal conditions, only a small portion of meningeal, perivascular dendritic cells and resident microglial cells may express low levels of Class II major histocompatibility complex (MHC) antigens. The expression of these antigens on various cell types seems to be related to the severity of the inflammatory response. In mild inflammation, Class II MHC antigen expression is upregulated mostly on microglia cells; only in severe inflammation can some expression of these antigens be seen on astrocytes. Gamma interferon (IFN-γ) is known

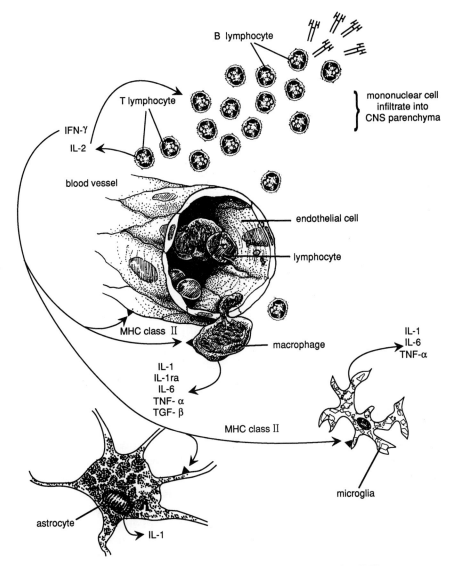

Fig. 1 Elements of the inflammatory response within the CNS.

to stimulate *in vitro* the expression of Class II MHC antigens on endothelial cells, microglial cells, and astrocytes (Wong *et al.*, 1984; Hirsch *et al.*, 1983; Fierz *et al.*, 1985). The nonhematogenous cells that are native to the CNS have a very limited role in CNS inflammation. Neurons, oligodendroglia cells, and ependymal cells, if not affected directly by an infectious agent, appear to be inert bystanders, even in the midst of severe inflammation.

Astrocytes perform a variety of functions within the CNS. Astrocytic processes are a vital part of the BBB, and the cells themselves maintain the homeostasis of the neuropil (Figure 2). Astrocytic cells are the main cells involved in scar formation following CNS injury. They are now considered an accessory cell to the immune system of the CNS (Hertz *et al.*, 1990; Yong *et al.*, 1991; Rodriguez *et al.*, 1987). They express MHC antigens, may act as antigen-presenting cells (APCs), and secrete cytokines. In inflammation, astrocytic cells (especially type 1) may be stimulated by LAF- and ICAM-1, by cytokines from T cells, macrophages, microglial cells, and/or other astrocytes. IL-2 stimulates proliferation of astroglia in experimental brain injury. *In vitro*, IL-1, tumor necrosis factor (TNF), and IFN-γ stimulate proliferation of astrocytes. IFN primes astrocytic cells to the effect of IL-2 by secretion of TNF, IL-1, IL-3, IL-6, and lymphotoxin.

The endothelial cells are not only an anatomical and functional barrier between the blood and the brain; they are also pivotal cells in inflammation. ECs not only regulate the influx of cells and solutes, but they may also act as APCs, and the luminal surface of ECs may be the site of antigen presentation and recognition. Class I MHC molecules necessary for antigen recognition can be found on all cells constituting the BBB, whereas Class II MHC can be induced by IFN-γ stimulation. Class II MHC antigens expressed on ECs increase with the increased severity of inflammation, suggesting that the MHC expression is progressively turned on and may, under certain conditions, lead to amplification of local inflammation. ECs activation in chronic (and not necessarily severe) inflammatory processes may not be a secondary consequence of a local process but may, in fact, initiate and perpetuate the inflammation (Hertz *et al.*, 1990; Gimborne and Beviaqua, 1988; Montovani and Dejana, 1989; Cotran, 1987).

It also appears that the endothelial cell may be a pivotal cell in autoimmune inflammatory reaction (with local intrathecal antibody formation) without the involvement of extraneuronal antigens or infectious agents. ECs may present antigens that are specific for the CNS and attract sensitized T cells. T cells may attach to CNS antigens and perpetuate inflammation by secreting lymphokines (IFN, IL-2) and attract even more lymphocytes. This critical mass of lymphocytes and lymphokines may open the BBB, which allows T cells to enter the CNS parenchyma to recruit B cells, which then locally produce antibodies against the CNS antigens presented by endothelial cells.

Microglia cells are considered immune-competent cells that are native to the CNS but whose origin is still unclear (Graeber and Streit, 1990). They are found throughout the CNS and constitute from 5 to 20% of all CNS cells (Figure 3). Microglia cells share common surface antigens with monocytes and macrophages but not with neuroectodermal cells. The functions of microglial cells include phagocytosis, presentation of antigens, production of IL-1, and stripping of synaptic buttons (deafferentation) from dis-

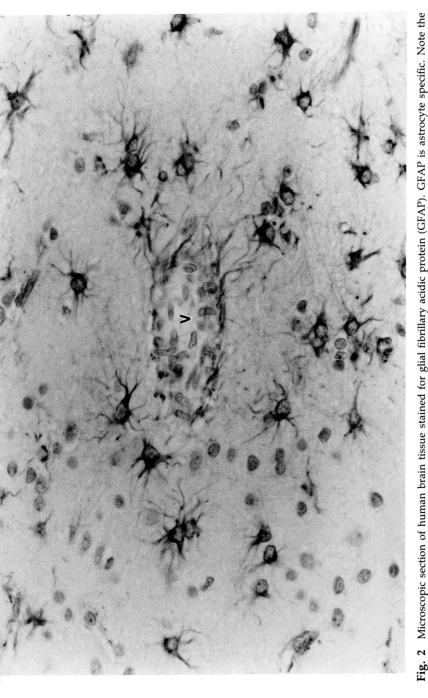

Fig. 2 Microscopic section of human brain tissue stained for glial fibrillary acidic protein (GFAP). GFAP is astrocyte specific. Note the cytoplasmic stain and long slender nonbranching processes (suction feet) running toward the wall of the blood vessel (v). The pale, oblong nuclei of endothelial cells are counterstained with hematoxylin. Anti-GFAP monoclonal antibody, Avidin-Biotin Technique, 70-μm-thick vibratome section, ×470.

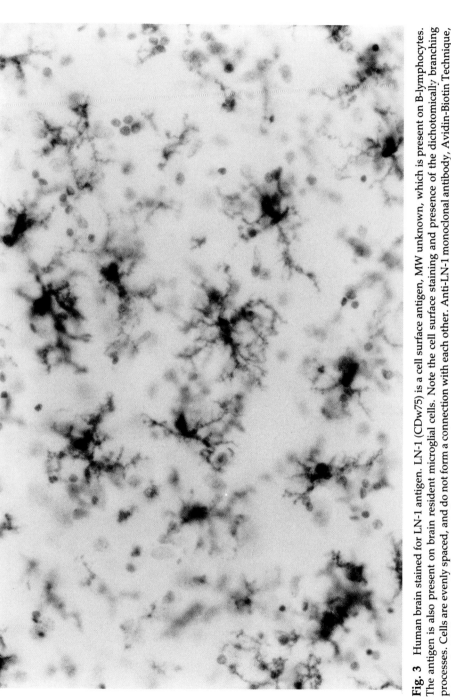

Fig. 3 Human brain stained for LN-1 antigen. LN-1 (CDw75) is a cell surface antigen, MW unknown, which is present on B-lymphocytes. The antigen is also present on brain resident microglial cells. Note the cell surface staining and presence of the dichotomically branching processes. Cells are evenly spaced, and do not form a connection with each other. Anti-LN-1 monoclonal antibody, Avidin-Biotin Technique, 70 µm thick vibratome section; nuclei were counterstained with hematoxylin, ×470.

tressed neurons. There is a low level of expression of Class II MHC antigens on microglial cells under normal conditions, and this expression can be dramatically increased with infusion of IFN-γ (Graeber and Streit, 1990; Tribolet de et al., 1984; Hayes et al., 1987; Hayes et al., 1988; Delisle et al., 1986; Hickey and Kimura, 1988; McGeer et al., 1987; McGeer et al., 1988). Microglia cells also express the CD4 molecule, which is considered an entry point for the human immunodeficiency virus (HIV) (Watkins et al., 1990; Bourdial et al., 1991; Levy, 1988; Michaels et al., 1988).

Yet another unique feature of the CNS is the presence of CNS-specific antigens such as myelin basic protein (MBP), glial fibrillary acidic protein (GFAP), or neuron-specific enolase (NSE). Such proteins can be the focus of autoimmune responses within the CNS. This autoimmune response can be a major contributing factor to pathology and clinical disease (see later discussions on viral-induced autoimmune response and experimental allergic encephalomyelitis).

II. Autoimmunity in the Central Nervous System

A strong body of evidence now suggests that some diseases of the CNS have an immunologic pathogenesis (Paterson, 1977, 1978, 1979, 1982). Examples include experimental allergic encephalomyelitis (EAE), acute disseminated encephalomyelitis (ADEM), and multiple sclerosis (MS). Acute and chronic relapsing EAE can be induced in laboratory animals by an injection of CNS tissue, CNS myelin, myelin basic protein, or more recently, T-cell lines specific for nervous system antigens. ADEM occurs in humans and animals after an antecedent virus infection (see later discussion on viral induced autoimmunity) or vaccination with a living virus or a vaccine containing nervous tissue. MS is an acute or chronic progressive remitting disorder of humans characterized by inflammatory cell infiltration and demyelination.

A. Experimental Allergic Encephalomyelitis

EAE is a useful autoimmune disease model for the study of mechanisms of cellular immune reactions in the CNS and has been considered an experimental model of MS since the earliest descriptions by Rivers et al. (1935). In recent years, reproducible small animal models of chronic EAE have become available (Stone and Lerner, 1965; Wisniewski and Keith, 1977; Massanari, 1980; Lubin et al., 1981; Brown et al., 1982). These small animal models cover the full spectrum of MS pathology (Wisniewski et al., 1982; Lassmann and Wisniewski, 1979) and allow the study of the pathogenesis of chronic inflammatory demyelinating plaque formation. Progress on the pathogenesis and treatment of EAE has been advanced by the selection and maintenance of permanent autoantigen MBP-specific T-cell lines. T cells can now be isolated from animals with EAE that will mediate EAE in the recipient animal. This isolation is possible as a result of progress in the characterization of immune cells subsets, using monoclonal antibodies, and the definition of their growth requirements (i.e., IL-2) (Ben-Nun *et al.*, 1981). It is not clear how the sensitized T cells present in the circulation of EAE animals, cross the BBB and recognize an antigen or antigens that are located in the major dense lines of the myelin sheath. One possible explanation of this phenomenon is that the low rate of physiological exchange of lymphocytes that appears to exist between the CNS and the circulation allows the entry of the sensitized T cells (Lassmann *et al.*, 1991; Wekerle *et al.*, 1986; Wekerle *et al.*, 1991).

Interaction between inflammatory cells and the endothelial cells lining the BBB is an important initial event during inflammation of the CNS. The expression of Ia and of the endothelial leukocyte adhesion molecule (ELAM-1) on endothelial cells in the CNS are some of the earliest changes detected to date in brains of animals with EAE (Rose *et al.*, 1991).

Although the etiology of MS is still unknown, the similarity of MS to remitting-relapsing EAE suggests that MS, like EAE, might be the consequence of either a direct or indirect autosensitization to myelin antigens (i.e., MBP and proteolipid apoprotein) (Rose *et al.*, 1991).

As a result of the application of advances in molecular biology, such as the polymerase chain reaction, and developments in cellular immunology, such as the ability to grow T-cell clones, great progress has been made in the pathogenesis and treatment of MS (Steinman, 1991). Recent reports that most encephalitogenic (BP-specific) T-cell clones derived from mice or rats use common variable region genes of the rearranged T-cell receptor (TCR) have intensified the search for analogous associations in humans (Burns *et al.*, 1989; Urban *et al.*, 1988). Steinman (1991) has recently reviewed the strong parallels between T- cell receptor (TCR) usage in the pathogenesis of EAE and TCR usage in MBP, and specific T cells in MS peripheral blood and T cells in demyelinated plaques in MS brains. The development of strategies for selective immunotherapy in EAE was based on these similarities. This therapy uses monoclonal antibodies on either Class II molecules of the MHC or TCR-variable regions or peptides that compete with HLA Class II molecules or vaccination against TCR-V regions. For example, vaccination of mice with appropriate TCR peptides is highly effective at inducing both cellular and humoral response to TCR and at inhibiting EAE (Howell *et al.*, 1989; Vanderbark *et al.*, 1989). Monoclonal antibodies that bind only the complex of BP and I-As inhibited EAE in H-2s mice when injected within −2 to +10 days of disease induction (Aharoni *et al.*, 1991). Sriram and Carroll (Sriram and Carroll, 1991) have shown that *in vivo* treatment with I-A antibodies at the earliest sign of EAE results in decreased homing of radiolabeled cells to the brain. These data suggest that Class II antigens play an important role in cellular migration across the BBB.

Other potential therapies for EAE include the use of cytokines (see cytokine section) and suppressor T cells. Although mechanisms involved in EAE remission are unclear, suppressor T cells have been postulated to play a role in the prevention of autoimmunity (Ofosu-Appiah and Mokhtarian, 1991). An adaptively transferred suppressor T-cell line, obtained from spleens of mice that recovered from EAE, was able to downgrade EAE in mice subsequently challenged with MBP-activated T cells.

III. Cytokines in the Central Nervous System

Immunologically important cytokines are produced chiefly by lymphocytes and macrophages. Inflammation in the nervous system is likely to be the same as in other organ systems, with a few modifications. Because of the BBB and the macromolecular nature of cytokines, some of these important inflammatory molecules are likely to be CNS resident derived. Recent studies have also indicated astrocytes, microglia, and endothelial cells as possible additional sources of CNS-derived cytokines (Fontana *et al.*, 1982; Frei *et al.*, 1985; Giulian *et al.*, 1985; Frei *et al.*, 1989; Sawada *et al.*, 1989). Immunocytochemical techniques have demonstrated the presence of a variety of cytokines (see earlier discussion) (i.e., MIF, IFN-γ, TNFα, IL-1,2,3) during chronic relapsing EAE (Baker *et al.*, 1991). IL-1, IL-2, TNFα, and IL-6 have also been shown in the serum and/or CSF of EAE animals and/or MS patients (Merril *et al.*, 1989; Gallo *et al.*, 1988; Gijbels *et al.*, 1990).

A. TGF-β1 and IL-1

Transforming growth factor β (TGF-β) has pleotrophic effects. Evidence to date includes the possible role of down-regulation of the IFN-γ induction of Class II MHC expression on the inductive phase of the immune response, as well as inhibition of cytotoxic T-cell development and antagonism of TNF at the effector end of the immune response (Racke *et al.*, 1991; Wahl *et al.*, 1988; Rook *et al.*, 1986; Ranges *et al.*, 1987; Czarniecki *et al.*, 1988; Schluesener, 1990; Shalaby and Ammann, 1988). When administered during EAE induction, TGF-β1 slightly delays the onset of disease (Kuruvilla *et al.*, 1991). However, when given during remission, TGF-β1 prevents the occurrence of relapses in relapsing EAE, suggesting an anti-inflammatory effect of TGF-β1. When TGF-β1 was preincubated *in vitro*, activation and proliferation of myelin basic protein-specific lymph node cells *in vitro* were decreased and severity of the clinical course was reduced (Racke *et al.*, 1991).

Recent data indicate that IL-1 may promote CNS inflammation, and that blocking IL-1 activity may prove beneficial in the treatment of CNS inflammatory disease. For example, EAE in the Lewis rat has been shown to be exacerbated by IL-1α. In addition, the disease was significantly delayed and attenuated by IL-1 receptor antagonist (IL-1ra) (Jacobs *et al.*, 1991).

IL-1 receptor antagonists have been used to ameliorate other inflammatory diseases such as rheumatoid arthritis and septic shock, and colitis in a rabbit model (Cominelli *et al.*, 1990; Ohlsson *et al.*, 1990; Wakabayashi *et al.*, 1991; Arend and Dayer, 1990; Higgins and Postlethwaite, 1991). Several structural variants of IL-1ra have been described (Arend, 1991) that might be of interest in exploring the therapeutic potential of IL-1ra. Administration of IL-1ra into the lateral ventricle of rabbit brains has been reported to block IL-1-induced non-rapid-eye movement sleep as well as IL-1-induced fever (Opp and Krueger, 1991).

The similarities of macrophages and microglia are striking (Merz *et al.*, 1987). For example, IL-1, IL-6, and TNFα are known to be produced by monocytes and macrophages. In the CNS, microglia have been implicated as a major contributor to the production of IL-1, IL-6, and TNF (Woodroofe *et al.*, 1991). Using a continuous microdialysis probe, Woodroofe *et al.* (1991) showed a 15-fold increase in IL-1 over a 24 to 48 hr period and a slight increase in IL-6 at day 1, as a result of mechanical trauma to the brain. Another potential cellular source of IL-1 is the astrocyte. However, the authors have immunocytochemical evidence that in this model the astrocyte response appears much later—at day 7. An increase in peripheral benzodiazepine receptors after local injection of IL-1 and TNFα has been demonstrated on glial cells, but not on neurons (Bourdial *et al.*, 1991), raising the possibility of a sequential mechanism involving the activation of microglia, the release of IL-1 and TNFα, and the promotion by these cytokines of the astroglial reaction.

Administration of human serum amyloid A to mice inhibited fever induced by rIL-1β or rTNFα *in vivo*, whereas the addition of human serum amyloid A to murine hypothalamic slices inhibited IL-1β- or TNFα-induced prostaglandin E2 production. These data suggest a possible feedback relationship between serum amyloid A and cytokines (Shainkin-Kestenbaum *et al.*, 1991).

Injection of IL-1 results in an increased release of corticotropin-releasing factor (Ohgo *et al.*, 1992; Besedovsky *et al.*, 1986; Sapolsky *et al.*, 1987; Uehara *et al.*, 1987). In addition, IL-1α injected into the third ventricle of castrated rats inhibited the pulsatile release of luteinizing hormone (Rettori *et al.*, 1991). In a recent report, Palazzolo *et al.* (1990) suggest that the central and neuroendocrine effects of IL-1 are most likely produced through changes in neurotransmitter metabolism in the brain. In another report, Mohankumai *et al.* (1991) provide evidence that IL-1 stimulates the release of catecholamines (e.g., dopamine and its metabolite, dihydroxyphenylacetic acid (DOPAC) from discrete hypothalamic nuclei of conscious, freely moving rats. The precise role that IL-1 may play in neuroimmunomodulation is still not clear. The important known role of the hypothalamic–pituitary–adrenocortical (HPA) axis in regulating inflammation mandates further studies of the role of IL-1 as a neuroimmunomodulator.

Another potential interaction of the nervous system and the immune system is the involvement of cytokines in neurogenic inflammation (Kimball, 1991). In the Kimball model, substance P, a neuropeptide, is at the center, interacting with fibroblasts, mast cells, B cells, and macrophages. In addition to substance P, other neuropeptides, neurotransmitters, and other vasoactive amines act in concert with cytokines to affect immunologic mechanisms.

B. IL-2, IL-6, TNFα, and IFN-γ

The roles of established monokines (IL-6 and TNFα) and T-cell products (IFN-γ and IL-2) on CNS pathology and physiology are stimulating areas of ongoing research. TNF appears to be a major cytokine involved in cellular injury. Axon and myelin abnormalities have been demonstrated *in vitro* by TNF (Selmaj and Raine, 1988). After IL-2 perfusion in rats, TNF was noted to coincide with myelin damage. Interestingly, IL-2 perfusion has been shown to compromise the BBB (Ellison and Merchant, 1991). Several structural variants of IL-1ra have been described (Arend, 1991) that might be of interest in exploring the therapeutic potential of IL-1ra. Several phosphodiesterase inhibitors (e.g., theophylline, pentoxifylline, and 3-isobutyl-1-methylxanthine) have been shown to suppress TNFα synthesis (Endres *et al.*, 1991). High TNF levels have been reported to be associated with several manifestations of malaria (Kremsner *et al.*, 1991; Shaffer *et al.*, 1991), and decreasing TNF, levels with recovery. In a murine model of cerebral malaria, pentoxifylline, which reduces TNF, given for 10 days after infection, protected the mice from development of cerebral malaria (Kremsner *et al.*, 1991).

One of the pleotrophic effects of IL-6 is a neurotrophic effect that has been described in viral diseases (Frei, 1989) and improved survival of mesencephalic catachoaminergic and septal cholinergic neurons (Hama *et al.*, 1991). Mice infected with lethal lymphocytic choriomeningitis (LCM) virus as well as LCM carrier mice have been shown to be correlated with high levels of secretion of IL-6 (Maskophidis *et al.*, 1991). Of interest is the possible role of IL-6 in the formation of Alzheimer amyloid plaque (Baurer and Strauss, 1991). Bauer *et al.* have shown a potent human proteinase inhibitor, α-2 macroglobulin (α2M), after stimulation with IL-6 (Ganter *et al.*, 1991). Subsequently, they examined whether α2M and IL-6 could be detected in Alzheimer disease (AD) brain. They report that AD cortical senile plaques display strong α2M and IL-6 immunoreactivity, with no such immunoreactivity found in age-matched control brains. The data indicate that neuronal cells are the site of α2M synthesis in AD brains.

Among the best known pleotrophic effects of IFN-γ is its ability to induce the expression of Class II MHC molecules on several cell types. Class II MHC antigens are known to be essential in antigen presentation. Studies have shown that IFN-γ can induce expression of Class II MHC molecules on astroglia (Sedgwick *et al.*, 1991). However, Sedgewick *et al.* (1991) were unable to show that astroglial cells act as stimulators of CD4+ T cells and therefore postulated another cell type as the major antigen-presenting cell in CNS inflammation. Infection with mouse hepatitis virus (MHV), has been shown to block expression of MHC molecules on murine cerebral endothelial cells (see later discussion) (Joseph *et al.*, 1991). Joseph *et al.* postulate possible release of cytokines by endothelial cells as a mechanism for blocking IFN-induced Class II antigens.

C. Other Cytokines

Several additional cytokines have been reported that may play a role in CNS pathology and physiology. Growth factors and, to some extent, IL-1β and TNFα appear to increase nerve growth factor synthesis and secretion by astrocytes (Yoshida and Gage, 1992). Cultured astrocytes have been reported to express macrophage colony-stimulating factor activity at a high level, which may be important in the replication of microglial precursors (Alliot *et al.*, 1991).

Growth differentiation factor-1, a recently described member of the transforming growth factor β superfamily, has been reported to be restricted almost exclusively to the CNS (Lee, 1991). This extracellular signaling factor is postulated to play a general role in nervous system maintenance and function. Of interest is one of two platelet-activating factor (PAF) antagonists, which has been shown to also inhibit IL-1β-induced ACTH secretion (Rougeot *et al.*, 1991). This suggests that IL-1 HPA secretion may be mediated, at least in part, by the production of PAF.

IV. Virus Infections of the Central Nervous System

Virus infection of the CNS can result in a wide range of pathogenic outcomes: a rapid, severely acute form; a chronic, progressive form; a reversible, nonproductive, latent type; or various intermediate stages. Disease is a direct result of interaction between host and infecting virus. Host parameters include age, genetic makeup, and immune competency, whereas viral factors include class and strain of agent, target specificity, and genomic variation. The phenotypic expression of disease is a complex multifactorial interaction among these parameters.

A. Viral Entry

The first step in the disease process involves entry of the virus into the CNS. Various host protective barriers prevent direct viral entry into the CNS and force indirect routes of infection. Agents that cause viremia can enter by replication in the endothelial cells that line the blood vessels. Viruses known to enter by this route include the togaviruses, enteroviruses, and certain retroviruses. Viruses can also invade from the bloodstream by entering the stroma and the choroid plexus through the fenestrated capillary and endothelium and either infecting or being transported across the choroid plexus into the CSF. Recently, it has been demonstrated that fibroblast-like cells isolated from the human choroid plexus can be infected with HIV (Harouse et al., 1989). Once in the CSF, the virus can infect ependymal cells lining the ventricles and invade the underlying CNS tissue. The virus can also enter through "Trojan horse" mechanisms, being transported within circulating leukocytes such as lymphocytes or macrophages/monocytes, which can contain such viruses as measles, mumps, canine distemper, lentiviruses, or togaviruses. Viruses can also infect peripheral neurons at such sites as the neuromuscular junction and can be axonally transported toward the CNS. Rabies and herpes simplex may utilize such a route (Johnson, 1984). Herpes simplex may also gain entrance to the CNS by means of the sensory neurons of the olfactory system.

B. Target Specificity

Once within the CNS, viruses encounter a differentiated cell population with complex, functionally integrated cell-to-cell interactions. The highly specialized cytoplasmic membranes of this cell population allow for great variation in virual receptor sites and in the abilities of cells to support viral replication. Viral tropism to cells within the CNS involves both cell and viral receptor molecules (Kascsak and Wisniewski, 1989). Polioviruses display a particular affinity for anterior horn motor neurons, whereas the rabies virus normally prefers neurons of the limbic system (Johnson, 1980). Infections with orthomyxoviruses or paramyxoviruses usually involve the selective infection of ependymal cells (Wolinsky et al., 1976). The polyomavirus, which is the causative agent of progressive multifocal leukoencephalopathy (see later discussion), produces a lytic infection of oligodendrocytes and a nonpermissive infection of astrocytes (Richardson, 1961). The Ia antigen receptors present on a variety of cell types have been implicated as viral receptors (Inada and Mims, 1990). Cellular CD4 protein interacts with HIV gp 120 and is the receptor for this virus on lymphocytes and monocytes (Wigdahl and Kunsch, 1990). Several studies suggest the presence of the CD4 receptor on cells within the CNS (Dewhurst *et al.*, 1987). The specific affinity of rabies virus to acetylcholine receptors serves to facilitate uptake and transfer of virus to the CNS and to determine neuronal specificity (Lentz and Burrage, 1982).

C. Viral-Mediated Immune Reaction

As stated earlier, one potential outcome of CNS viral infection is rapid acute disease, usually including encephalitis and/or meningoencephalitis. This can be accompanied by perivascular inflammation involving polymorphonuclear cells followed later by macrophages, lymphocytes, and microglia. During infection by certain viruses, i.e., poliovirus, the inflammatory response consists of a meningeal reaction, perivascular cuffing, and parenchymal infiltration. Polymorphonuclear leukocytes are seen early, with a later shift to predominantly mononuclear cells. Microglial cell infiltration and neuronophagia are also seen (Johnson, 1982).

Pathogenesis is normally a two-step process consisting of viral-mediated cell destruction as well as immune-mediated, viral-induced cellular destruction. Viral antigens are normally good immunogens, and host immune surveillance directs a T-cell-dependent immune response (Burns, 1975). Such a response is directed primarily against infected cells that express viral or altered cell surface proteins. Antibodies can function as intermediaries in the destruction of infected cells by means of complement-mediated cytotoxicity or antibody-dependent cellular cytotoxicity or by serving as opsinizing factors. Cytotoxic T cells can destroy such cells directly or release lymphokines to recruit, activate, and/or sensitize other lymphoreticular elements. Cytolytic T lymphocytes (CTLs) are an important effector in antiviral immunity (Zinkernagel and Doherty, 1986). Such cells can recognize foreign viral antigens on cell surfaces only in the context of self MHC structures. Until recently, the HLA Class I molecules were thought to be the primary, if not the only, HLA recognition structure for CTLs. Studies of measles and Epstein-Barr virus (EBV) infection suggest that HLA Class II molecules can also serve as recognition sites, further expanding the potential action of CTLs. Viral antigens recognized by CTLs have also been expanded beyond the traditional cell surface molecules (Braciale and Braciale, 1986). Preliminary data indicate that recognition of internal viral polypeptides and perhaps even nonstructural gene products may be a common feature of antiviral CTLs. Coronavirus MHV-4 can selectively block gamma-interferon-induced Class II antigen expression on cerebral endothelial cells (Joseph *et al.*, 1991). Studies by other investigators have shown Class I modulation on mouse glial cells by other related coronaviruses (Suzumura *et al.*, 1986). In such a manner, viruses may be able to evade immune-mediated events that occur at the level of the BBB. The virus is able to avoid host immune surveillance and to enter the CNS. Such events probably also prevent late immune-mediated demyelinating disease, which is absent in MHV-4 virus infection (see later discussion).

Immunodeficiency states, such as AIDS or iatrogenic immunosuppression in transplant recipients, may sometimes modify the inflammatory response of the CNS to pathogens. In AIDS, especially at the terminal stage of disease, the picture of CNS inflammation, i.e., in toxoplasma gondii encephalitis or in progressive multifocal leukoencephalopathy caused by JC virus, can differ from that seen in nonimmuno-suppressed individuals. The inflammation seems muted, and the destructive component of the process (fulminant necrosis) may dominate. This may serve as another example that the inflammatory response within the CNS is partly dependent on the peripheral immune system.

D. Virus-Induced Autoimmunity

As discussed earlier, immune surveillance in response to viral infections can lead to virus-induced immune response to normal host components. During acute infections, this response can lead to increased tissue damage. During chronic or persistent infections, such responses can perpetuate or be the primary cause of the disease process. Involvement can take the form of humoral response (autoantibodies) as well as cell-mediated autoimmune (CMAI) response (Ter Meulen, 1989). Such autoimmunity may involve a phenomenon known as molecular mimicry (Srinvasappa et al., 1986), an immune process in which molecules coded for by dissimilar genes share similar structures. In such a manner, antiviral antibodies may bind to host antigens as well as to antigens of the virus. Many examples of such mimicry have now been identified: measles virus phosphoprotein and keratin (Fujinami et al., 1983); vaccinia virus hemagglutin and vimentin (Dales et al., 1983); fusion protein of measles and heat shock protein (Shesheberadarin and Norby, 1984); HIV gp120 and neuroleukin (Mizarachi, 1989). In an analysis of monoclonal antibodies to 11 different viruses, 4% of such antibodies cross-reacted with host cell determinants (Srinvasappa et al., 1986). Generation of cytotoxic cross-reactive effector lymphocytes or antibodies would recognize "self proteins" located at target cells. The virus need not be present for such events to take place. Myelin basic protein exhibits a significant degree of homology with several viral proteins, including hepatitis B virus polymerase. Inoculation of hepatitis B virus polymerase peptide into rabbits caused perivascular infiltration localized to the CNS, reminiscent of EAE (Fujinami and Oldstone, 1985).

Several other mechanisms are potentially operational in virus-induced autoimmune disease. Viruses may disrupt normal immune regulation by direct interaction with cells of the reticuloendothelial system (RES). As discussed earlier, many viruses can replicate in these cell types, leading to destruction of lymphocyte subpopulations or stimulation of autoreactive clones. Viruses may incorporate host molecules into their envelope or coat, or they may insert, modify, or expose other cellular components on the cell surface. Immune pathological events may also be triggered by induction of Class II MHC antigens on the surface of infected CNS cells. MHC antigens are expressed only at low levels or not at all on the majority of CNS cells (Hart and Fabre, 1981). Astrocytes exposed *in vitro* to measles or coronavirus JHM begin to express MHC Class II antigens, which are further enhanced in the presence of TNF (Massa *et al.*, 1987). An analogous situation *in vivo* would certainly facilitate CTL-mediated autoimmune response.

Postinfectious encephalomyelitis has been associated with a wide range of virus infections including measles, mumps, rubella, vaccinia, and herpes zoster and certain respiratory viral infections (Johnson and Griffin, 1986). Neuropathological changes resemble those seen in EAE and appear to be a direct result of an MBP-directed immune response (Ter Meulen, 1989). Coronavirus JHM causes acute demyelinating encephalitis by selective infection of oligodendrocytes. Lymphocytes from sick animals that are passively transferred to syngeneic animals produce lesions in the recipients that resemble those in individuals with allergic encephalomyelitis (Ter Meulen, 1989). Viral infection of oligodendrocytes appears capable of inducing an autoimmune response against the myelin proteins produced by these cells. In measles-induced encephalomyelitis, there is little evidence that virus invades the CNS. Deregulation of autoreactive cells may occur secondarily to viral infection of lymphoid cells. Demyelinating disease caused by Theiler's murine encephalomyelitis virus (TMEV), a nonbudding enterovirus, may result from a virus-specific, delayed-type hypersensitivity (DTH) (Clatch *et al.*, 1986). Lymphokines produced by MHC Class II-restricted, TMEV-specific, DTH T cells primed by interaction with TMEV-infected macrophages would recruit and activate additional macrophages, leading to nonspecific macrophage-induced damage.

E. Viral Persistence

In contrast to the autoimmune mechanisms described above, persistent viral infections can be a consequence of the ability of the virus to avoid immune surveillance. In the face of excessive viral antigen, both virus-specific antibodies and CTLs are suppressed or rendered ineffective. Viruses may be able to down regulate appropriate recognition molecules on the surface of immune cells. Expression of virus surface proteins involved in immune recognition may also be reduced. Reduced expression of glycoprotein has been observed during persistent infections with arenaviruses, paramyxoviruses, retroviruses, and rhabdoviruses (Oldstone, 1989). Antibody-induced antigenic modulation can lead to measles virus persistent infection in the CNS (Fujinami and Oldstone, 1984). Presumably, this modulation can occur in body compartments that are devoid of the effector molecules of complement such as the CNS. Subacute sclerosing panencephalitis (SSPE) results from a persistent CNS infection with defective measles virus (Wechsler and Meissner, 1982). A defect in viral envelope genes prevents expression of viral antigen on cell surfaces. Infection is propagated by cell-to-cell transmission of virus, allowing the agent to avoid immune surveillance. Viruses can also replicate in the cellular constituents of the immune system and in such a way disable specific immune responsiveness. Viruses thus persist within cells that are ordinarily utilized to provide clearance. Viruses such as measles and HIV can infect lymphocytes and/ or macrophages, resulting in generalized immunosuppression. Such immunosuppression leaves the host susceptible to infection by a wide range of other microorganisms, leading to the opportunistic infections often associated with HIV and other such viruses.

F. Viral Latency

Viruses can also avoid immune surveillance through latency, a state of reversible, nonproductive infection. Viral genetic information can remain within the host in either an integrated or an episomal state. Retroviruses such as HIV use reverse transcriptase to insert their DNA proviral form into host-cell DNA; this integration step is a prerequisite for the replication of these RNA viruses (Mahry, 1985). Herpes simplex virus (HSV), which resides in sensory ganglion cells, integrates its DNA directly into host nuclear DNA. The DNA of other DNA viruses such as EBV or JC agent, the polyomavirus that causes progressive multifocal leukoencephalopathy, remains latent in a nonintegrated episomal form. Latent infections established by these viruses may result from a lack of host factors that are critical for the expression of viral early gene products (Garcia-Blanco and Cullen, 1991). The subsequent activation of specific cellular transcription factors in response to extracellular stimuli can induce the expression of virus and lead to CNS disease. Herpesviruses such as HSV-1, HSV-2, or VZV cause initial acute peripheral infection followed by a latent infection of neurons. In this environment, sheltered from immune surveillance, the virus can remain for the life of the host. HSV-1 can be activated by a number of seemingly unrelated stimuli such as physical or emotional stress or damage to adjacent tissue. Reactivation probably results from a signal transduction event that directly or indirectly induces HSV-1 gene transcription (Leib *et al.*, 1989). Latently EBV-infected B cells can also persist for the life of the individual. If immediate early viral gene expression does not occur, EBV may establish a latent infection (Miller, 1985). Both activated T lymphocytes and nondividing macrophages are able to support the synthesis and integration of HIV-1 proviruses (Fauci, 1988). Resting T cells are nonpermissive and do not support replication or integration. Resultant unintegrated viral intermediates may persist in a viable yet transcriptionally inert form for extended periods of time. In quiescent macrophages or in T cells in a resting state, cellular factors critical for proviral transcription may not be active. Postintegration latency in HIV-1 may result from inefficient proviral transcription and from a suboptimal amount of REV, a viral-coded transactivation regulatory protein (Pomerantz *et al.*, 1990). Stimulation of these cells in some manner could induce cellular transcription factors increasing REV which leads to productive virus replication. The rare demyelinating disorder, progressive multifocal leukoencephalopathy (PML) (see earlier discussion), is caused by the reactivation of latent polyomavirus (JCV) in the oligodendroglia cells of affected individuals (Mazlo and Tariska, 1980). This disease is usually associated with an underlying disorder of the RES system in which immune responsiveness is impaired. Loss of immune surveillance allows reexpression of virus and cytocidal effects on oligodentrocytes, leading to demyelination.

G. Chronic Progressive Noninflammatory Infection

The final type of interaction of virus within the CNS is a chronic persistent infection that does not elicit an immune response. Wild mouse ecotropic immune leukemia virus (MuLv) induces a progressive form of hind limb paralysis in a natural population of mice as well as in laboratory animals (Gardner *et al.*, 1973). Pathologically, the disease is characterized by the absence of host inflammatory response at the site of tissue destruction and by a picture of neuronal degeneration, spongiform gray matter lesions, and gliosis. Paralysis is a direct result of viral replication, most notably in anterior horn motor neurons, but virus can also infect endothelial and glial cells. There is no virus-mediated CTL or antibody response. The CNS is devoid of inflammatory infiltrates or deposits of IgG or complement. In genetically susceptible laboratory strains of mice, ability to induce disease is age dependent and involves tolerance to the virus. Passive immunization with antibodies to MuLv virus can prevent paralysis. Neuronal destruction and spongiosis may be a direct result of the interaction of viral gene expression in the neuron. Recent evidence suggests that a posttranscriptional step in virus envelope protein synthesis is impaired and that neurological disease may be a consequence of abortive replication of virus within neurons (Sharpe *et al.*, 1990). Such abortive infections can make the presence of virus difficult to detect. Analogies to other retrovirus CNS infections, notably HIV and HTLV-1, suggest that similar mechanisms may be operational in CNS disease caused by these agents.

Another group of infectious agents that establish CNS disease in the absence of inflammatory response are the agents of the transmissible spongiform encephalopathies (TSEs) or prion diseases (Carp *et al.*, 1989). Unlike the retroviral disease described above, in which immune response to virus is age dependent and the disease process may include tolerance, there is no evidence for the ability of the host to generate any immune response to the agents of TSE. These agents cause Creutzfeldt–Jakob disease (CJD), Gerstmann–Straussler–Scheinker syndrome (GSS), and kuru in humans and are associated with scrapie, bovine spongiform encephalopathy (BSE), chronic wasting disease, and transmissible mink encephalopathy (TME) in animals. The agents that cause these diseases are poorly characterized, but it is certain that they do not exhibit properties of known viruses or virus-like agents. These agents replicate peripherally in the RES system, notably in spleen and lymph nodes. Agent crosses into the CNS, leading to spongiosis, gliosis, and neuronal destruction in the absence of any inflammatory response, similar to that described above for the retroviruses. Modulation of the immune system only affects the agent given peripherally. Immunological compounds, given close to the time of peripheral infection, that stimulate the immune response shorten incubation periods, whereas compounds that suppress the immune response extend the incubation period. Treatment with dextran sulfate (Farkuhar and Dickinson, 1986) extends disease and may mediate its effect through interaction with macrophages. Recent studies suggest the importance of follicular dendritic cells (Kitamoto et al., 1991) in agent peripheral replication. Similar dendritic cells are involved in antigen presentation and virus replication in infections caused by other viruses. Similar to evidence described for the neurotropic retroviruses, pathology within the CNS may include abnormal protein processing, in this case, the production of an abnormal host-coded protein termed PrP (Prusiner, 1991). Both agent replication and spongiform change are associated with the presence of this protein within the CNS.

V. Conclusion

In conclusion, the inflammatory response within the CNS appears to have several aspects. First, the CNS itself is unique from other organs in the presence of BBB with specialized endothelial cells, the presence of CNS-specific cells (e.g., microglia or astrocytes), and the presence of CNS-specific antigens. Second, infectious agents such as viruses comprise a wide spectrum of agents with varied neural tissue virulence and varied specificity of agents to certain CNS cell types. Some of these agents may produce fulminant disease with severe, if not lethal, CNS damage, whereas others may persist for decades, resulting in chronic or latent effects. The interactions among the cells and environment of the CNS, infectious agents, and the immune response are quite complex. Studying the unique aspects of the CNS-immune response provides us the window of opportunity to view fascinating and diverse aspects of these responses that otherwise would not be available.

References

Aharoni, R., Teitelbaum, D., Arnon, R., and Puri, J. (1991). Immunomodulation of experimental allergic encephalomyelitis by antibodies to the antigen-Ia complex. *Nature (London)* **351**, 147–150.

Alliot, F., Lecain, E., Grima, B., and Pessac, B. (1991). Microglial progenitors with a high proliferative potential in the embryonic and adult mouse brain. *Proc. Natl. Acad. Sci. U.S.A.* **88**, 1541–1545.

Arend, W. P. (1991). Interleukin-1 receptor antagonist. *J. Clin. Invest.* **88**, 1445–1449.

Arend, W. P., and Dayer, J. M. (1990). Cytokines and cytokine inhibitors or antagonists in rheumatoid arthritis. *Arthritis Rheum.* **33**, 305–315.

Azarelli, B., Mirkin, L. D., Goheen, M., Muller, J., and Crockett, C. (1984). The leptomeningeal vein. A site for re-entry of leukemic cells into the systemic circulation. *Cancer* **54**, 1333–1343.

Baker, D., O'Neill, J. K., and Tuch, J. L. (1991). Cytokines in the central nervous system of mice during chronic relapsing experimental allergic encephalomyelitis. *Cell. Immunol.* **134**, 505–510.

Baurer, J., and Strauss, S. (1992). Interleukin-6 and alpha 2-macrogroleutin indicate an acute phase state in Alzheimer's disease cortices. *FEBS Lett.* **285**, 111–114.

Ben-Nun, A., Wekerle, H., and Cohen, I. R. (1981). The rapid isolation of clonable antigen specific T lymphocyte lines capable of mediating autoimmune encephalomyelitis. *Eur. J. Immunol.* **11**, 195–199.

Besedovsky, H., Del Rey, A., Sorkin, E., and Dinarello, C. A. (1986). Immunoregulatory feedback between interleukin-1 and glucocorticoid hormones. *Science* **233**, 652–654.

Bourdial, F., Toulmond, S., Surana, A., Benavides, J., and Scatton, B. (1991). Increase in W3 (peripheral type benzodiazepine) binding sites in the rat cortex and striatum after local injection of interleukin-1, tumor necrosis factor-alpha and lipopolysaccharide. *Brain Res.* **543**, 194–200.

Braciale, T. J., and Braciale, V. L. (1986). CTL recognition of transfected H-2 gene and viral gene products. *In* "Concepts in Viral Pathogenesis" (A. L. Notkins and M. B. A. Oldstone, eds.), pp. 174–181. Springer-Verlag, New York.

Bradbury, M. (1979). "The Concept of a Blood-Brain Barrier." John Wiley and Sons, Chichester, New York.

Brierley, J. B., and Graham, D. I. (1992). Hypoxia and vascular disorders at the central nervous system. *In* "Greenfields Neuropathology" (J. H. Adams, J. A. N. Corsellis, and L. W. Duchen, eds.), p. 127. John Wiley and Sons, New York.

Brightman, M. W. (1989). The anatomic basis of the blood-brain barrier. *In* "Implications of the Blood-Brain Barrier and Its Manipulation" (E. A. Neuwelt, ed.), pp. 53–83. Plenum, New York.

Broadwell, R. D. (1989). Transcytosis of macromolecules through the blood-brain barrier: A cell biological perspective and critical appraisal. *Acta Neuropathol.* **79**, 117–128.

Brown, A., McFarlin, D. E., and Raine, C. S. (1982). Chronologic neuropathology of relapsing experimental allergic encephalomyelitis in the mouse. *Lab. Invest.* **46**, 171–185.

Burns, W. H. (1975). Viral antigens. *In* "Viral Immunology and Immunopathology" (A. L. Notkins, ed.), pp. 43–56. Academic Press, New York.

Burns, F. R., Li, X., Shen, N., Offner, H., Cou, Y. K., Vandenbark, A. A., and Heber-Katz, E. (1989). Both rat and mouse T-cell receptors specific for encephalitogenic determinant of myelin basic protein use similar V-alpha and V-beta-chain genes even though the major histocompatibility complex and encephalitogenic determinants being recognized are different. *J. Exp. Med.* **169**, 27–39.

Carp, R. I., Kascsak, R. J., Wisniewski, H. M., Merz, P. A., Rubenstein, R., Bendheim, P., and Bolton, D. C. (1989). The nature of the unconventional slow infection agents remains a puzzle. *Alzheimer Dis. Assoc. Disord.* **3**, 79–99.

Clatch, R. J., Lipton, H. L., and Miller, S. D. (1986). Characterization of Theiler's murine encephalomyelitis virus (TMEV) specific delayed type hypersensitivity responses in TMEV induced demyelinating disease: Correlation with clinical signs. *J. Immunol.* **136**, 920–927.

Cominelli, F., Nast, C. C., Clark, B. D., Schindler, R., Llerena, R., Eysselein, V. E., Thompson, R. C., and Dinarello, C. A. (1990). Interleukin 1 (IL-1) gene expression, synthesis, and effect of specific IL-1 receptor blockade in rabbit immune complex colitis. *J. Clin. Invest.* **86**, 972–980.

Cotran, R. S. (1987). New roles for the endothelium in inflammation and immunity. *Am. J. Pathol.* **129**, 407–413.

Czarniecki, C. W., Chiu, H. H., Wong, G. H. W., McCabe, S. M., and Palladino, M. A. (1988). Transforming growth factor beta1 modulates the expression of class II histocompatibility antigens on human cells. *J. Immunol.* **140**, 4217–4223.

Dales, S., Fujinami, R. S., and Oldstone, M. B. A. (1983). Serologic relatedness between Thy-1.2 and actin revealed by monoclonal antibody. *J. Immunol.* **131**, 1332–1338.

Delisle, M. B., Bouissou, H., and Saidi, A. (1986). What's new in cerebral pathology in acquired immune deficiencies? *Pathol. Res. Pract.* **181**, 85–92.

Dewhurst, S., Stevenson, M., and Volsky, D. J. (1987). Expression of the T4 molecule (AIDS virus receptor) by human brain-derived cells. *FEBS Lett.* **213**, 133–137.

Dustin, M. L., and Springer, T. A. (1988). Lymphocyte-function-associated antigen-1 (LFA-1) interaction with intercellular adhesion molecule-1 (ICAM-1) is one of at least three mechanisms for lymphocyte adhesion to cultured endothelial cells. *J. Cell. Biol.* **107**, 321–331.

Ellison, M. D., and Merchant, R. E. (1991). Appearance of cytokine-associated central nervous system myelin damage coincides temporarily with serum tumor necrosis factor induction after recombinant interleukin-2 infusion in rats. *J. Neuroimmunol.* **33**, 245–251.

Endres, S., Fulle, H. J., Sinha, B., Stall, D., Dinarello, A., Gerzer, R., and Weber, P. C. (1991). Cyclic nucleotides differentially regulate the synthesis of tumor necrosis factor alpha- and interleukin-1beta by human mononuclear cells. *Immunology* **72**, 56–60.

Farkuhar, C. F., and Dickinson, A. G. (1986). Prolongation of scrapie incubation period by an injection of dextran sulfate 500 within the month before or after injection. *J. Gen. Virol.* **67**, 463–476.

Fauci, A. S. (1988). The human immunodeficiency virus: Infectivity and mechanisms of pathogenesis. *Science* **239**, 617–622.

Fierz, W., Endler, B., Reske, K., Wekerle, H., and Fontana, A. (1985). Astrocytes as antigen presenting cells: Induction of Ia antigen expression on astrocytes by T cells via immune interferon and its effects on antigen presentation. *J. Immunol.* **134**, 3785–3793.

Fontana, A., Kristensen, F., Dubs, R., Gemsa, D., and Weber, E. (1982). Production of prostaglandin E and interleukin-1 like factor by cultured astrocytes and C6 glioma cells. *J. Immunol.* **129**, 2413–2419.

Fontana, A., Fierz, W., and Wekerle, H. (1984). Astrocytes present myelin basic protein to encephalitogenic T-cell lines. *Nature (London)* **307**, 273–276.

Frei, K., Bodmer, S., Schwerdel, C., and Fontana, A. (1985). Astrocytes of the brain synthesize interleukin 3-like factor. *J. Immunol.* **135**, 4044–4047.

Frei, K., Malipiero, U., Leist, T., Zinkernagel, R. M., Schwab, M. E., and Fontana, A. (1989). On the cellular source and function of IL-6 produced in the central nervous system in viral disease. *Eur. J. Immunol.* **19**, 689–694.

Fujinami, R. S., and Oldstone, M. B. A. (1984). Antibody initiates virus persistence: Immune modulation and measles virus infection. *In* "Concepts in Viral Pathogenesis" (A. L. Notkins, and M. B. A. Oldstone, eds.), pp. 187–193. Springer-Verlag, New York.

Fujinami, R. S., and Oldstone, M. B. A. (1985). Amino acid homology and immune responses between the encephalitogenic site of myelin basic protein and virus: A mechanism for autoimmunity. *Science* **230**, 1043–1045.

Fujinami, R. S., Oldstone, M. B. A., Wroblewska, Z., Frankel, M. E., and Koprowski, H. (1983). Molecular mimicry in viral infection: Cross-reaction of measles phosphoprotein or of herpes simplex virus protein with human intermediate filaments. *Proc. Natl. Acad. Sci. U.S.A.* **80**, 2346–2350.

Gallo, P., Piccino, M., Pagni, S., and Tavolato, B. (1988). Interleukin-2 levels in serum and cerebrospinal fluid of multiple sclerosis patients. *Ann. Neurol.* **24**, 795–797.

Ganter, U., Strauss, S., Jonas, U., Weidemann, A., Beyreuther, K., Volk, B., Berger, M., and Bauer, J. (1991). Alpha 2-macroglobulin synthesis in interlukin-6 stimulated human neuronal (SH-SY5Y neuroblastoma) cells: Potential significance for the processing of Alzheimer beta-amyloid precursor protein. *FEBS Lett.* **282**, 127–131.

Garcia-Blanco, M. A., and Cullen, B. R. (1991). Molecular basis of latency in pathogenic human viruses. *Science* **254**, 815–820.

Gardner, M. B., Henderson, B. E., Officer, J. E., Rongey, R. W., Parker, J. C., Oliver, C., Estes, J. D., and Huebner, R. J. (1973). A spontaneous lower motor neuron disease apparently caused by indigenous type C RNA virus in wild mice. *J. Natl. Cancer Inst.* **51**, 1243–1249.

Gijbels, K., Damme, J. V., Proost Put, W., Carton, H., and Biliau, A. (1990). Interleukin-6 production in the central nervous system during experimental autoimmune encephalomyelitis. *Eur. J. Immunol.* **20**, 233–235.

Gimborne, M. A., Jr., and Beviaqua, M. P. (1988). Vascular endothelium. Functional modulation at the blood interface. *In* "Endothelial cell biology" (N. Simionescu, and M. Simionescu, eds.), pp. 255–273. Plenum, New York.

Giulian, D., Baker, T. J., Shih, L. C., and Lachman, L. B. (1985). Interleukin-1 of the central nervous system is produced by ameboid microglia. *J. Exp. Med.* **164**, 594–604.

Graeber, M. B., and Streit, W. J. (1990). Microglia: Immune network in the CNS. *Brain Pathol.* **1**, 2–5.

Hama, T., Kushima, Y., Miyamoto, M., Kubota, M., Takii, N., and Hatanaka, H. (1991). Interleukin-6 improves the survival of mesencephalic catecholaminergic and septal cholinergic neurons from postnatal two-week old rats in cultures. *Neuroscience (Oxford)* **40**, 445–452.

Harlan, J. M. (1985). Leukocyte-endothelial interactions. *Blood* **65**, 513–525.

Harouse, J. M., Wroblewska, Z., Laughlin, M. A., Hickey, W. F., Schonwetter, B. S., and Gonzalez-Scarano, F. (1989). Human choroid plexus cells can be latently infected with human immunodeficiency virus. *Ann. Neurol.* **25**, 406–411.

Hart, D. N. J., and Fabre, J. W. (1981). Demonstration and characterization of IA positive dendritic cells in the interstitial tissues of rat heart and other tissues but not brain. *J. Exp. Med.* **154**, 347–361.

Hayes, G. M., Woodroofe, M. N., and Cuzner, M. L. (1987). Microglia are the major cell type expressing MHC class II in human white matter. *J. Neurol. Sci.* **80**, 25–37.

Hayes, G. M., Woodroofe, M. N., and Cuzner, M. L. (1988). Characterisation of microglia isolated from adult human and rat brain. *J. Neuroimmunol.* **19**, 177–189.

Hertz, L., McFarlin, D. E., and Waksman, B. H. (1990). Astrocytes: Auxiliary cells for immune responses in the central nervous system? *Immunol. Today* **11**, 265–268.

Hickey, W. F., and Kimura, H. (1988). Privascular microglial cells of the CNS are bone marrow-derived and present antigen in vivo. *Science* **239**, 290–292.

Higgins, G. C., and Postlethwaite, A. E. (1991). Interleukin-1 inhibitors and their significance in rheumatoid arthritis. *In* "Monoclonal Antibodies, Cytokines and Arthritis" (T. F. Kresina, ed.), pp. 133–172. Marcel Dekker, New York.

Hirano, A., Dembitzer, H. M., Becker, N. H., Levine, S., and Zimmerman, H. M. (1970).

Fine structural alterations of the blood-brain barrier in EAE. *J. Neuropathol. Exp. Neurol.* **29**, 432–440.

Hirsch, M. R., Wietzerbin, J., Pierres, M., and Goridis, C. (1983). Expression of Ia antigens by cultured astrocytes treated with gamma interferon. *Neurosci. Lett.* **41**, 199–204.

Howell, M. D., Winters, S. T., Olee, T., Powell, H. C., Carlo, D. J., and Brostoff, S. W. (1989). Vaccination against experimental allergic encephalomyelitis with T cell receptor peptides. *Science* **246**, 668–670.

Inada, T., and Mims, C. A. (1990). Ig antigen and Fc receptors of mouse peritoneal macrophages as determinants of susceptibility of lactic dehydrogenase virus. *J. Gen. Virol.* **37**, 1–40.

Jacobs, C. A., Baker, P. O., Raux, E., Picha, K. S., Toivola, B., Waugh, S., and Kennedy, M. K. (1991). Experimental autoimmune encephalomyelitis is exacerbated by IL-1alpha and suppressed by soluble IL-1 receptor. *J. Immunol.* **146**, 2983–2989.

Johnson, K. P. (1984). The pathogenesis of viral infections of the nervous system. *Neurol. Clin.* **2**, 179–185.

Johnson, R. T. (1980). Selective vulnerability of neural cells to viral infections. *Brain* **103**, 447–472.

Johnson, R. T. (1982). "Viral Infections of the Nervous System," pp. 87–128. Raven Press, New York.

Johnson, R. T., and Griffin, D. (1986). Virus induced autoimmune demyelinating disease of the CNS. In "Concepts in Viral Pathogenesis II" (A. L. Notkins, and M. B. A. Oldstone, eds.), pp. 203–209. Springer-Verlag, New York.

Joseph, J., Knobler, R. L., Lublin, F. D., and Hart, M. N. (1991). Mouse hepatitis virus (MHV-4, JHM) blocks gamma interferon-induced major histocompatibility complex class II antigen expression on murine cerebral endothelial cells. *J. Neuroimmunol.* **33**, 181–190.

Kascsak, R. J., and Wisniewski, H. M. (1989). Pathogenesis of virus-induced and autoimmune nervous system injuries. In "Child Neurology and Developmental Disabilities" (J. H. French, S. Harel, P. Casaer, M. I. Gottlieb, I. Rapin, and D. C. De Vivo, eds.), pp. 89–98. Paul H. Brookes, Baltimore.

Kimball, E. S. (1991). Involvement of cytokines in neurogenic inflammation. In "Cytokines and Inflammation" (E. S. Kimball, ed.), pp. 169–189. CRC Press, Boca Raton, Florida.

Kitamoto, T., Muramoto, T., Mohri, S., Doh-Ura, K., and Tateishi, J. (1991). Abnormal isoform of prion protein accumulates in follicular dendrite cells in mice with Creutzfeldt Jacob disease. *J. Virol.* **65**, 6292–6295.

Kremsner, P. G., Grundmann, H., Neifer, S., Sliwa, K., Sahlmüller, G., Hegenscheid, B., and Bienzle, U. (1991). Pentoxifylline prevents murine cerebral malaria. *J. Infect. Dis.* **164**, 605–608.

Kuruvilla, A. P., Shah, R., Hochwald, G. M., Liggitt, H. D., Palladino, M. A., and Thorbecke, G. J. (1991). Protective effect of transforming growth factor beta1 on experimental autoimmune diseases in mice (experimental allergic encephalomyelitis/collagen-induced arthritis). *Proc. Natl. Acad. Sci. U. S. A.* **88**, 2918–2921.

Lassmann, H., and Wisniewski, H. M. (1979). Chronic relapsing experimental allergic encephalomyelitis. Clinicopathological comparison with multiple sclerosis. *Arch. Neurol. (Chicago)* **36**, 490–497.

Lassmann, H., Rossler, K., Zimprich, F., and Vass, K. (1991). Expression of adhesion molecules and histocompatibility antigens at the blood-brain barrier. *Brain Pathol.* **1**, 115–123.

Lee, S. J. (1991). Expression of growth/differentiation factor 1 in the nervous system: Conservation of bierstronic structure. *Proc. Natl. Acad. Sci. U.S.A.* **88**, 4250–4254.

Leib, D. A., Coen, D. M., Bogard, C. L., Hicks, K. A., Yager, D. R., Knipe, D. M., Tyler, K. L., and Schaffer, P. (1989). Immediate early regulatory gene mutants define different stages in establishment and reactivation of herpex simplex virus latency. *J. Virol.* **63**, 759–768.

Lentz, T. L., and Burrage, T. G. (1982). Is the acetylocholine receptor a rabies virus receptor? *Science* **215**, 182–185.

Levy, J. A. (1988). The human immunodeficiency virus and its pathogenesis. *Infect. Dis. Clin. North Am.* **2**, 285–297.

Lossinsky, A. S., Badmajew, V., Robson, J. A., Moretz, R. C., and Wisniewski, H. M. (1989). Sites of egress of inflammatory cells and horseradish peroxidase transport across the blood-brain barrier in a murine model of chronic relapsing experimental allergic encephalomyelitis. *Acta Neuropathol.* **78**, 359–371.

Lublin, F. D., Maurer, P. H., Berry, R. G., and Tippett, D. (1981). Delayed, relapsing experimental allergic encephalomyelitis in mice. *J. Immunol.* **126**, 819–822.

Mahry, B. W. J. (1985). Strategies of virus persistence. *Br. Med. Bull.* **41**, 50–56.

Maskophidis, D., Frei, K., Lahler, J., Fontana, A., and Zinhernagel, R. (1991). Production of random classes of immunoglobulins in brain tissue during persistent viral infection paralleled by secretion of interleukin-6 (IL-6) but not IL-4, IL-5 and gamma interferon. *J. Virol.* **65**, 1364–1369.

Massa, P. T., Schimpl, A., Wecker, E., and Ter Meulen, V. (1987). Tumor necrosis factor amplifies measles virus-mediated Ia induction on astrocytes. *Proc. Natl. Acad. Sci. U.S.A.* **84**, 7242–7245.

Massanari, R. M. (1980). A latent-relapsing neuroautoimmune disease in Syrian hamsters. *Clin. Immunol. Immunopathol.* **16**, 211–220.

Mazlo, M., and Tariska, I. (1980). Morphological demonstration of the first phase of polyomavirus replication in oligodendroglia cells of human brain in progressive multifocal leukoencephalopathy (PML). *Acta Neuropathol.* **49**, 133–143.

McGeer, P. L., Itagaki, S., Tago, H., and McGeer, E. G. (1987). Reactive microglia in patients with senile dementia of the Alzheimer type are positive for the histocompatibility glycoprotein HLA-DR. *Neurosci. Lett.* **79**, 195–200.

McGeer, P. L., Itagaki, S., and McGeer, E. G. (1988). Expression of the histocompatibility glycoprotein HLA-DR in neurological disease. *Acta Neuropathol.* **76**, 550–557.

Merril, J. E., Strom, S. R., Ellison, G. W., and Meyers, L. W. (1989). In vitro study of mediators of inflammation in multiple sclerosis. *J. Clin. Immunol.* **9**, 84–96.

Merz, G. S., Schwenk, V., Schuller-Levis, G., Gruca, S., and Wisniewski, H. M. (1987). Isolation and characterization of macrophages from scrapie-infected mouse brain. *Acta Neuropathol.* **72**, 240–247.

Michaels, J., Price, R. W., and Rosenblum, M. K. (1988). Microglia in the giant cell encephalitis of acquired immunodeficiency syndrome:proliferation, infection and fusion. *Acta Neuropathol.* **76**, 373–379.

Miller, G. (1985). Epstein Barr virus. In "Virology" (B. N. Fields, ed.), pp. 563–589. Raven Press, New York.

Mizarachi, Y. (1989). Neurotropic activity of monomeric glucophosphoisomerase was blocked by human immunodeficiency virus and peptides from HIV-1 envelope glycoproteins. *J. Neurosci. Res.* **23**, 217–224.

Mohankumai, P. S., Thyagarajan, S., and Quadri, S. K. (1991). Interleukin-1 stimulates the release of dopamine and dihydroxyphonyacetic acid from hypothalamus in vivo. *Life Sci.* **48**, 925–930.

Montovani, A., and Dejana, E. (1989). Cytokines as communication signals between leukocytes and endothelial cells. *Immunol. Today* **10**, 370–375.

Ofosu-Appiah, W., and Mokhtarian, F. (1991). Characterization of a T-suppressor cell line that downgrades experimental allergic encephalomyelitis in mice. *Cell. Immunol.* **135**, 143–153.

Ohgo, S., Nakatsuru, K., Oki, Y., Ishikawa, E., and Matsukura, S. (1992). Stimulation by interleukin-1 (IL-1) of the release of rat corticotropin-releasing factor (CRF), which is independent of the cholinergic mechanism, from superfused rat hypothalomaneurohypophysial coplexes. *Brain Res.* **550**, 213–219.

Ohlsson, K., Björk, P., Bergenfeldt, M., Hageman, R., and Thompson, R. C. (1990). Interleukin-1 receptor antagonist reduces mortality from endotoxin shock. *Nature (London)* **348**, 550–552.

Oldstone, M. B. A. (1989). Viral persistence. *Cell* **56**, 517–520.

Opp, M. R., and Krueger, J. M. (1991). Interleukin-1 receptor antagonist blocks interleukin-1 induced sleep and fever. *Am. J. Physiol.* **260**, R453–R457.

Palazzolo, D. L., and Quadri, S. K. (1990). Interleukin-1 stimulates catecholamine release from the hypothalamus. *Science* **47**, 2105–2109.

Paterson, P. (1982). Molecular and cellular determinants of neuroimmunologic inflammatory disease. *FASEB J.* **41**, 2569–2576.

Paterson, P. Y. (1977). Autoimmune neurological disease: Experimental animal systems and implications for multiple sclerosis. In "Autoimmunity. Genetics, Immunologic, Virologic and Clinical Aspects" (N. Talal, ed.), pp. 643–692. Academic Press, New York.

Paterson, P. Y. (1978). The demyelinating diseases: Clinical and experimental studies in animals and man. In "Immunological Diseases" (M. Samter, N. Alexander, B. Rose, W. B. Sherman, D. W. Talmage, and J. H. Vaughn, eds.), pp. 1400–1435. Little Brown, Boston.

Paterson, P. Y. (1979). Neuroimmunologic diseases of animals and humans. *Rev. Infect. Dis.* **1**, 468–482.

Pomerantz, R. J., Trono, D., Feinberg, M. B., and Baltimore, D. (1990). Cells nonproductively infected with HIV-1 exhibit an aberrant pattern of viral RNA expression: A molecular model of latency. *Cell* **61**, 1271–1276.

Powell, H. C., Myers, R. R., Mizisin, A. P., Olee, T., and Brostoff, S. W. (1991). Response of the axon and barrier endothelium to EAN induced by autoreactive T cell lines. *Acta Neuropathol.* **82**, 364–377.

Prusiner, S. B. (1991). Molecular biology of prion diseases. *Science* **252**, 1515–1522.

Racke, M. D., Khib-Jalbut, S., Cannella, B., Albert, P. S., Raine, C. S., and McFarlin, D. C. (1991). Prevention and treatment of chronic relapsing experimental allergic encephalomyelitis by transforming growth factor - beta1. *J. Immunol.* **146**, 3012–3017.

Raine, C. S., Canella, B., Duivestijn, A. M., and Cross, A. H. (1990). Homing to central nervous system vasculature by antigen-specific lymphocytes. II Lymphocyte/endothelial cell adhesion during the initial stages of autoimmune demyelination. *Lab Invest.* **63**, 476–489.

Ranges, G. E., Figari, I. S., Espevik, T., and Palladino, M. A. (1987). Inhibition of cytotoxic T cell development by transforming growth factor-beta and reversal by recombinant tumor necrosis factor-A. *J. Exp. Med.* **166**, 991.

Reese, T. S., and Karnovsky, M. J. (1967). Fine structural localization of a blood-brain barrier to exogenous peroxidase. *J. Cell. Biol.* **34**, 207–217.

Rettori, V., Gimeno, M. F., Karara, A., Gonzales, M. C., and McCann, S. M. (1991). Interleukin-1 alpha inhibits prostaglandin E-2 release to suppress pulsatile release of luteinizing hormone but not follicle-stimulating hormone. *Proc. Natl. Acad. Sci. U.S.A.* **88**, 2763–2767.

Richardson, E. (1961). Progressive multifocal leukoencephalopathy. *N. Engl. J. Med.* **265**, 815–822.

Rivers, T. M., Sprint, D. H., and Berry, G. P. (1935). Encephalomyelitis accompanied by myelin destruction experimentally produced in monkeys. *J. Exp. Med.* **61**, 689–702.

Rodriguez, M., Pierce, M. L., and Howie, E. A. (1987). Immune response gene products (Ia antigens) on glial and endothelial cells in virus-induced demyelination. *J. Immunol.* **138**, 3438–3442.

Rook, A. H., Kehrl, J. H., Wakefield, L. M., Roberts, A. B., Sporn, M. B., Burlington, D. B., Lane, H. C., and Fauci, A. S. (1986). Effects of transforming growth factor-beta on the functions of natural killer cells: Depressed cytolytic activity and blunting of interferon responsiveness. *J. Immunol.* **136**, 3916–3920.

Rose, L. M., Richards, T. L., Petersen, R., Peterson, J., Hruby, S., and Alvord, Jr., E. C. (1991). Short analytical review: Remitting-relapsing EAE in nonhuman primates: A valid model of multiple sclerosis. *Clin. Immunol. Immunopathol.* **59**, 1–15.

Rougeot, C., Tiberghien, C., Minary, P., and Dray, F. (1991). Basal and PAF-, interleukin 1-, ether stress-induced hypothalamic pituitary adrenal secretion of conscious rat: Modulation by PAF antagonists. *J. Lipid Mediators* **4**, 45–60.

Sapolsky, R., Rivier, C., Yamamoto, G., Plotsky, P., and Vale, W. (1987). Interleukin-1 stimulates the secretion of hypothalamic corticotropin-releasing factor. *Science* **238**, 522–524.

Sawada, M., Kondo, N., Suzumura, A., and Marunouchi, T. (1989). Production of tumor necrosis factor-alpha by microglia and astrocytes in culture. *Brain Res.* **491**, 394–397.

Schluesener, H. J. (1990). Transforming growth factors type B1 and B2 suppress rat astrocyte autoantigen presentation and antagonize hyperinduction of class II major histocompatibility complex antigen expression by interferon-gamma and tumor necrosis factor-a. *J. Neuroimmunol.* **27**, 41–47.

Sedgwick, J. D., Mossner, R., Schwender, S., and Ter Meulen, V. (1991). Major histocompatibility complex-expressing nonhematoporetic astroglial cells prime only CD8+ T lymphocytes: Astroglial cells as perpetrators but not initiators of CD4+ T cell responses in the central nervous system. *J. Exp. Med.* **173**, 1235–1246.

Selmaj, K. W., and Raine, C. S. (1988). Tumor necrosis factor mediates myelin and oligodendrocyte damage in vitro. *Ann. Neurol.* **23**, 339–346.

Shaffer, N., Grau, G. E., Hedberg, K., Davachi, F., Lyamba, B., Hightower, A. W., Breman, J. G., and Ngayen-Dinh, P. (1991). Tumor necrosis factor and severe malaria. *J. Infect. Dis.* **163**, 96–101.

Shainkin-Kestenbaum, R., Berlyne, G., Zimlichman, S., Sorin, H. R., Nyska, M., and Danon, A. (1991). Acute phase protein, serum amyloid A, inhibits IL-1 and TNF-induced fever and hypothalamic PGE2 in mice. *Scand. J. Immunol.* **34**, 179–183.

Shalaby, J. R., and Ammann, A. J. (1988). Suppression of immune cell function in vitro by recombinant human transforming growth factor-beta. *Cell. Immunol.* **112**, 343–350.

Sharpe, A. H., Hunter, J. J., Chassler, P., and Jaenish, R. (1990). Role of abortive retroviral infection of neurons in spongiform CNS degeneration. *Nature (London)* **346**, 181–183.

Shesheberadarin, H., and Norby, E. (1984). Three monoclonal antibodies against measles F protein cross-react with the cellular stress proteins. *J. Virol.* **52**, 995–999.

Srinivasappa, J., Saegusa, T., Prabhakar, B. S., Gentry, M. K., Buchmeier, M. J., Wilktor, T. J., Koprowski, H., Oldstone, M. B. A., and Notkins, A. L. (1986). Molecular mimicry: Frequency of reactivity of monoclonal antibodies with normal tissues. *J. Virol.* **571**, 397–401.

Sriram, S., and Carroll, L. (1991). Haplotype-specific inhibition of homing of radiolabeled lymphocytes in experimental allergic encephalomyelitis following treatment with anti-Ia antibodies. *Cell. Immunol.* **135**, 222–231.

Staunton, D. E., Dustin, M. L., Erickson, H. P., and Springer, T. A. (1990). The arrangement of the immunoglobulin-like domains of ICAM-1 and the binding sites of LFA-1 and rhinovirus. *Cell* **61**, 243–254.

Steinman, L. (1991). The development of rational strategies for selective immunotherapy against autoimmune demyelinating disease. *Adv. Immunol.* **49**, 357–379.

Stone, S. H., and Lerner, E. M. (1965). Chronic disseminated allergic encephalomyelitis in guinea pigs. *Ann. N. Y. Acad. Sci.* **122**, 227–241.

Suzumura, A., Lavi, E., Weiss, S. R., and Silberberg, D. H. (1986). Coronavirus infection induces H-2 antigen expression on oligodendrocytes and astrocytes. *Science* **232**, 991–993.

Ter Meulen, V. (1989). Virus-induced cell mediated immunity. *In* "Concepts in Viral Pathogenesis III" (A. L. Notkins, and M. B. A. Oldstone, eds.), pp. 297–303. Springer-Verlag, New York.

Tribolet de, N., Hamov, M. F., Mach, J. P., Carrel, S., and Schreyer, M. (1984). Demonstration of HLA-DR in normal human brain. *J. Neurol. Neurosurg. Psychiatry* **47**, 417.

Uehara, A., Gottschall, P. E., Dahl, R. R., and Arimura, A. (1987). Interleukin-1 stimulates ACTH release by an indirect action which requires endogenous corticotropin releasing factor. *Endocrinology* **121**, 1580–1582.

Urban, J. L., Kuman, V., Kono, D. H., Gomez, C., Horvath, S. J., Clayton, J., Ando, D. G., Sercarz, E. E., and Hood, L. (1988). Restricted use of T-cell receptor V genes in murine autoimmune encephalomyelitis raises possibilities for antibody therapy. *Cell* 54, 577–592.

Vanderbark, A. A., Hashim, G., and Offner, H. (1989). Immunization with a synthetic T-cell receptor V-region peptide protects against experimental allergic encephalomyelitis. *Nature (London)* 341, 541–544.

Wahl, S. M., Hunt, D. A., Wong, H. L., Dougherty, S., McCartney-Francis, N., Wahl, L. M., Ellingsworth, L., Schmidt, J. A., Hall, G., Roberts, A. B., and Sporn, M. B. (1988). Transforming growth factor-beta is a potent immunosuppressive agent that inhibits IL-1-dependent lymphocyte proliferation. *J. Immunol.* 140, 3026–3032.

Wakabayashi, G., Gelfand, J. A., Burke, J. F., Thompson, R. C., and Dinarello, C. A. (1991). A specific receptor antagonist for interleukin-1 prevents Escherichia coli-induced shock in rabbits. *FASEB J.* 5, 338–343.

Watkins, B. A., Dorn, H. H., Kelly, W. B., Armstrong, R. C., Potts, B. J., Michaels, F., Kufta, C. V., and Dubois-Dalcq, M. (1990).Specific tropism of HIV-1 for microglial cells in primary human brain cultures. *Science* 249, 549–553.

Wechsler, S. L., and Meissner, H. C. (1982). Measles and SSPE: Similarities and differences. *Prog. Med. Virol.* 28, 65–95.

Wekerle, H., Linington, C., Lassmann, H., and Meyermann, R. (1986). Cellular immune reactivity within the CNS. *Trends Neurosci.* 9, 271.

Wekerle, H., Engelhardt, B., Risau, W., and Meyermann, R. (1991). Interaction of T-lymphocytes with cerebral endothelial cells in vitro. *Brain Pathol.* 1, 107–114.

Wolinsky, J. S., Klassen, T., and Baringer, J. R. (1976). Persistence of neuroadapted mumps virus in brains of newborn hamsters after intraperitoneal inoculation. *J. Infect. Dis.* 133, 260–267.

Wigdahl, B., and Kunsch, C. (1990). Human immunodeficiency virus infection and neurologic dysfunction. *Prog. Med. Virol.* 37, 1–46.

Wisniewski, H. M., and Keith, A. B. (1977). Chronic relapsing EAE an experimental model of multiple sclerosis. *Ann. Neurol.* 1, 144–148.

Wisniewski, H. M., Lassmann, H., Brosnan, C. F., Mehta, P. D., Lidsky, A. A., and Madrid, R. E. (1982). Multiple sclerosis: Immunological and experimental aspects. In "Recent Advances in Clinical Neurology" (M. Glaser, ed.), pp. 95–125. Churchill/Livingstone, Edinburgh.

Wong, G. H., Bartlett, P. F., Clark-Lewis, I., Battye, F., and Schrader, J. W. (1984). Inducible expression of H-2 and Ia antigens on brain cells. *Nature (London)* 310, 688–691.

Woodroofe, M. N., Saina, G. S., Wadhiva, M., Hayes, G. M., Laughlin, A. J., Tinker, A., and Cuzner, M. L. (1991). Detection of interleukin-1 and interleukin-6 in adult rat brain, following mechanical injury, by in vivo microanalysis: Evidence of a role for microglia in cytokine production. *J. Neuroimmunol.* 33, 227–236.

Yednock, T. A., Butcher, E. C., Stoolman, L. M., and Rosen, S. D. (1985). Lymphocyte homing receptor: Relationship between the Mel-14 antigen and cell surface lectin. *J. Cell. Biol.* 101, 233a.

Yong, V. W., Yong, F. P., Ruijs, T. C. G., Antel, J. P., and Kim, S. U. (1991). Expression and modulation of HLA-DR on cultured human adult astrocytes. *J. Neuropathol. Exp. Neurol.* 50, 16–28.

Yoshida, K., and Gage, F. H. (1992). Fibroblast growth factors stimulate nerve growth factor synthesis and secretion by astrocytes. *Brain Res.* 538, 118–126.

Zinkernagel, R. M., and Doherty, P. C. (1986). MHC restricted cytotoxic T cells: Studies on the biological role of polymorphic major transplantation antigens determining T-cell restriction specificity, function and responsiveness. *Adv. Immunol.* 27, 51–177.

Index

Acetaminophen
  hepatotoxicity, 301, 309
  inflammatory effects, 11, 13
Acquired immunodeficiency syndrome, *see
  also* Human immunodeficiency virus
  clinical course, 110–111
  patient classification, 112–113
  tumor necrosis factor α levels in patients,
    112–113
Acrodermatitis enteropathica, zinc role, 198
Acute phase proteins
  dimethylnitrosoamine acute response,
    183–184
  functions, 72–73
  genes
    glucocorticoid response elements, 83
    promoters, 82–83
    regulation, 82–83
  response mediation by cytokines
    interactive effects of cytokines, 79–80,
      87–88
    receptor signal transduction, 81–82
    specific, 75–79
  role in homeostasis, 73–74
  synthesis
    mediators, 71–72
    rates, 72–74
    sites, 71–72
  types, 72–73, 80, 183
Addressins
  control of expression, 322
  types, 322
Adenosine
  efficacy, 128–129
  as tumor necrosis factor α inhibitor,
    128–129
ADP ribosylation
  inhibitors, 127
  role in tumor necrosis factor toxicity, 127

Adrenocorticotropic hormone
  HIV effect on production, 112
  induction by cytokines, 45, 79
Adult respiratory stress syndrome
  characterization, 108
  incidence, 108
  mortality, 108
  platelet-activating factor role, 109
  sepsis association, 108
  tumor necrosis factor α role, 108–110
Airway hyperreactivity
  induction by ozone, 260
  inflammation, 260, 268
  inhibitors, 260
  mechanism, 268
Alzheimer's disease, role of interleukin 6,
  331–332
Ampicillin, skin toxicity, 218
Amyloid A, cytokine feedback, 330
Antigens, *see specific antigens*
Antioxidants, dietary prevention of LDL
  oxidation, 242
Apolipoprotein B
  modification in oxidized LDL, 235–
    236
  mutation in atherosclerosis, 235
Arachidonic acid, metabolic pathways,
  25–26
Arthritis, rheumatoid, *see* Rheumatoid
  arthritis
Asbestos
  effect on lung cells
    endothelial cells, 286
    epithelial cells, 286, 288
    macrophages, 270, 285–287
  fibrosis induced by
    cytokine response, 291
    mechanism, 270, 285–288
    role of immune response, 288